Dietary Supplements

Dietary Supplements

SECOND EDITION

Edited by

Pamela Mason
BSc, MSc, PhD, MRPharmS
Independent Pharmaceutical Consultant
London, UK

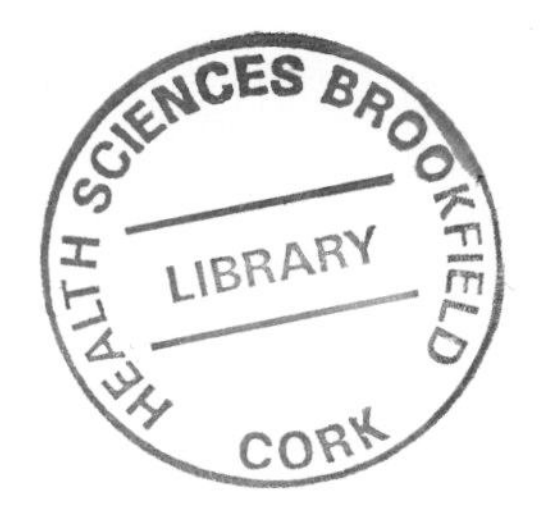

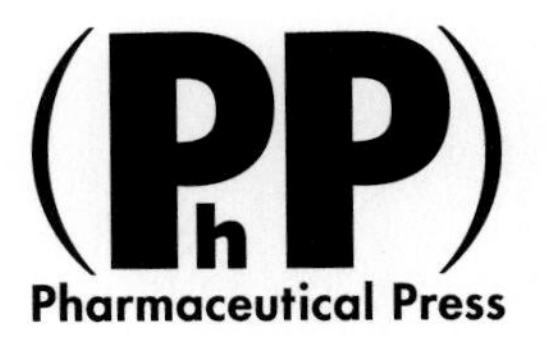

Published by the Pharmaceutical Press
1 Lambeth High Street, London SE1 7JN, UK

First edition published by Blackwell Science Ltd 1995
Reprinted 1998
Second edition 2001

Text design by Barker/Hilsdon, Lyme Regis, Dorset
Typeset by Type Study, Scarborough, North Yorkshire
Printed in Great Britain by The Bath Press, Bath

ISBN 0 85369 459 1

A catalogue record for this book is available from the British Library

Contents

Preface

SINCE THE FIRST EDITION of this book was published six years ago, the UK market for dietary supplements has almost doubled. The general public's interest in these products – either as additions to the diet or as an aid to the prevention or management of certain conditions – continues to grow.

As a result, health professionals are often asked questions about supplements, but frequently feel they have not got the confidence or the knowledge, or both, to answer them effectively. Given the abundance of spurious information, of which a great deal can be found on the Internet, this lack of confidence is not surprising, and there are relatively few sources of sound, unbiased information on this topic.

Development of an evidence base for dietary supplements has, at least until recently, been hampered by the lack of good-quality research, although fortunately that is now starting to change; a number of credible, peer-reviewed studies have been published since the first edition of this book. However, there are still a large number of unanswered questions in relation to both the efficacy and the safety of these products, and the inevitable 'more research needed' will apply to many dietary supplements for some time to come. In spite of this, these uncertainties should not prevent health professionals from giving advice and information on these products, and the aim of this book is to help them to do that.

Both the breadth and the depth of information provided have been considerably expanded for this edition. The number of supplements has increased by half to include substances that have become more popular during recent years: aloe vera, creatine, glucosamine, green tea, isoflavones, probiotics, etc. In addition, the information included has also increased, mainly due to the increase in published studies.

The easy-to-use format of the first edition has been retained, and it is my intention that this book can be used as a reference source or as a text which can be read. Moreover, in this edition, I have included recommended intakes of nutrients and some aspects of the law relating to supplements, not only for the UK but also for Europe and the United States. I hope that the book will be useful to colleagues in many countries round the world.

Pamela Mason
March 2001

Introduction

THERE IS NOW considerable interest in dietary supplements and increasing numbers of people are using them. In the UK, sales of dietary supplements in 2000 were approximately £346 million (see Table 1).[1]

While there is a great deal of information about these substances – increasingly so on the Internet – not all of it is reliable. Indeed, there are probably few areas associated with healthcare where such confusion exists. This confusion extends to health professionals as well as the general public. Because dietary supplements are not medicines, pharmacists are often unfamiliar with them and, because they are not foods (in the sense of being part of a normal diet), dietitians are (understandably) wary of recommending them. Doctors typically receive little nutritional education and may not have the knowledge or the time to give informed advice.

In addition, supplements are a topic about which there is a great deal of disagreement even between nutrition experts. Some say they are largely unnecessary because a balanced diet provides all the required vitamins and minerals, others say that supplements make a worthwhile contribution to a healthy diet, while increasingly some experts say that optimal health cannot easily be achieved without them.

Table 1 Sales of different types of supplements in the UK (2000 figures[1])

Total	£346m
Fish oils	£72m
Multivitamins	£77m
Single vitamins	£51m
Evening primrose oil and other GLA products	£29m
Garlic	£13m
Other	£104m

GLA = gamma-linolenic acid.

[1]Source: Information Resources, Eagle House, The Ring, Bracknell, RG12 1HB. http://www.infores.com

Given the growth in sales of dietary supplements, it is appropriate to ask what evidence there is of their efficacy. Are there rigorous trials to show that these products work? Until the early 1990s, there were relatively few well-conducted trials involving vitamins and minerals, and fewer still on substances such as garlic, fish oils, ginseng, etc. Evidence was largely limited to anecdotal reports and single case studies or poorly conducted intervention trials. The argument was frequently made that controlled trials could not be conducted with supplements, because they often contain a range of natural ingredients whose effects are difficult to separate. However, such arguments are often misguided, and an increasing body of evidence is now emerging from double-blind, randomised, placebo-controlled trials, and also from systematic reviews and meta-analyses. Some of these suggest that some supplements (e.g. folic acid, fish oils) are effective in some groups of the population in certain circumstances. However, for other supplements (e.g. royal jelly) there is little evidence of benefit.

What are dietary supplements?

Definition

Various definitions for dietary supplements exist world-wide. In the UK, they have been defined as

'foods in unit dosage form, e.g. tablets, capsules and

> elixirs, taken to supplement the diet. Most are products containing nutrients normally present in foods which are used by the body to develop cells, bone, muscle, etc., to replace co-enzymes depleted by infection and illness, and generally to maintain good health'.[a]

In addition to vitamins and minerals, this definition also covers ingredients such as garlic, fish oils, evening primrose oil and ginseng, which can be taken to supplement dietary intake or for their suggested health benefits.

Similarly, one definition in Europe states

> 'food supplements are preparations including tablets, capsules, powders and liquids which are composed of, or contain, nutrients, micronutrients and/or other edible substances consumed in unit quantities in addition to the normal food intake. Food supplements can be composed of vitamins, minerals and trace elements; peptides, amino acids and similar nitrogen-containing compounds; oils and fatty acids and their esters; fibres and other materials of plant or animal microbial origin as well as fermentation products, including those in dehydrated, concentrated or extracted form'.[b]

In the United States, the Dietary Supplement Health Education Act (DSHEA) 1994 defines a dietary supplement as

> 'a product (other than tobacco) that is intended to supplement the diet which bears or contains one or more of the following dietary ingredients: a vitamin, a mineral, a herb or other botanical, an amino acid, a dietary substance for use by man to supplement the diet by increasing the total daily intake, or a concentrate, metabolite, constituent, extract or combinations of these ingredients. It is intended for ingestion in pill, capsule, tablet or liquid form, is not represented for use as a conventional food or as the sole item of a meal or diet and is labelled as a dietary supplement'.

This definition, like those in the UK and Europe, also expands the meaning of dietary supplements beyond essential nutrients to include such substances as ginseng, garlic, fish oils, psyllium, enzymes and mixtures of these.

One of the key points in these definitions is that dietary supplements are products consumed in unit quantities in addition to normal food intake. This differentiates supplements from other foods, such as fortified foods and functional foods, to which nutrients are added. However, a major difference in the US definition is the explicit inclusion of 'herbs or other botanicals' in the list of dietary ingredients.

In Europe, due to existing laws relating to herbal preparations in most member states, the definition of supplements is less precise and refers only to other 'materials of plant, animal or microbial origin'. Moreover, in several countries of the European Union (EU), many herbal preparations are considered to be medicines requiring registration, and are not sold as food supplements.

In the UK, herbal products are currently marketed under a variety of arrangements – either as fully licensed medicines, 'medicines exempt from licensing' under section 12 of the 1968 Medicines Act or as cosmetics or foods, so they do not fall entirely in the food supplements category.

Enteral feeds (e.g. Complan and Ensure) and slimming aids are also classified as dietary supplements by nutritionists and dietitians, but for the purposes of this book, these products will be ignored.

Classification

Dietary supplements fall into several categories. These are:

1 Vitamins and minerals
   - Multivitamins and minerals. These normally contain around 100% of the Recommended Daily Amount (RDA) for vitamins, with varying amounts of minerals and trace elements.
   - Single vitamins and minerals. These may contain very large amounts, and when levels exceed ten times the RDA, they are often termed 'megadoses'.

a Definition developed by the Proprietary Association of Great Britain (PAGB), British Herbal Manufacturers' Association (BHMA) and the Health Food Manufacturers' Association (HFMA).

b Definition developed by the European Federation of Health Product Manufacturers (EHPM).

- — Combinations of vitamins and minerals. These may be marketed for specific population groups and lifestyles, e.g. athletes, children, pregnant women, slimmers, teenagers, vegetarians, etc.
- — Combinations of vitamins and minerals with other substances, such as evening primrose oil and ginseng.

2 'Unofficial' vitamins and minerals, for which a requirement and a deficiency disorder in humans has not, so far, been recognised, e.g. boron, choline.
3 Natural oils containing fatty acids for which there is some evidence of beneficial effects, e.g. evening primrose oil, fish oils and flaxseed.
4 Natural substances containing ingredients with recognised pharmacological actions but whose composition and effects have not been fully defined, e.g. garlic, ginkgo biloba and ginseng.
5 Natural substances whose composition and effects are not well defined but which are marketed for their 'health-giving properties', e.g. *Chlorella*, royal jelly and *Spirulina*.
6 Enzymes with known physiological effects, but of doubtful efficacy when taken by mouth, e.g. superoxide dismutase.
7 Amino acids or amino acid derivatives, e.g. carnitine, *N*-acetyl cysteine, *S*-adenosylmethionine.

Uses of supplements

Individuals buy supplements for many different reasons, which may include the following:

- As an insurance policy to supplement what an individual may consider to be a poor diet (e.g. no time or inclination to eat regular meals).
- To improve overall health and fitness.
- To prolong vitality and delay the onset of age-associated problems.
- As a tonic or 'pick-me-up' when feeling run-down or after illness.
- For symptoms of stress.
- Recommended by an alternative health practitioner or health professional.
- Pregnancy.
- Slimming.
- Smoking.
- To improve performance and body building in sports and athletics.
- To prevent or treat various signs and symptoms (e.g. colds, cardiovascular disease, cancer, poor sight, skin problems, arthritis, premenstrual syndrome, etc).

There are three main approaches to the use of supplements. They can be used to:

- treat or prevent nutritional deficiency;
- reduce the risk of 'non-deficiency' disease (e.g. cardiovascular disease, cancer, cataract); and
- promote optimal health.

When vitamins were first discovered during the early years of the 20th century, their only indication was for the prevention and treatment of deficiency diseases such as scurvy, beri-beri, pellagra, etc. This concept of preventing deficiency led to the development of dietary standards such as RDAs and, more recently, to the Dietary Reference Values.[1] These values were based on amounts of nutrients required to prevent deficiency, and even though subject to various limitations, they are still the best measure of dietary adequacy.

After the Second World War, it was thought that nutritional deficiencies had largely disappeared and, as a consequence, scientific interest in vitamins and minerals waned. However, with the increase in various chronic diseases such as cardiovascular disease and cancer, vitamins once again became an area of growing interest, and it was suggested that supplements might help to reduce the risk of developing such conditions. Now, there is growing concern among the public to improve quality of life, and supplements are increasingly used to promote so-called optimum health.

Furthermore, despite the idea that nutritional deficiency had largely disappeared, recent UK nutrition surveys have shown that there is no room for complacency. Although average dietary intakes may appear adequate, some groups of the surveyed populations are clearly at risk of marginal deficiencies.

Thus, the National Diet and Nutrition Survey in pre-school children[2] showed that 8% of the surveyed youngsters aged 1½ to 4½ years were anaemic, a further 12% were mildly iron deficient, and 15% had a poor intake of zinc. Vitamin A deficiency was present in 8%, vitamin B_2 deficiency in 23%, and vitamin C deficiency in 3%.

A similar nutritional survey of older children[3] again showed that average nutrient intakes were largely fine, but anaemia was present in 1.5% of boys and 5% of girls, with respective totals of 13% and 27% having low serum ferritin – an indication of iron deficiency. In addition, zinc was found to be low in the diets of 10% of boys and 20% of girls. Also of concern were calcium intakes, which were below the Lower Reference Nutrient Intake (LRNI) in 6% of boys and 12% of girls. For magnesium the respective figures were 12% and 27% and for vitamin A 10% and 11%. Furthermore, some of the surveyed youngsters also appeared to have poor status for vitamin B_{12}, vitamin C, vitamin D, folate, riboflavin and thiamine.

The National Diet and Nutrition Survey of people aged 65 years and over[4] followed a similar pattern, showing that there were nutritional problems in some individuals. Up to 38% of the surveyed population were deficient in vitamin D, up to 38% were deficient in vitamin C, up to 18% in folate, up to 15% in vitamin B_{12} and up to 30% in iron. Of the free-living individuals, 11% of men and 9% of women were anaemic.

It is therefore clear that deficiency is not a thing of the past. Various groups of the population could be at risk of nutrient deficiency and could benefit from supplementation. These include:

- People in a particular demographic category, e.g. infants and children, adolescents, women during pregnancy and lactation and throughout the reproductive period, the elderly and ethnic minorities.

- People whose nutritional status may be compromised by lifestyle (enforced or voluntary), e.g. smokers, alcoholics, drug addicts, slimmers, strict vegetarians (i.e. vegans), food faddists, individuals on low incomes and athletes.

- People whose nutritional status may be compromised by surgery and/or disease, e.g. malabsorption syndromes, hepatobiliary disorders, severe burns and wounds and inborn errors of metabolism.

- People whose nutritional status may be compromised by long-term drug administration (e.g. anticonvulsants may increase the requirement for vitamin D).

Increasingly, people are taking supplements for reasons other than prevention of deficiency and at amounts higher than the RDA. Moreover, evidence is increasing that, at least for some nutrients (e.g. folic acid, vitamin E), there may be benefits in achieving higher intakes than the RDA.

However, while there is agreement about the beneficial effects of nutrients in the prevention of deficiency disease and the amounts required to achieve such effects, there is controversy about amounts required for reduction in risk of chronic disease and so-called 'optimum health'. Some would argue that higher amounts are required, and that basing requirements for nutrients only on the prevention of deficiency disease is inadequate. But what other endpoints should be used is open to debate; longevity, increased resistance to cancer and coronary heart disease, improved athletic performance, and so on. Higher levels of intake cannot always easily be obtained from diet alone, and supplementation is required. However, excessive intake of some nutrients can lead to toxicity, and it is with this in mind that several committees world-wide have established or are planning to establish safe upper limits for supplement intake.

In addition, there is a growing number of supplements which are not officially recognised vitamins or minerals, but various related substances (e.g. glucosamine, shark cartilage) proposed to have benefits for health. In many cases, appropriate doses for these substances have not been established and are at best estimates.

Legal status

The UK

In the UK, the majority of dietary supplements are classified legally as foods, and sold under food law. There are just a few exceptions (e.g. Abidec, Pregaday, Epogam, Efamast, Maxepa and some generic vitamin and mineral preparations), which are licensed medicines. Deciding whether a product is a medicine or not is the role of the Medicines Control Agency (MCA). A medicine is defined by law as 'any substance or combination of substances presented for treating or preventing disease and/or which may be administered with a view to restoring, correcting or modifying physiological functions'.

There is, however, no definition of a food. Nevertheless, if an ingested product is not a medicine, it is a food, and no product can be both a food and a medicine at the same time.

Unlike medicines, most supplements are not subject to the controls of the Medicines Act (1968) and the European Commission (EC) Directive on Medicines for Human Use, 65/65. Because supplements classed as foods do not require product licences, they do not have to go through such rigorous clinical trials, and are therefore much cheaper to put on the market than medicines.

Dietary supplements are not controlled by quite the same strict conditions of dosage, labelling, purity criteria and levels of ingredients as medicines. The retail supply of those vitamins which have product licences (i.e. medicines) are subject to limitations which depend on their strength and maximum daily dose as shown in Table 2.

Dietary supplements containing levels of vitamins in excess of those in prescription-only medicines are available to the public. However, in recognition of the fact that consumers are increasingly using high-dose products, the Department of Health is setting maximum limits of intake for vitamins and minerals.

Table 2 Limitations on the sale or supply of licensed medicines containing certain vitamins

Vitamin	Legal status
Vitamin A	Up to 2250 μg (7500 units) GSL
	Over 2250 μg (7500 units) POM
Vitamin D	Up to 10 μg (400 units) GSL
	Over 10 μg (400 units) P
Cyanocobalamin	Up to 10 μg GSL
	Over 10 μg POM
Folic acid	Up to 200 μg GSL
	200–500 μg P
	Over 500 μg POM

GSL = subject to control under the Medicines (General Sales List) Order, 1977.
POM = subject to control under the Medicines (Prescriptions Only) Order, 1977.
P = Pharmacy-only products.

Europe

In the European Union (EU), the diversity in the way supplements are regulated is wide. There are three main approaches to regulating vitamin and mineral supplements:

1 The RDA is considered to be the regulatory dividing line between a food and a medicine. This approach is used in countries (e.g. France) which consider that supplements sold as foods should only be sold for preventing clinical deficiencies.

2 A more complex approach creates a middle category between foods and medicines. Products containing the RDA or less are classified as foods, while higher dose products do not necessarily become medicines, but require some sort of pre-marketing authorisation (e.g. Belgium, Greece).

3 Supplements are regulated by existing food law, which places upper limits on dosage when there are genuine safety concerns for consumers. This approach is used in countries that operate a philosophy of freedom of choice for the consumer (e.g. the UK, the Netherlands, Sweden).

As an illustration, a 60 mg vitamin C supplement – 60 mg being the EU RDA for vitamin C – can be sold as a food in all countries, but a 250 mg product can be sold according to the law as a food only in the Netherlands and the UK. However, in many cases actual practice is different from the law, and it is only in Belgium where it would be unlikely to find vitamin C 250 mg as a food supplement. A summary of the current legal framework for dietary supplements in the EU is provided in Table 3.

However, the regulatory environment in Europe is changing rapidly. The EC has adopted a draft Directive aimed at harmonising the marketing of food supplements in EU member states. The Directive includes a 'positive list' of vitamins and minerals permitted in food supplements, and a second list identifying the chemical substances which can be used in their manufacture. Other substances such as amino acids, essential fatty acids, fibre, ginseng, etc., may be addressed later and included in the list.

These proposals also seek to establish maximum upper intakes in addition to preserving the status of the RDAs. This is because increasing numbers of people take high-dose supplements and there is a need to stipulate upper safe levels. The Scientific Committee for Food (SCF) is being asked to give its opinion on upper safe levels for vitamins and minerals, which will then be set by the European Commission.

The Directive also pays attention to labelling of content and dosage. It states that labelling should not imply that a varied and adequate diet cannot provide sufficient quantities of nutrients. In addition, claims relating to the prevention, treatment or cure of disease in the labelling, advertising or promotion of food supplements will be prohibited. The consultation process is expected to take between two and four years (2000–2004), at the end of which time the Directive will be formally adopted.

The USA

In the United States, the Food and Drug Administration (FDA) regulates dietary supplements according to the DSHEA 1994. Under this law, supplements are regulated in a similar manner to food products, and they cannot be marketed as medicines or food additives. This Act includes a framework for safety, guidelines for third-party literature provided at the point of sale, guidance on good manufacturing practice (GMP) and labelling standards. Under DSHEA, manufacturers are responsible for marketing safe and properly labelled products, but the FDA bears the burden of proving that a product is unsafe or improperly labelled. However, it appears that the FDA has insufficient resources for doing this, and there is concern that not all supplements in the USA are marketed according to best standards of practice.

Quality assurance

Medicines are subject to rigorous quality control, including disintegration and bioavailability tests, and precision as to levels of ingredients and contaminants, and must be produced according to GMP standards. However, in the UK, no such legally binding standards exist for food supplements, and there is some evidence from the USA that amounts of vitamins and minerals in food supplements vary somewhat from levels stated on product labels.[5]

However, two UK trade organisations – the Council for Responsible Nutrition (CRN) and the Health Food Manufacturers' Association (HFMA) – have published their own standards of GMP.[6,7] Although these guidelines are voluntary and not legally binding, member companies of the organisations are encouraged to abide by them. How many do is not clear, but increasing numbers of companies are becoming more responsible and operating to high standards in this area.

Labels

Supplements marketed under food law in the UK are subject to the Food Labelling Regulations (1996), while those that are medicines must be labelled according to the provisions of the Medicines Act and EC 65/65. The Food Labelling Regulations require a full list of ingredients, both active and inactive, in decreasing order by weight, on the label.

As required by EU regulations, labels on dietary supplements must express their nutrient content in terms of RDAs. EU RDAs are based on the requirements of adult men and are said to apply to average adults. They take no account of differences in nutritional requirements according to age, sex and other factors,

Table 3 National regulations on vitamins, minerals and supplements in the EU

Austria	Food supplements are regulated under Austrian Food Law and fall within a special category of products, the so-called 'Verzehrprodukte'. Products in this category must be notified with the Ministry of Health. The acceptable levels for vitamins and minerals are evaluated on a case-by-case basis. Health claims must also be approved.
Belgium	Food supplements in unit dose form (e.g. tablets) must be notified. They are classified as nutrients if they do not exceed specific RDA levels: — 1.5 × RDA for vitamins A, D and some minerals — 3 × RDA for vitamins B, C, E, H, K and F — 2 × RDA for various other minerals A special marketing authorisation can be given by the control authorities on a case-by-case basis for products in excess of these levels.
Denmark	There are two categories of supplements: — Products containing less than approximately 1–2 × RDA can be sold freely following registration with the National Food Authority — Products containing above 1–2 × RDA are defined as 'strong vitamins' and must demonstrate that they are used for the treatment of a deficiency
Finland	Vitamin and mineral supplements can be sold freely up to the levels of approximately 1 × RDA without notification. Above the RDA they must be registered with the National Bureau of Health.
France	There is no specific law on vitamin and mineral supplements, but the authorities tend to regard them as medicines if they exceed the RDA. However, various higher dose products are freely available without approval.
Germany	There is no specific regulation on vitamin and mineral supplements in either food or medicines law. They are generally classified according to their nutrient levels, presentation and claims: — up to 1 × RDA, products are regarded as foods — 1–3 × RDA, products can be foods, dietetic foods or medicines, depending on the claims and presentation of the product — >3 × RDA, products are regarded as medicines — Minerals are normally regarded as medicines if they exceed 1 × RDA
Greece	There is a special category for food supplements. Products coming from EU countries and containing nutrient levels below 1–3 × RDA can be marketed after fulfilling the requirements of a notification procedure. Products coming from non-EU countries or containing nutrients in excess of 1–3 × RDA must follow an authorisation procedure, which takes a maximum of 120 days.
Ireland	There is no specific law on food supplements. The Ministry of Health restricts products sold as foods to 1 × RDA, but the authorities tolerate higher doses if safety can be demonstrated.
Italy	There is no specific law on food products, but the Ministry of Health generally considers products above 1.5 × RDA as medicines. However, high-dose supplements are accepted on the market without authorisation as long as they make no medicinal or dietetic claims.
Luxembourg	There is no specific law on vitamin and mineral supplements. However, products which exceed 2–3 × RDA are generally considered to be medicines and need to be registered. Products below or equal to 1 × RDA are regarded as foods. There is no notification or registration required for these products.
Netherlands	A specific limit of 1.5 × RDA is set for vitamins A and D. All other food supplements can be sold freely as long as they are safe and no medicinal claims are made. Health claims are permitted if they can be backed up by reliable evidence. There is a list of permitted claims and new ones are evaluated.

Table 3 Continued

Portugal	There is no specific law on supplements, but products are normally notified prior to marketing. The authorities normally consider products with doses above 0.5–1 × RDA to be medicines. Specific restrictions are in place for vitamins A, D, folic acid and certain minerals (e.g. iron).
Spain	There is no specific law on food supplements, but products are subject to evaluation by the authorities. Products with doses exceeding the RDA are generally regarded as medicines, while those below the RDA are regarded as foods. However, many products exceeding the RDA are sold widely without registration.
Sweden	A specific limit is set for vitamins A, D, B_6, folic acid, iron, zinc, iodine and selenium. Other supplements can be sold freely as long as they are safe and make no medicinal claims.
UK	Dietary supplements are regarded as foods as long as they are safe and no medicinal claims are made. Under the Food Safety Act 1990, the supplier is responsible for controlling product safety.

and are therefore simple approximations used for labelling purposes only.

Claims

Claims are one of the most confusing and contentious areas in relation to dietary supplements. What can be claimed in law is fairly clear, but in the past the law has frequently been broken, with illegal and extravagant claims being made, if not on the product itself, then often on accompanying literature. In addition, it is often not just a matter of what is said about a product, but the impression that the words create. Efforts are being made world-wide to tighten up the claims that can be made about supplements and ensure that they are truthful and based on good evidence.

There are two main types of claims: medicinal claims and health claims.

Medicinal claims

A medicinal claim is a claim that states or implies that a product has the property of treating, preventing or curing human disease, or makes any reference to such property. Dietary supplements, unless licensed as medicines, may not be promoted for medicinal use, and they may not make medicinal claims. Thus, no claim may be made that a dietary supplement is capable of curing, treating or preventing a human disease or adverse condition or interfering with the normal operation of a physiological function of the human body.

In the UK, guidance on what constitutes a medicinal claim is provided in Medicines Act Leaflet 8 (MAL 8), a document published by the MCA. Wording such as 'this product prevents heart disease' or 'this product lowers blood pressure' is illegal and constitutes an offence. However, the situation is not always so clear-cut. Thus, in some contexts, 'protect' or 'avoid' may have the same meaning as 'prevent' and are therefore not allowed. Depending on the product, particular words that the MCA may also regard as medicinal include: restores, repairs, eliminates, controls, counteracts, combats, alleviates, clears, stops, removes, heals, cures, remedies, treats, avoids, protects, prevents, fights, reduces, lowers, strengthens, checks, ends, calms and detoxifies. However, providing they are not made in connection with or in the context of a disease or illness, words such as beneficial, revitalising, relaxing (except sedatives), refreshing, invigorating, uplifting or soothing, are not usually regarded as implying a medicinal claim.

Maintenance claims may also be regarded as medicinal when made for a product targeted at a vulnerable section of the population if there is an implication that the product will restore, or help to restore, a specific physiological function or organ to a normal healthy state. In addition, stress, anxiety and nervous tension are regarded as adverse conditions, and claims to cope with or manage them are regarded as medicinal.

Health claims

A health claim is a direct, indirect or implied claim used in product labelling, advertising and promotion that consumption of the product carries a specific health benefit or avoids a specific health detriment. Health claims include nutrient function claims describing the physiological role of nutrients in growth, development and normal functioning of the body (e.g. calcium helps in the development of strong teeth and bones), but they do not include nutrient content claims (e.g. that a product is high in fibre or low in fat).

In the UK, health claims are subject to the general provision of the Food Safety Act, 1990 which makes it a criminal offence to describe falsely a food or to mislead as to its nature, substance, or quality. Health claims are also subject to the Trade Descriptions Act, 1968 which makes it unlawful to apply a false or misleading trade description to goods; this prohibition extends to indirect or implied health claims.

Dietary supplements are allowed to make health claims, but what constitutes a health claim is often unclear. Health claims are not allowed to name diseases, but they can name body organs, body systems, and also risk factors which may adversely affect good health. Wording such as 'this product may help to maintain a healthy heart' or 'this product helps to keep your cholesterol levels healthy' are acceptable according to the law. However, such claims may be interpreted by consumers to mean that such a product will definitely prevent heart attacks. Moreover, names, packaging, imagery, advertorials, and testimonials by well-known personalities can also be extremely influential in forming an impression about a supplement.

However, the fact that supplements cannot make clear claims in some areas also causes confusion. For example, there is now good evidence that increased intake of folic acid preconceptually and during early pregnancy can reduce the incidence of neural tube defects such as spina bifida. However, unless such products are licensed as medicines, they cannot make such a claim.

This issue of health claims is now being tackled in various parts of the world. The USA was one of the first countries to develop legislation in this area. In Europe, there is currently no legal definition of health claims at either EU or member state level, and this lack of clarity has led to the development of several national voluntary codes including the Joint Health Claims Initiative (JHCI; see p. xviii) in the UK. However, in 1999 *Codex Alimentarius*[c] developed draft guidelines for health claims, and it is possible that these might provide a basis for future EU recommendations.

The USA

In the United States, the DSHEA regulates the labelling of supplements and the claims that can be made. This Act includes permissible statements describing the link between a nutrient and a deficiency or between a nutrient and its effect on the body's structure or function, or its effect on well-being. Examples include 'promotes relaxation' or 'builds strong bones'. But to make these claims, the supplement label must also carry the disclaimer: 'This statement has not been validated by the Food and Drug Administration. This product is not intended to diagnose, treat, cure or prevent any disease'.

Under the US Nutrition Labelling and Education Act of 1990, a number of specific health claims are also permitted. These describe the link between a specific nutrient and the reduction in risk of a particular disease or condition, and they are based on significant scientific agreement. Claims applicable to dietary supplements include those in relation to calcium and osteoporosis, folic acid and neural tube defects, soluble fibre (from oat bran and psyllium seed) and coronary heart disease (CHD) and soya and CHD.

---

c *Codex Alimentarius* is the international standard-setting body for food and related feeds. It was created in 1962 to implement the Food Standards Programme of the Food and Agriculture Organisation (FAO) and the World Health Organization (WHO).

Codex Alimentarius

Codex Alimentarius defines health claims as: 'any claim establishing a relation between a food or a constituent of that food and health, or any claim which suggests that a food or a constituent of that food has an impact on health'. The general principles established by *Codex Alimentarius* for making a health claim are as follows:

1. Health claims should be scientifically substantiated. They should be truthful, not misleading, not exaggerated, and not deceptive.
2. The company is responsible for their justification on the basis of sound scientific evidence, and the evidence must be available to the authorities.
3. The food or ingredient must be subject to validation. Amounts need to be indicated and efficacy guaranteed within the period of the shelf life.
4. Claims must be justified in the context of the whole diet and applicable to the amount of the food normally consumed.

Codex Alimentarius distinguishes two types of health claims:

1 Enhanced function claims: these concern specific beneficial effects of the consumption of foods and their constituents on physiological (and psychological) functions or biological activities. They do not include nutrient function claims.

2 Reduction of disease risk claims: these relate to the consumption of a food or food component (in the context of the total daily diet) that might help to reduce the risk of a specific disease or condition.

The UK Joint Health Claims Initiative

In 1997, the UK Joint Health Claims Initiative (JHCI) was set up as a joint venture between consumer organisations, enforcement authorities and industry trade association bodies to address concerns relating to health claims, and to develop a code of practice for regulating the use of health claims on foods. The Code was launched in December 2000 and details are available on the JHCI web site.[8]

The aims of the Code are to stop the use of misleading and unsubstantiated claims, and to encourage accurate and responsible information. The Code attempts to clarify and augment the existing legislation and to complement – but not replace – existing codes and guidelines. The Code is monitored by an administrative body, with a governing council and secretariat, which has access to independent scientific expertise that can be used to help companies who wish to make health claims.

The JHCI distinguishes two types of health claims:

1 Generic health claims: these are health claims based on well-established, generally accepted knowledge from evidence in the scientific literature and/or recommendations from national or international public health bodies such as the Committee on Medical Aspects of Food Policy (COMA), now superseded by the Scientific Advisory Committee on Nutrition (SACN), the US FDA or the EU Scientific Committee for Food (SCF). The Code Administration Body is responsible for developing a list of generic claims for consideration by the Expert Committee, and the list will be reviewed regularly in the light of new evidence and scientific consensus. Further scientific substantiation by companies wishing to use such claims will not be required.

2 Innovative health claims: these are health claims other than generic health claims. They have to be substantiated in accordance with the Code, and must be based on a systematic review of all the available scientific evidence (not just data which support the health claim). Evidence used should preferably be based on results from controlled clinical trials in humans, but additional information from epidemiological, animal and laboratory-based studies may be used. All innovative health claims have to stand up to peer review and be fully documented.

Provided that they are not used in such a way as to create an implication of disease prevention and are not used in connection with, or in the context of, a disease, the following words/claims are not generally regarded as indicating or implying that a product is capable of treating, preventing or curing a disease. In the context of the JHCI, these are therefore acceptable as health claims:

- 'Helps maintain normal cholesterol levels. Healthy cholesterol levels are known to play a part in maintaining a healthy heart'. (*Note*: claims to 'lower or reduce cholesterol' are common in advertising through custom and practice. The legality of such claims has not been tested in the courts.)
- 'Maintains bowel regularity which can help to ensure healthy digestion and bowel'.
- 'Is beneficial to the health of the stomach and digestion system'.
- 'Contributes to healthy metabolism and blood circulation which keeps the heart and blood vessels clear and healthy'.
- 'Helps maintain normal blood flow to the brain, which is particularly important in old age'.
- 'Provides nutrients to convalescents that are needed to ensure a healthy immune system'.
- 'Good for your blood pressure which helps to maintain the heart and normal blood flow to the body. This is particularly important for people who are overweight or smoke'. (Such a health claim should not infer that diet is a substitute for lack of exercise or can compensate for smoking.)
- 'Important – Doctors recommend that women trying to become pregnant, and in the first 12 weeks of pregnancy, take an extra 400 μg supplement of folic acid a day for the normal development of the baby's spinal cord'.
- 'Folic acid contributes to the normal growth of the fetus/unborn baby/baby in the womb'.
- 'Folic acid is good for fetal development/the development of the fetus'.

Law enforcement

In the UK, enforcement of food law, including health claims, is the responsibility of the local authorities trading standards departments. The local authority associations are in turn coordinated by LACOTS (Local Authorities Co-ordinating Body on Food and Trading Standards). LACOTS is responsible for improving the quality of trading standards and food enforcement by promoting coordination, consistency and good regulation. It provides advice and guidance to trading standards authorities, but it does not have the force of law, and any LACOTS advice is not binding on a local authority.

The MCA has no jurisdiction over the sale of products classified as foods. The MCA can only determine whether a product is a medicine or not. Other EU countries have various arrangements for enforcing the law, while in the USA it is the responsibility of the FDA.

Role of the health professional

When asked about supplements, health professionals should emphasise the importance of consuming a diet based on healthy eating guidelines. This is a diet rich in starchy, fibrous carbohydrates, including fruit and vegetables, and low in fat, sugar and salt. Dietary supplements do not convert a poor diet into a good one.

Health professionals should be aware of dietary standards and good food sources for nutrients. They should be able to assess an individual's risk of nutrient deficiency and need for further referral by asking questions to detect cultural, physical, environmental and social conditions which may predispose to inadequate intakes.

There is a need to be aware of the potential for adverse effects with supplements. Thus, when a client or patient presents with any symptoms, questions should be asked about the use of dietary supplements. Individuals will not always volunteer this information without prompting because they believe that supplements are 'natural' and therefore safe.

Health professionals should make their clients aware of the existence of badly worded claims and advertisements and of the dangers of supplement misuse.

Pharmacists have a particular responsibility, simply because they sell these products. When supplying any supplement with perceived health benefits, pharmacists must be careful to avoid giving their professional authority to a product which may lack any health or therapeutic benefit and has risks associated with its use. In accordance with the Code of Ethics of the Royal Pharmaceutical Society of Great Britain, this may involve not stocking or selling the product. Pharmacists must not give the impression that any dietary supplement is efficacious when there is no evidence for such efficacy.

However, provided that a product is not harmful for a particular individual, the freedom to use it should be respected. What is important is that consumers are able to make informed and intelligent choices about the products they buy.

Patient/client counselling

The following questions may be used by health professionals before making any recommendations about supplement use:

1. Who is the supplement for? The individual buying the product may not be the consumer; requirements for vitamins and minerals vary according to age and sex.
2. Why do you think you need a supplement? The individual may have misconceptions about the need for and benefits of supplements that should be addressed.
3. What are your symptoms (if any) and how long have you had them? The individual could have a serious underlying disorder that should be referred for appropriate diagnosis and treatment.
4. What do you eat? A simple dietary assessment should be undertaken to give some indication as to whether vitamin and mineral deficiency is likely.
5. Is your diet restricted in any way? Slimming, vegetarianism or religious conviction could increase the risk of nutritional deficiency.
6. Do you take any prescription or over-the-counter medicines? This information can be used to assess possible drug–nutrient interactions.
7. Do you take other supplements? If so, which ones? This information can be used to assess potential overdosage of supplements which could be toxic.
8. Do you suffer from any chronic illness, e.g. diabetes, epilepsy, Crohn's disease? Nutrient requirements in patients with chronic disease may be greater than in healthy individuals.
9. Are you pregnant or breast-feeding? Nutrient requirements may be increased.
10. Do you take part in sports or other regular physical activity?
11. Do you smoke? Requirements for some vitamins (e.g. vitamin C) may be increased.
12. How much alcohol do you drink? Excessive alcohol consumption may lead to deficiency of the B vitamins.

Guidelines for supplement use

The following guidelines may be useful in making recommendations:

- Compare labels with dietary standards (usually RDAs).
- In the absence of an indication for a specific nutrient, a balanced multivitamin/mineral product is normally preferable to one which contains one or two specific nutrients.
- Use a product that provides approximately 100% of the RDA for as wide a range of vitamins and minerals as possible.
- Avoid preparations containing unrecognised nutrients or nutrients in minute amounts; this increases the cost, but not the value.
- Avoid preparations which claim to be natural, organic, or high potency; this increases the cost and, in the case of high-potency products, the risk of toxicity.
- Distinguish between credible claims and unsubstantiated claims.
- If there is uncertainty about product quality, check with the companies concerned. Ask about quality assurance. For example, is the final product analysed to guarantee that the contents in the bottle match the label declarations? Are tests for disintegration, dissolution or other tests for bioavailability conducted?

References

1 Department of Health. *Dietary Reference Values for food energy and nutrients for the United Kingdom.*

Report on Health and Social Subjects No 41. London: HMSO, 1991.

2 Office of Population Censuses and Surveys Social Survey Division and Department of Health. *National Diet and Nutrition Survey: Children aged 1½ to 4½ years*. London: HMSO, 1995.

3 Office for National Statistics Social Survey Division. *National Diet and Nutrition Survey: Young people aged 4 to 18 years*. London: Stationery Office, 2000.

4 Ministry of Agriculture, Fisheries and Food. *National Diet and Nutrition Survey: People aged 65 years and over*. Report of the diet and nutrition survey. London: Stationery Office, 1998.

5 Consumerlab. Independent tests of herbal, vitamin and mineral supplements. http://www.consumerlab.com (accessed 12 December 2000).

6 Council for Responsible Nutrition. *Guidelines for Good Manufacturing Practice for Manufacturers of Food Supplements*. Thames Ditton, Surrey: CRN, 1997.

7 Health Food Manufacturers' Association. *Guidelines for Good Manufacturing Practice for Manufacturers of Food Supplements*. Thames Ditton, Surrey: HFMA, 1997.

8 Joint Health Claims Initiative. http://www.jhci. org.uk (accessed 15 December 2000).

How to use this book

THIS BOOK COVERS 72 commonly available dietary supplements, including vitamins, minerals, trace elements and other substances, such as garlic, ginseng and fish oils. Herbal products such as Echinacea and St John's wort are not included. For ease of reference, they are arranged in alphabetical order and provide information, where appropriate, under the following standard headings.

Description

States the type of substance; e.g. a vitamin, mineral, fatty acid, amino acid, enzyme, plant extract, etc.

Nomenclature

Lists names and alternative names in current usage.

Units

Includes alternative units and conversion factors.

Constituents

Lists active ingredients in supplements that are not pure vitamins or minerals (e.g. evening primrose oil contains gamma-linolenic acid).

Human requirements

Lists for different ages and sex (where established):

- UK Dietary Reference Values (including LRNI, EAR, RNI, safe intakes).
- US Recommended Dietary Allowances (RDAs), Adequate Intakes (AIs), Tolerable Upper Intake Levels (ULs).
- World Health Organization (WHO) Reference Nutrient Intakes.
- European Population Reference Intakes (PRIs).
- European Union Recommended Daily Amounts (RDAs).

Definitions

The UK

Dietary reference values (DRVs) were established in 1991 to replace RDAs.

- EAR: Estimated Average Requirement. An assessment of the average requirement for energy or protein or a vitamin or mineral. About half the population will need more than the EAR, and half less.

- LRNI: Lower Reference Nutrient Intake. The amount of protein, vitamin or mineral which is considered to be sufficient for the few people in a group who have low needs. Most people will need more than the LRNI and if people consistently consume less they may be at risk of deficiency of that nutrient.

- RNI: Reference Nutrient Intake. The amount of protein, vitamin or mineral which is sufficient for almost every individual. This level of intake is much higher than many people need.

- Safe Intake: A term used to indicate intake or range of intakes of a nutrient for which there is not enough information to estimate RNI, EAR or LRNI. It is considered to be adequate for almost everyone's needs, but not large enough to cause undesirable effects.

- DRV: Dietary Reference Value. A term

used to cover LRNI, EAR, RNI and safe intake.

The USA

RDAs were revised in 1989 and jointly produced by the Food and Nutrition Board, the National Academy of Sciences and the National Research Council. However, the Institute of Medicine and the Food and Nutrition Board are currently establishing a set of reference values to replace the previous RDAs for the USA and Canada. The new dietary Reference Intakes will encompass EARs, RDAs, adequate intakes (AIs) and ULs. RDAs and AIs are set at levels that should decrease the risk of developing a nutritional deficiency disease.

- RDA: Recommended Dietary Allowance. The average amount of energy or a nutrient recommended to cover the needs of groups of healthy people.

- AI: Adequate Intake. Defined as a recommended intake value based on observed or experimentally determined approximations or estimates of nutrient intake by a group (or groups) of healthy people that are assumed to be adequate. Used when an RDA cannot be determined.

- UL: Tolerable Upper Intake Levels. Defined by the Food and Nutrition Board of the US National Academy of Sciences as the highest total level of a nutrient (diet plus supplements) which could be consumed safely on a daily basis, that is unlikely to cause adverse health effects to almost all individuals in the general population. As intakes rise above the UL, the risk of adverse effects increases. The UL describes long-term intakes, so an isolated dose above the UL need not necessarily cause adverse effects. The UL defines safety limits, and is not a recommended intake for most people most of the time.

Europe

- PRI: Population Reference Intake = mean requirement + 2 Standard Deviations (SDs).

- Acceptable Range: range of safe values given where insufficient information is available to be more specific.

- RDA: Recommended Daily Amount. Provides sufficient for most individuals. The EU RDA is used on dietary supplement labels.

The following points should be noted in relation to dietary standards:

- Dietary standards are intended to assess the diets of populations not of individuals. Thus, both the RDA and the UK RNI are set at 2 SDs above the average population requirement and are intended to cover the needs of 95% of the population. So, if an individual is typically consuming the RDA or the RNI for a particular nutrient, it can be assumed that his/her diet provides adequate amounts (or more than adequate amounts) of that nutrient to prevent deficiency. If intake is regularly below the RNI, it cannot necessarily be assumed that the diet is inadequate, because the person may have a lower requirement for that nutrient. However, if an individual is consistently consuming less than the LRNI for a nutrient, it can be assumed that the diet is deficient in that nutrient. Nevertheless, individuals differ from each other in the amounts of nutrients they need and the quantities they absorb and utilise, and although the dietary standards are the best figures currently available, they were never intended to assess the adequacy of individual diets.

- Dietary standards are estimates, which are assessed from a variety of epidemiological, biochemical and nutritional data, including:
  - The intake of a nutrient required to prevent or cure clinical signs of deficiency.
  - The intake of a nutrient required to maintain balance (i.e. intake – output = zero).
  - The intake of a nutrient required to maintain a given blood level, tissue concentration or degree of enzyme saturation.
  - The intake of a nutrient in the diet of a healthy population.

- Dietary standards apply only to healthy people, not to those with disease whose nutrient needs may be very different. Requirements may be increased in patients with disorders of the gastrointestinal tract, liver and kidney, and also in those with inborn errors of metabolism, cancer, severe infections, wounds, burns and following surgery. Drug administration may also alter nutrient requirements.

Intakes

States amounts of nutrients provided by the average adult diet in the UK.[1]

Action

Describes the role of the substance in maintaining physiological function and identifies pharmacological actions where appropriate.

Dietary sources

Lists significant food sources based on average portion sizes.[2] In addition, a food may be described as an 'excellent' or 'good' source of a nutrient. This does not describe any food as 'excellent' or 'good' overall; it defines only the amount of the nutrient (per portion or serving) in relation to the RNI of the nutrient for the average adult male. Thus, an excellent source provides ≥30% of the RNI, and a good source provides 15–30% of the RNI.

Where no RNI has been set for a particular nutrient, 'excellent' and 'good' are defined numerically.

Metabolism

Discusses absorption, transport, distribution and excretion.

Bioavailability

Includes the effects of cooking, processing, storage methods, and substances in food which may alter bioavailability.

Deficiency

Lists signs and symptoms of deficiency.

Possible uses

Discusses potential indications for use of the substance with evidence from the literature. Evidence for use of supplements is obtained from several types of studies:

- Epidemiological studies. These are population-based studies, and early evidence for the potential value of a nutrient usually comes from epidemiological research. For example, the idea that antioxidant supplements could reduce the risk of cancer came from studies in populations where high intake of fruit and vegetables was associated with a low risk of cancer.

- *In vitro* (laboratory) studies and animal studies. Data from these studies can be used to support evidence, but are not enough on their own. Although both types of study allow for good control of variables such as nutrients and more aggressive intervention, each suffers from the uncertainties connected with extrapolating any observed effects to humans.

- Observational studies. These may be prospective and retrospective and include in decreasing order of persuasiveness, cohort studies, case-control studies and uncontrolled studies. In prospective studies subjects are recruited and observed prior to the occurrence of the outcome. In retrospective studies, investigators review the records of subjects and interview subjects after the outcome has occurred. Retrospective studies are more vulnerable to recall bias and measurement error but less likely to suffer from the subject selection bias that can occur in prospective studies. In all observational studies, the investigator has no control of the intervention.

- Intervention studies. The investigator controls whether subjects receive an intervention or not. The randomised controlled trial (RCT) is the 'gold standard'. Intervention trials with supplements differ from those with drugs. Unlike studies with drugs, those with foods and nutrients may have additional confounders secondary to the intervention itself. For example, results from intervention studies with antioxidant supplements (e.g. vitamins A, C and E) in the prevention of cancer are inconsistent, even though epidemiological studies have consistently shown that diets high in these nutrients are associated with reduced cancer risk. This could be because such diets contain a range of other substances apart from those in the tested supplements and the antioxidants are merely acting as markers for a type of diet which is protective. Moreover, chronic disease (e.g. cancer, coronary heart disease) develops over many years, and to investigate the effect of a supplement on disease risk therefore requires a prolonged study period (e.g. 20–30 years) as well as a huge number of subjects, and this makes such studies difficult and expensive to conduct. However, without such trials, evidence for efficacy of many supplements will remain sparse.

Precautions/contraindications

Lists diseases and conditions in which the substance should be avoided or used with caution.

Pregnancy and breast-feeding

Comments on safety or potential toxicity during pregnancy and lactation.

Adverse effects

Describes the risks that may accompany excessive intake, and signs and symptoms of toxicity.

Interactions

Lists drugs and other nutrients which may interact with the supplement. This includes drugs that affect vitamin and mineral status and supplements which influence drug metabolism.

Dose

Gives usual recommended dosage (if established).

References

1 Gregory J, Foster K, Tyler H, Wiseman M. *The Dietary and Nutritional Survey of British Adults*. London: HMSO, 1990.
2 Holland B, Welch AA, Unwin ID, *et al. McCance and Widdowson's. The Composition of Foods*. 5th edn. London: Royal Society of Chemistry and Ministry of Agriculture, Fisheries and Food, 1991.

Aloe vera

Description

Aloe vera is the mucilaginous substance obtained from the central parenchymatous tissues of the large blade-like leaves of *Aloe vera*. It should not be confused with aloes, which is obtained by the evaporation of water from the bitter yellow juice that is drained from the leaf.

Constituents

Aloe vera contains polysaccharides, tannins, sterols, saponins, vitamins, minerals, cholesterol, gamma-linolenic acid and arachidonic acid. Unlike aloes, aloe vera does not contain anthraquinone compounds and does not therefore exert a laxative action.

Action

Used externally, aloe vera acts as a moisturiser and reduces inflammation. Internally, it may act as a hypoglycaemic and hyperlipidaemic agent.

Possible uses

Topical aloe vera has been investigated for its effects on wound healing and psoriasis, while oral aloe vera has been investigated in patients with diabetes mellitus and hyperlipidaemia.

A review in 1987 concluded that topical application of aloe vera gel reduces acute inflammation, promotes wound healing, reduces pain and exerts an antipruritic effect.[1] A further review in 1999[2] stated that research had continued to confirm these benefits.

A double-blind, placebo-controlled study of 60 people with psoriasis of mean duration 8.5 years found that applying aloe vera to skin lesions three times a day for eight months led to significant improvement in 83% of aloe vera patients, but in only 6% of those who used placebo.[3]

In rabbits, aloe vera cream was found to be better than placebo and as effective as oral pentoxifylline in improving tissue survival after frostbite.[4]

In a study of 27 patients, aloe vera gel healed burns faster than Vaseline gauze,[5] and in rats enhanced wound healing in second-degree burns.[6]

A recent systematic review of 10 studies[7] showed that oral aloe vera might be useful as an adjunct for lowering blood glucose concentrations in diabetes and for reducing blood lipid levels in hyperlipidaemia.

Conclusion

A huge number of *in vitro* and animal studies have examined aloe vera over the past 30 years. However, few studies have been conducted in humans, and most have been poorly controlled. Topical aloe vera may be helpful in psoriasis, but whether it is useful for wound healing is unclear. There is some (albeit limited) evidence that oral aloe vera may be useful for lowering blood glucose levels in diabetes and reducing blood lipid levels in hyperlipidaemia.

Precautions/contraindications

None established, although the potential hypoglycaemic effect means that it should be used with caution in patients with diabetes mellitus.

Pregnancy and breast-feeding

No problems have been reported, but there have not been sufficient studies to guarantee the safety of aloe vera in pregnancy and breast-feeding.

Adverse effects

None reported apart from occasional allergic reactions. However, there are no long-term studies investigating the safety of aloe vera.

Interactions

None reported.

Dose

Aloe vera is available in the form of creams, gels, tablets, capsules and juice. The International Aloe Science Council operates a voluntary approval scheme which gives an official seal ('IASC-certified') on products containing certified raw ingredients processed according to standard guidelines.

Used internally, there is no established dose. Product manufacturers suggest ½ to ¾ cup of juice or one to two capsules three times a day. The juice in the product should ideally contain at least 98% aloe vera, and no aloin.

Used externally, aloe vera should be applied liberally as needed. The product should contain at least 20% aloe vera.

References

1 Heggers JP, Kucukcelebi A, Listengarten B, *et al.* Beneficial effects of aloe in wound healing in an excisional wound model. *J Altern Complement Med* 1996; 2: 271–277.
2 Reynolds T. Aloe vera leaf gel: A review update. *J Ethnopharmacol* 1999; 68: 3–37.
3 Syed TA, Ahmad SA, Holt AH, *et al.* Management of psoriasis with aloe vera extract in a hydrophilic cream: A placebo controlled double blind study. *Trop Med Int Hlth* 1996; 1: 505–509.
4 Miller MB. Treatment of experimental frostbite with pentoxifylline and aloe vera cream. *Arch Otolaryngol Head Neck Surg* 1995; 121: 678–680.
5 Visuthikosol V, Chowchuen B, Sukwanarat Y, *et al.* Effect of aloe vera gel to healing of burn wound: A clinical and histological study. *J Med Assoc Thai* 1995; 78: 403–409.
6 Somboonwong J, Thanamittramanee S, Jariyapongshul A, Patumraj S. Therapeutic effects of aloe vera on cutaneous microcirculation and wound healing in second degree burn model in rats. *J Med Assoc Thai* 2000; 83: 417–425.
7 Vogler BK, Ernst E. Aloe vera: A systematic review of its clinical effectiveness. *Br J Clin Pract* 1999; 49: 823–828.

Alpha-lipoic acid

Description

Alpha-lipoic acid is a naturally occurring sulphur-containing co-factor. It is synthesised in humans.

Nomenclature

Alternative names include alpha-lipoate, thioctic acid, lipoic acid, 2-dithiolane-3 pentatonic acid, 1,2-dithiolane-3 valeric acid.

Action

Alpha-lipoic acid functions as a potent antioxidant and as a co-factor for various enzymes (e.g. pyruvate dehydrogenase and alpha-ketoglutarate dehydrogenase) in energy-producing metabolic reactions of the Krebs cycle.

In addition, it appears to improve recycling of other antioxidant compounds, including vitamins C and E,[1] co-enzyme Q[2] and glutathione.[3] It may also protect against arsenic,[4] cadmium,[5] lead[6] and mercury[7] poisoning.

Dietary sources

Alpha-lipoic acid is present in foods, such as spinach, meat (especially liver) and brewer's yeast, but it is difficult to obtain amounts used in clinical studies (i.e. possibly therapeutic amounts) from food.

Metabolism

Alpha-lipoic acid is both fat-soluble and water-soluble, and this facilitates its diffusion into lipophilic and hydrophilic environments. It is metabolised to dihydrolipoic acid (DHLA), which also demonstrates antioxidant properties.

Possible uses

As a dietary supplement, alpha-lipoic acid is claimed to improve glucose metabolism and insulin sensitivity in diabetes, and to reduce replication of the human immunodeficiency virus (HIV). It has been investigated for possible use in patients with diabetes mellitus, glaucoma, HIV and hypertension.

Diabetes mellitus

Alpha-lipoic acid appears to increase muscle cell glucose uptake and increase insulin sensitivity in individuals with type 2 diabetes mellitus. *In vitro*, alpha-lipoic acid has been found to stimulate glucose uptake by muscle cells in a manner similar to insulin.[8]

In an uncontrolled study, patients with type 2 diabetes given 1000 mg lipoic acid intravenously experienced a 50% improvement in insulin-stimulated glucose uptake.[9] In a further uncontrolled pilot study,[10] 20 patients with type 2 diabetes were given 500 mg lipoic acid intravenously for 10 days. Glucose uptake increased by an average of 30%, but there were no changes in either fasting blood glucose or insulin levels.

In a study involving 10 lean and 10 obese patients with type 2 diabetes,[11] alpha-lipoic acid improved glucose effectiveness and prevented hyperglycaemia-induced increases in serum lactate and pyruvate. In the lean diabetic patients, but not the obese patients, alpha-lipoic acid resulted in improved insulin sensitivity and lower fasting glucose.

In a placebo-controlled, multicentre pilot study,[12] 74 patients with type 2 diabetes were randomised to receive either alpha-lipoic acid 600 mg either once, twice or three times a day, or placebo. When compared with placebo, significantly more subjects had an increase in insulin-stimulated glucose disposal. As there was no dose-related effect, all three treatment groups were combined into one active group and compared with placebo. The increase in insulin-stimulated glucose disposal was then statistically significant, suggesting that oral administration of alpha-lipoic acid can improve insulin sensitivity in patients with type 2 diabetes.

Alpha-lipoic acid has been used extensively in Germany for the treatment of diabetic neuropathy. An *in vitro* study showed that alpha-lipoic acid reduced lipid peroxidation of nerve tissue.[13] A study in rats with diabetes induced by streptozotocin showed that alpha-lipoic acid reversed the reduction in glucose uptake which occurs in diabetes, and that this change was associated with an improvement in peripheral nerve function.[14]

In a randomised, double-blind, placebo-controlled multicentre trial, 73 patients with non-insulin-dependent diabetes mellitus (NIDDM) were randomised to receive oral alpha-lipoic acid 800 mg daily or placebo for four months. Of the total patients, 17 dropped out of the study, but the results suggested that alpha-lipoic acid might slightly improve cardiac autonomic neuropathy (assessed by measures of heart rate variability) in NIDDM patients.[15]

In a randomised, placebo-controlled study involving 24 patients with type 2 diabetes,[16] oral treatment with 600 mg alpha-lipoic acid three times a day for three weeks appeared to reduce the chief symptoms of diabetic neuropathy. A further placebo-controlled, randomised, double-blind trial showed that oral alpha-lipoic acid 600 mg once or twice daily appeared to have a beneficial effect on nerve conduction in patients with both type 1 and type 2 diabetes.[17]

A review[18] of the evidence of the effect of alpha-lipoic acid in the treatment of diabetic neuropathy concluded that short-term treatment with oral or *in vitro* alpha-lipoic acid appears to reduce the chief symptoms of diabetic neuropathy, but this needs to be confirmed by larger studies.

Glaucoma

In a study involving 75 patients with open-angle glaucoma,[19] lipoic acid was administered in a dose of either 75 mg daily for two months or 150 mg daily for one month. Improvements in biochemical parameters and visual function were found, particularly in the group receiving 150 mg lipoic acid.

Human immunodeficiency virus

Alpha-lipoic acid blocks activation of NF-kappa B, which is required for HIV transcription, and has also been noted to improve antioxidant status, T-helper lymphocytes, and the T-helper/ suppressor cell ratio in HIV infected T-cells.[20] However, it is not known whether supplementation would improve survival in individuals who are HIV-positive.

Miscellaneous

Results of preliminary studies suggest that alpha-lipoic acid may lower blood pressure,[21] improve the symptoms of burning mouth syndrome[22] and improve T-cell functions *in vitro* in advanced stage cancer patients.[23]

> **Conclusion**
> There is preliminary evidence that alpha-lipoic acid might have a role in patients with diabetes mellitus in improving glucose utilisation, insulin sensitivity and neuropathy. Very limited evidence also exists that alpha-lipoic acid may be helpful in glaucoma and hypertension and slow replication of HIV and cancer cells, but evidence of benefit in all these conditions, including diabetes, is too limited to make recommendations for supplementation.

Precautions/contraindications

Alpha-lipoic acid should be used with caution in patients predisposed to hypoglycaemia, including patients taking antidiabetic agents.

Pregnancy and breast-feeding

No problems have been reported, but there have not been sufficient studies to guarantee the safety of alpha-lipoic acid in pregnancy and breast-feeding.

Adverse effects

None reported, apart from occasional skin rashes. However, there are no long-term studies assessing the safety of alpha-lipoic acid.

Interactions

Drugs

Oral hypoglycaemics and insulin: Theoretically, alpha-lipoic acid could enhance the effects of these drugs.

Dose

Alpha-lipoic acid is available in the form of tablets and capsules.

The dose is not established. Studies have used 150–600 mg daily. Dietary supplements provide 50–300 mg daily.

References

1 Scholich H, Murphy ME, Sies H. Antioxidant activity of dihydrolipoate against microsomal lipid peroxidation and its dependence on α-tocopherol. *Biochim Biophys Acta* 1989; 1001: 256–261.

2 Kagan V, Serbinova E, Packer L. Antioxidant effects of ubiquinones in microsomes and mitochondria are mediated by tocopherol recycling. *Biochem Biophys Res Commun* 1990; 169: 851–857.

3 Busse E, Zimmer G, Schopohl B, *et al.* Influence of alpha-lipoic acid on intracellular glutathione in vitro and in vivo. *Arzneimittelforschung* 1992; 42: 829–831.

4 Grunert RR. The effect of DL-α-lipoic acid on heavy metal intoxication in mice and dogs. *Arch Biochem Biophys* 1960; 86: 190–194.

5 Muller L, Menzel H. Studies on the effect of lipoate and dihydrolipoate in the alteration of cadmium toxicity in isolated hepatocytes. *Biochim Biophys Acta* 1990; 1052: 386–391.

6 Gurer H, Ozgunes H, Oztezcan S, Ercal N. Antioxidant role of alpha-lipoic acid in lead toxicity. *Free Radic Biol Med* 1999; 27: 75–81.

7 Keith RL, Setiarahardjo I, Fernando Q, *et al.* Utilization of renal slices to evaluate the efficacy of chelating agents for removing mercury from the kidney. *Toxicology* 1997; 116: 67–75.

8 Estrada DE, Ewart HS, Tsakiridis T, *et al.* Stimulation of glucose uptake by the natural co-enzyme alpha-lipoic acid/thioctic acid: participation of elements of the insulin signaling pathway. *Diabetes* 1996; 45: 1798–1804.

9 Jacob S, Henricksen EJ, Schiemann AL, *et al.* Enhancement of glucose disposal in patients with type 2 diabetes by alpha-lipoic acid. *Arzneimittelforschung* 1995; 45: 872–874.

10 Jacob S, Henricksen EJ, Tritschler HJ, *et al.* Improvement of insulin-stimulated glucose disposal in type 2 diabetes after repeated parenteral administration of thioctic acid. *Exp Clin Endocrinol Diabetes* 1996; 104: 284–288.

11 Konrad T, Vicini P, Kusterer K, *et al.* Alpha-lipoic acid treatment decreases serum lactate and pyruvate concentrations and improves glucose effectiveness in lean and obese patients with type 2 diabetes. *Diabetes Care* 1999; 22: 280–287.

12 Jacob S, Ruus P, Hermann R, *et al.* Oral administration of RAC-alpha-lipoic acid modulates insulin sensitivity in patients with type 2 diabetes mellitus: A placebo-controlled pilot trial. *Free Radic Biol Med* 1999; 27: 309–314.

13 Nickander KK, McPhee BR, Low PA, *et al.* Alpha-lipoic acid: Antioxidant potency against lipid peroxidation of neural tissues in vitro and implications for diabetic neuropathy. *Free Radic Biol Med* 1996; 21: 631–639.

14 Kishi Y, Schmeizer JD, Yao JK, *et al.* Alpha-lipoic acid: effect of glucose uptake, sorbitol pathway, and energy metabolism in experimental diabetic neuropathy. *Diabetes* 1999; 48: 2045–2051.

15 Ziegler D, Schatz H, Conrad F, *et al.* Effects of treatment with the antioxidant alpha-lipoic acid on cardiac autonomic neuropathy in NIDDM patients. A 4-month randomized controlled multicenter trial (DEKAN Study). Deutsche Kardiale Autonome Neuropathie. *Diabetes Care* 1997; 20: 369–373.

16 Ruhnau KJ, Meissner HP, Finn JR. Effects of a 3-week oral treatment with the antioxidant thioctic acid (alpha-lipoic acid) in symptomatic diabetic polyneuropathy. *Diabetes Med* 1999; 16: 1040–1043.

17 Reljanovic M, Reichel G, Rett K, *et al.* Treatment of diabetic polyneuropathy with the antioxidant thioctic acid (alpha-lipoic acid): A two year multicenter randomized double-blind placebo-controlled trial (ALADIN II). Alpha lipoic acid in diabetic neuropathy. *Free Radic Res* 1999; 31: 171–179.

18 Ziegler D, Reljanovic M, Mehnert H. Alpha-lipoic acid in the treatment of diabetic polyneuropathy in Germany: Current evidence from clinical trials. *Exp Clin Endocrinol Diabetes* 1999; 107: 421–430.

19 Filina AA, Davydova NG, Endrikhovskii SN, *et al.* Lipoic acid as a means of metabolic therapy of open-angle glaucoma. *Invest Ophthalmol* 1995; 111: 6–8.

20 Baur A, Harrer T, Peukert M, *et al.* Alpha-lipoic acid

is an effective inhibitor of human immunodeficiency virus (HIV-1) replication. *Klin Wochenschr* 1991; 69: 722–724.

21 Vasdev S, Ford CA, Parai S, *et al*. Dietary alpha-lipoic acid supplementation lowers blood pressure in spontaneously hypertensive rats. *J Hypertens* 2000; 18: 567–573.

22 Femiano F, Gombos F, Scully C, *et al*. Burning mouth syndrome (BMS): Controlled open trial of the efficacy of alpha-lipoic acid (thioctic acid) on symptomatology. *Oral Dis* 2000; 6: 274–277.

23 Mantovani G, Maccio A, Melis G, *et al*. Restoration of functional defects in peripheral blood mononuclear cells isolated from cancer patients by thiol antioxidants alpha-lipoic acid and *N*-acetyl cysteine. *Int J Cancer* 2000; 86: 842–847.

Antioxidants

Description

Various antioxidant systems have evolved to offer protection against free radicals and prevent damage to vital biological structures such as lipid membranes, proteins and DNA. Antioxidant capacity is a concept which is used to describe the overall ability of tissues to inhibit free-radical-mediated processes.[1] It is dependent on the concentrations of individual antioxidants and the activity of protective enzymes. The most common and important antioxidant defences are shown in Table 1.

The antioxidant vitamins can be divided into those that are water-soluble and exist in aqueous solution – primarily vitamin C – and those that are fat-soluble and exist in membranes or lipoproteins – vitamin E and beta-carotene. Lipid membranes are particularly vulnerable to oxidative breakdown by free radicals. Vitamin E protects cell membranes from destruction by undergoing preferential oxidation and destruction. Some quinones, such as ubiquinone (co-enzyme Q) also appear to have antioxidant properties. All these substances can act as free radical scavengers and can react directly with free radicals.

Some trace elements act as essential components of antioxidant enzymes; copper, magnesium or zinc for superoxide dismutase and selenium for glutathione peroxidase.

Table 1 Antioxidant defences

- Intracellular antioxidants
  Enzymes
  — catalase
  — glutathione peroxidase
  — superoxide dismutase
- Extracellular antioxidants
  Vitamin C
  Sulphydryl groups
- Membrane antioxidants
  Carotenoids
  Ubiquinone
  Vitamin E
- Substances essential for synthesis of antioxidant enzymes
  Copper
  Manganese
  Selenium
  Zinc

Action

Antioxidants are believed to protect against certain diseases by preventing the deleterious effects of free-radical-mediated processes in cell membranes and by reducing the susceptibility of tissues to oxidative stress.

Free radicals

Each orbital surrounding the nucleus of an atom is occupied by a pair of electrons. If an orbital in the outer shell of a molecule loses an electron, the molecule becomes a free radical. As a result of the unpaired electron, the molecule becomes unstable and, therefore, highly reactive. The free radical may then react with any other nearby molecule, also converting that molecule to a free radical which can then initiate another reaction. Some free radicals are capable of causing severe damage to cells.

Theoretically, a single free radical can ultimately cause an endless number of reactions. This chain reaction is terminated either by the free radical's reaction with another free radical, resulting in the formation of a covalently bound molecule, or by the free radical's reaction with an antioxidant, an antioxidant enzyme, or both. Fortunately, many enzyme systems have evolved to provide protection against free radical production.

Because antioxidant defences are not completely efficient, increased free-radical formation in the body is likely to increase damage. The term 'oxidative stress' is often used to refer to this effect. If mild oxidative stress occurs, tissues often respond by increasing their antioxidant defences. However, severe oxidative stress can cause cell injury and cell death.

There is growing evidence that free-radical damage is involved in the development of many diseases, such as atherosclerosis, cancer, Parkinson's disease and other neurodegenerative disorders, inflammatory bowel disease and lung disease.

Possible uses

Epidemiological evidence suggests that low plasma levels of antioxidant nutrients and low dietary intakes are related to an increased risk of diseases such as coronary heart disease (CHD) and cancer. There is also increasing evidence that these diseases can be prevented or delayed to some extent by dietary changes, in particular by increased consumption of fruits and vegetables. Several substances in fruit and vegetables (e.g. betacarotene, vitamin C and vitamin E) may act to diminish oxidative damage *in vivo* and, because endogenous antioxidant defences are not completely effective, dietary antioxidants may be important in diminishing the cumulative effects of oxidative damage in the human body.

A question of particular current interest is whether supplementation of adequately nourished subjects with antioxidant nutrients will reduce the incidence of such diseases. The few intervention trials of antioxidants reported so far have shown little evidence for the value of supplements. However, further large trials are still in progress.

Cardiovascular disease

Experimental studies suggest an inverse association between CHD mortality and vitamins C, E and betacarotene, and argue strongly in favour of a protective role of antioxidants in the development of atherosclerosis.

In a cross-cultural study of middle-aged men representing 16 European populations,[1] differences in mortality from ischaemic heart disease were primarily attributable to plasma levels of vitamin E. Twelve of the 16 populations had similar blood cholesterol levels and blood pressure, but differed greatly in tocopherol levels and heart disease death rates. For vitamin E, mean plasma levels lower than 25 μmol/l were associated with a high risk of CHD, whereas plasma levels above this value were associated with a lower risk of the disease. In the case of vitamin C, mean plasma levels <22.7 μmol/l were found in those regions that had a moderate to high risk of CHD, whereas plasma levels in excess of this level tended to be found in those areas at low risk.

In a large case control study in Scotland,[2] 6000 men aged 35–54 years were studied for a possible association between antioxidant status and risk of angina pectoris. Highly significant correlations were found between low plasma concentrations of betacarotene, vitamin C, vitamin E and risk of angina.

The Health Professionals Study,[3] a large prospective investigation, which looked at 39 910 US male health professionals aged 40–75 years, showed that men who took more than 100 units of vitamin E daily for over two years had a 37% reduction in risk of heart disease. The Nurses' Health Study,[4] in which 87 245 female nurses aged 34–59 years took part, showed that women who took more than 200 units of vitamin E daily for more than two years had a 41% reduction in risk of CHD.

The first intervention trial published was a study of 333 male physicians aged between 40 and 84 years with angina pectoris and/or coronary revascularisation, and it showed that 50 mg of betacarotene on alternate days resulted in a 44% reduction in major coronary events.[5]

However, another study[6] tested aspirin, vitamin E and betacarotene in the prevention of cardiovascular disease and cancer in 39 876 women aged 45 years and older. Among those randomly assigned to receive 50 mg betacarotene or a placebo every other day, there were no statistically significant differences in incidence of cardiovascular disease, cancer or overall death rate after a median of two years of treatment and two years of follow-up.

In a study of 1862 men aged 50–59 years,[7] who were followed for a median of 5.3 years, dietary supplements of alpha tocopherol (50 mg a day), betacarotene (20 mg a day), both, or a placebo were given. There were significantly more deaths from CHD among those who took betacarotene supplements, and a non-significant trend towards more deaths in the vitamin E group.

A double-blind clinical trial[8] found that taking high doses of vitamin C (500 mg twice a day) and E (700 units twice a day) and betacarotene (30 000 units twice a day) did not reduce the risk of arteries re-blocking after balloon coronary angioplasty. The patients took either probucol, probucol plus three antioxidants, the antioxidants alone, or placebo. All the patients also received aspirin. After six months the rates of repeated angioplasty were 11% in the probucol group, 16.2% in the combined treatment group, 24.4% in the multivitamin group, and 26.6% in the placebo group.

Cancer

There is now good evidence linking high intake of fruit and vegetables with lower incidence of certain cancers, and it is presumed that the protective nutrients are some or all of the antioxidant nutrients.

In a study of 25 802 volunteers in Washington County, Maryland,[9] pre-diagnostic blood samples from 436 cancer cases at nine cancer sites were compared with 765 matched control cases. Serum betacarotene levels showed a strong protective association with lung cancer, suggestive protective associations with melanoma and bladder cancer, and a suggestive but non-protective association with lung cancer. Serum vitamin E levels showed a protective association with lung cancer, but none of the other cancer sites studied showed impressive associations. Low levels of serum lycopene (a carotenoid occurring in ripe fruits) were strongly associated with pancreatic cancer and less strongly associated with cancer of the bladder and rectum.

The Basel study from Switzerland[10] demonstrated that patients who had died from all cancers, including cancer of the bronchus and the stomach, had statistically lower mean carotene levels compared with a matched group of healthy survivors.

In a Finnish study,[11] individuals with low serum levels of vitamin E had about a 1.5-fold risk of cancer compared with those with a higher serum level of vitamin E. The strength of the association between serum vitamin E level and cancer risk varied for different cancer sites, and was strongest for some gastrointestinal cancers and for the combined group of cancers unrelated to smoking.

An intervention trial in Linxian, China[12] provided some of the earliest clinical data on the effects of specific vitamin-mineral supplementation on cancer incidence and disease-specific mortality. Linxian County has one of the world's highest rates of oesophageal and gastric cancers. Combined daily doses of 15 mg betacarotene, 30 mg vitamin E and 50 µg selenium taken over five years were associated with a 13% reduction in deaths from cancer, and an overall reduction in mortality of 9%. These results, although impressive, might have been achieved because the population studied had low intakes and were deficient in the nutrients investigated. A similar study is required in a well-nourished population.

Not all studies have shown positive results. The Alpha Tocopherol Beta-Carotene (ATBC) study in Finland[13] found no reduction in the incidence of lung cancer among male smokers after five to eight years of dietary supplementation with either vitamin E or betacarotene; incidence of lung cancer increased by 18% and overall death rate by 8% in the group receiving betacarotene. However, these results should be considered in the context of the population studied – the subjects had smoked an average of 20 cigarettes a day for 36 years. Most studies with antioxidants suggest that their protective properties are associated with the early stages of cancer and it is likely that this intervention took place too late in the carcinogenic process. In addition, the study could have employed too low a dose (50 mg vitamin E and/or 20 mg betacarotene were used) or was of too short a duration.

Nevertheless, another trial,[14] which tested a combination of betacarotene and vitamin A, was terminated after four years because it appeared that those taking the supplements and who also smoked had a 28% higher incidence of lung cancer and a 17% higher death rate.

More recently, a study conducted in ferrets (which metabolise betacarotene in a similar way to humans) may help to explain why high doses of betacarotene appeared to increase the risk of lung cancer in these studies.[15] The study found that excessive amounts of betacarotene stored in the lungs were oxidised into substances that decreased the activity of a tumour suppressor but increased that of a tumour promoter in ferret lung. The animals were divided into four groups: one group received betacarotene and was exposed to cigarette smoke equivalent to a human smoking 1.5 packs a day; two other groups received either the supplement or smoke exposure; and a control group received neither. The first group had the strongest pre-cancerous changes.

In the Nurses' Health Study,[16] large intakes of vitamin C or E did not protect women from breast cancer. In contrast, there was a significant inverse association of vitamin A intake with risk of this disease. The authors concluded, however, that vitamin A supplements are unlikely to influence the risk of breast cancer among women whose dietary intake of this vitamin is already adequate.

In the Polyp Prevention Study[17] there was no evidence that supplements of either betacarotene or vitamins C and E reduced the incidence of colorectal adenomas.

Cataract

Antioxidants are also being investigated for a possible protective effect in cataract. Low vitamin C intakes have been associated with increased risk of cataract.[18] Increased levels of supplementary vitamins C and E correlated with a 50% reduction in the risk of cataracts.[19] The Nurses' Health Study[20] found that dietary carotenoids, although not necessarily betacarotene, and long-term vitamin C supplementation may reduce the risk of cataracts.

Age-related macular degeneration

Research is being conducted to determine whether taking supplements or consuming foods rich in antioxidants can protect against age-related macular degeneration (AMD), a disease in which the central portion of the retina deteriorates so that only peripheral vision remains. A study following 3654 individuals aged 49 years or older found no statistically significant association between AMD and dietary intake of either carotene, zinc or vitamins A or C, either from diet, supplements or both.[21] An earlier study involving 156 subjects with AMD showed that neither serum alpha tocopherol nor betacarotene was significantly associated with age-related maculopathy (ARM).[22]

In 29 000 smoking males aged 50–69 years and assigned randomly to alpha tocopherol (50 mg a day), betacarotene (20 mg a day), placebo or both, no beneficial effect of supplementation on the occurrence of ARM was found.[23] However, in a study involving 21 120 male physicians,[24] those who used vitamin E supplements or multivitamins had a possible but non-significant reduced risk of AMD, the authors concluding that large reductions in the risk of AMD were unlikely.

A Cochrane review[25] (which included one study) concluded that there is no evidence to date that people without AMD should take

Conclusion

Biochemical evidence suggests that oxidative stress caused by accumulation of free radicals is involved in the pathogenesis of several diseases. Appropriate levels of antioxidant nutrients might therefore be expected to delay or prevent these diseases. Several epidemiological studies have found lower serum levels of antioxidant nutrients in patients with cardiovascular disease, cancer and cataract, but there is (as yet) little evidence that supplements of antioxidant nutrients prevent disease. Further intervention trials are needed. In the meantime, the best advice to give is to eat plenty of fruit and vegetables (five or more servings a day).

antioxidant vitamin and mineral supplements to prevent or delay the onset of the disease.

References

1 Gey KF, Puska P, Jordan P, Moser UK. Inverse correlation between plasma vitamin E and mortality from ischaemic heart disease in cross-cultural epidemiology. *Am J Clin Nutr* 1991; 53: 326S–334S.
2 Riemersma RA, Wood DA, MacIntyre CCA, *et al.* Risk of angina pectoris and plasma concentrations of vitamins A, C and E and carotene. *Lancet* 1991; 337: 1–5.
3 Rimm EB, Stampfer MJ, Ascherio A, *et al.* Vitamin E consumption and the risk of coronary heart disease in men. *N Engl J Med* 1993; 328: 1450–1456.
4 Stampfer MJ, Hennekens CH, Manson JE, *et al.* Vitamin E consumption and the risk of coronary heart disease in women. *N Engl J Med* 1993; 328: 1444–1449.
5 Gaziano JM, Manson JE, Ridker PM, *et al.* Beta carotene therapy for chronic stable angina. *Circulation* 1990; 82 (suppl. III): 201 (abstract 0796).
6 Rapola JM, Virtamo J, Ripatti S, *et al.* Randomised trial of alpha-tocopherol and beta-carotene supplements on incidence of major coronary events in men with previous myocardial infarction. *Lancet* 1997; 349: 1715–1720.
7 Hennekens CH, Buring JE, Manson JE, *et al.* Lack of effect of long term supplementation with betacarotene on the incidence of malignant neoplasms and cardiovascular disease. *N Engl J Med* 1996; 334: 1145–1149.
8 Tardif JC. Probucol and multivitamins in the prevention of restenosis after coronary angioplasty. *N Engl J Med* 1997; 337: 365–372.
9 Comstock GW, Helzlsouer KJ, Bush T. Prediagnostic serum levels of carotenoids and vitamin E as related to subsequent cancer in Washington County, Maryland. *Am J Clin Nutr* 1991; 53: 260S–264S.
10 Stahelin HB, Gey KF, Eichholzer M, Ludin E. β-carotene and cancer prevention: the Basel study. *Am J Clin Nutr* 1991; 53: 265S–269S.
11 Knekt P, Aromaa A, Maatela J, *et al.* Vitamin E and cancer prevention. *Am J Clin Nutr* 1991; 53: 283S–286S.
12 Blot WJ, Li JY, Taylor PR. Nutrition intervention trials in Linxian, China: Supplementation with specific vitamin/mineral combinations, cancer incidence, and disease-specific mortality in the general population. *J Natl Cancer Inst* 1993; 85: 1483–1492.
13 The Alpha Tocopherol, Beta-Carotene Cancer Prevention Study Group. The effect of vitamin E and beta carotene on the incidence of lung cancer in male smokers. *N Engl J Med* 1994; 330: 1029–1035.
14 Omenn GS, Goodman GE, Thornquist MD, *et al.* Effects of a combination of betacarotene and vitamin A on lung cancer and cardiovascular disease. *N Engl J Med* 1996; 334: 1150–1155.
15 United States Department of Agriculture. Why megadoses of betacarotene may promote lung cancer. USDA Agricultural Research Service Food & Nutrition Research Briefs, January 1999, p. 1.
16 Hunter DJ, Manson JE, Colditz GA, *et al.* A prospective study of vitamins C, E and A and the risk of breast cancer. *N Engl J Med* 1993; 329: 234–240.
17 Greenberg ER, Baron JA, Tosteson TD, *et al.* A clinical trial of antioxidant vitamins to prevent colorectal adenoma. *N Engl J Med* 1994; 331: 141–147.
18 Jacques PF, Chylack LT. Epidemiologic evidence of a role for the antioxidant vitamins and carotenoids in cataract prevention. *Am J Clin Nutr* 1991; 53: 352S–355S.
19 Robertson J McD, Donner AP, Trevithick JR. A possible role for vitamins C and E in cataract prevention. *Am J Clin Nutr* 1991; 53: 346S–351S.
20 Hankinson SE, Stampfer MJ, Seddon JM, *et al.* Nutrient intake and cataract extraction in women: A prospective study. *Br Med J* 1992; 305: 335–339.
21 Smith W, Mitchell P, Webb K, Leeder SR. Dietary antioxidants and age-related maculopathy: The Blue Mountains Study. *Ophthalmology* 1999; 106: 761–767.
22 Smith W, Mitchell P, Rochester C, *et al.* Serum betacarotene, alpha tocopherol and age-related maculopathy: The Blue Mountain study. *Am J Ophthalmol* 1997; 124: 839–840.
23 Teikari JM, Laatikainen L, Virtamo J, *et al.* Six-year supplementation with alpha-tocopherol and beta-carotene and age-related maculopathy. *Acta Ophthalmol Scand* 1998; 76: 224–229.
24 Christen WG, Ajani UA, Glynn RG, *et al.* Prospective cohort study of antioxidant vitamin supplement use and the risk of age-related maculopathy. *Am J Epidemiol* 1999; 149: 476–484.
25 Evans JR, Henshaw K. Antioxidant vitamin and mineral supplementation for preventing age related macular degeneration. *Cochrane Database Syst Rev* 2000; 2: CD000253.

Bee pollen

Description

Bee pollen consists of flower pollen and nectar from male seed flowers. It is collected by the worker honey bee, mixed with secretions from the bee, such as saliva, which contains digestive enzymes, and is then carried back to the beehive on the hind legs of the bee. The pollen is harvested at the entrance to the beehive as bees travel through the wire mesh brushing their legs against a collecting vessel. Commercial qualities of pollen can also be collected directly from the flowers.

Constituents

Bee pollen consists of protein, carbohydrates, minerals, and essential fatty acids such as alpha-linolenic acid and linoleic acids. It also contains small amounts of B vitamins, vitamin C, flavonoids and various amino acids, hormones, enzymes and co-enzymes. In nutritional terms the amounts of vitamins and minerals are too small to be significant.

Action

Bee pollen may have antioxidant and anti-inflammatory activity.

Possible uses

Bee pollen has been claimed to be useful for improving prostatitis and benign prostatic hypertrophy, although all the studies conducted so far have been uncontrolled and none has been published in English. Bee pollen has also been claimed to be beneficial in reducing the risk of atherosclerosis, hypertension and varicose veins, but there are no clinical studies to support these claims.

Two double-blind, placebo-controlled trials in humans have investigated the effects of bee pollen in cross-country runners[1] and in elderly patients with memory deterioration.[2] However, there were no improvements in running speed or memory function in these two studies, respectively.

Precautions/contraindications

Bee pollen is contraindicated in people with a known history of atopy or allergy to pollen or plant products because of the risk of hypersensitivity.

Pregnancy and breast-feeding

No problems have been reported, but insufficient studies have been performed to guarantee the safety of bee pollen in pregnancy and breast-feeding.

Adverse effects

Bee pollen may cause allergic reactions, which include nausea, vomiting and anaphylaxis. One 19-year-old man with asthma had a fatal reaction to bee pollen.[3] Anecdotally, bee pollen has been shown to promote hyperglycaemia in diabetes.

Interactions

None documented.

Dose

Bee pollen is available in the form of capsules and powder.

The dose is not established. Product manufacturers tend to recommend doses of 500–1500 mg daily from capsules or ½ to one teaspoon of the powder.

References

1 Steben RE, Boudreaux P. The effects of pollen and protein extracts on selected blood factors and performance of athletes. *J Sports Med Phys Fitness* 1978; 18: 221–226.

2 Iversen T, Fiigaard KM, Schriver P, *et al*. The effects of NaO Li Su on memory functions and blood chemistry in elderly people. *J Ethnopharmacol* 1997; 56: 109–116.

3 Prichard M, Turner KJ. Acute hypersensitivity to ingested processed pollen. *Aust NZ J Med* 1985; 15: 346–347.

Betaine

Description

Betaine is a co-factor in various methylation reactions.

Action

Betaine works with choline, vitamin B_{12}, and also *S*-adenosyl methionine (SAMe), a derivative of the amino acid methionine, from which homocysteine is synthesised.

Possible uses

As a supplement, betaine is available in the form of the hydrochloride and as such contains 23% hydrochloric acid. It has been used as a digestive aid to treat people with achlorhydria.

Betaine has been reported to play a role in reducing plasma homocysteine levels, which may reduce the risk of heart disease. A study in 15 healthy men and women aged 18–35 years showed that betaine 6 g daily for three weeks reduced plasma homocysteine concentration after two weeks by 0.9 μmol/l, and after three weeks by 0.6 μmol/l.[1] However, the extent of the decrease was much smaller than that in patients with homocystinuria[2] and appears to be smaller than that established by interventions with folic acid.[3] There is, therefore, insufficient evidence to recommend betaine supplements for the prevention of coronary heart disease.

Precautions/contraindications

Betaine should be avoided in patients with peptic ulcer.

Pregnancy and breast-feeding

No problems have been reported, but there have not been sufficient studies to guarantee the safety of betaine in pregnancy and breast-feeding.

Adverse effects

Betaine may cause gastrointestinal irritation.

Interactions

None documented.

Dose

Betaine is available in the form of tablets and capsules.

The dose is not established. Dietary supplements provide 250–500 mg in each dose.

References

1 Brouwer IA, Verhoef P, Urgert R. Betaine supplementation and plasma homocysteine in healthy volunteers. *Arch Intern Med* 2000; 160: 911.
2 Wilcken DE, Wilcken B, Dudman NP, Tyrell PA. Homocystinuria: the effects of betaine in the treatment of patients not responsive to pyridoxine. *N Engl J Med* 1983; 309: 448–453.
3 Homocysteine Lowering Trialists' Collaboration. Lowering blood homocysteine with folic acid-based supplements: Meta-analysis of randomised trials. *Br Med J* 1998; 316: 894–898.

Biotin

Description

Biotin is a water-soluble vitamin and a member of the vitamin B complex.

Nomenclature

Biotin was formerly known as vitamin H or coenzyme R.

Human requirements

See Table 1 for Dietary Reference Values for biotin.

Intakes

In the UK, the average adult diet provides 33 µg daily. Biotin is also produced by colonic bacteria, but the effect of this on biotin requirements is not known.

Action

Biotin functions as an integral part of the enzymes that transport carboxyl units and fix carbon dioxide. Biotin enzymes are important in carbohydrate and lipid metabolism, and are involved in gluconeogenesis, fatty acid synthesis, propionate metabolism and the catabolism of amino acids.

Dietary sources

Biotin is ubiquitous in the diet. The richest sources of biotin are liver, kidney, eggs, soya beans and peanuts. Meat, wholegrain cereals, wholemeal bread, milk and cheese are also good sources. Green vegetables contain very little biotin.

Metabolism

Absorption

Biotin is absorbed rapidly from the gastrointestinal tract by facilitated transport (at low concentrations) and by passive diffusion (at high concentrations). Absorption is greater in the jejunum than the ileum and minimal in the colon.

Distribution

Biotin is bound to plasma proteins.

Table 1 Dietary Reference Values for biotin (µg/day)

EU RDA = 0.15 mg

Age	UK safe intake	USA AI	European acceptable range
0–6 months	–	5	–
7–12 months	–	6	–
1–3 years	–	8	–
4–8 years	–	12	–
Males and females			
11–50+ years	10–20	–	15–100
9–13 years	–	20	–
14–18 years	–	25	–
19–70+ years	–	30	–

AI = Adequate intake.

Elimination

Excess biotin is excreted largely unchanged in the urine. It also appears in breast milk.

Deficiency

Biotin deficiency is a risk only in those patients on prolonged parenteral nutrition (who will automatically be given multivitamin supplements). Deficiency has been induced by the ingestion of large amounts of raw egg white, which contain the biotin-binding protein, avidin, to a diet low in biotin.[1]

Symptoms of biotin deficiency include anorexia, nausea, vomiting, dry scaly dermatitis, glossitis, loss of taste, somnolence, panic and an increase in serum cholesterol levels and bile pigments.

Possible uses

Biotin has been claimed to be of value in the treatment of brittle finger nails, acne, seborrhoeic dermatitis, hair fragility and alopecia, but such claims need further confirmation by controlled clinical trials.

Biotin deficiency has been associated with sudden infant death syndrome (SIDS). In one study, the median biotin levels in the livers of infants who died from SIDS were significantly lower than those of infants who died from explicable causes.[2] However, evidence that biotin deficiency is an important contributory factor in SIDS is circumstantial and unequivocal proof is lacking. There is no requirement for biotin supplements in newborn or young infants. Supplements should *not* be sold to parents for this purpose.

Precautions/contraindications

No problems have been reported.

Pregnancy and breast-feeding

No problems have been reported.

Adverse effects

None reported.

Interactions

Drugs

Anticonvulsants (carbamazepine, phenobarbitone, phenytoin and primidone): requirements for biotin may be increased.

Dose

Biotin is available in the form of tablets and capsules. However, it is available mainly in multivitamin preparations.

The dose is not established. Dietary supplements provide 100–300 μg daily.

References

1 Baugh CM, Malone JW, Butterworth Jr, CE. Human biotin deficiency: A case history of biotin deficiency induced by raw egg consumption in a cirrhotic patient. *Am J Clin Nutr* 1968; 21: 173–182.
2 Heard GS, Hood RL, Johnson AR. Hepatic biotin and sudden infant death syndrome. *Med J Aust* 1983; 2: 305–306.

Boron

Description

Boron is an ultratrace mineral.

Human requirements

Boron is essential in plants and some animals, and evidence of essentiality is accumulating in humans; however, as yet requirements have not been defined.

Intakes

Most UK diets appear to provide about 2 mg daily.

Action

Boron appears to be important in calcium metabolism, and can affect the composition, structure and strength of bone. It may also influence the metabolism of calcium, copper, magnesium, phosphorus, potassium and vitamin D. In addition, boron affects the activity of certain enzymes. It also affects brain function; boron deprivation appears to depress mental alertness.

Dietary sources

Foods of plant origin, especially non-citrus fruits, leafy vegetables and nuts, are rich sources of boron, but there is little in meat, fish and poultry. Beer, wine and cider contain significant amounts.

Metabolism

Absorption

Dietary boron is rapidly absorbed. The mechanism of absorption from the gastrointestinal tract has not been elucidated.

Distribution

Boron is distributed throughout the body tissues; the highest concentrations are found in the bone, spleen and thyroid.

Elimination

Boron is excreted mainly in the urine.

Deficiency

No precise signs and symptoms of boron deficiency have been defined.

Possible uses

Boron has been claimed to prevent osteoporosis and to both prevent and relieve the symptoms of osteoarthritis, as well as to improve memory.

Bone

In a study of 12 postmenopausal women,[1] boron supplementation (3 mg daily) reduced the urinary excretion of both calcium and magnesium, and increased serum levels of oestradiol and ionized calcium.

A further study[2] has provided evidence that boron can both enhance and mimic some effects of oestrogen ingestion in postmenopausal women. In women receiving oestrogen therapy, an increase in boron intake increased serum oestradiol concentrations to higher levels than when boron intake was low. However, there is no evidence that boron supplements can relieve the symptoms of the menopause. The effects seen in this study did not occur in men or in women not receiving oestrogen therapy. However, another study[3] in men found that supplementation with boron (10 mg/day) significantly increased oestradiol concentrations, and there was also a trend for plasma testosterone levels to increase. These findings support the contention that, if oestrogen is beneficial to calcium metabolism, then boron might also be beneficial.

However, another study[4] in postmenopausal women showed that 3 mg boron daily had no effect on bone mineral absorption and excretion, plasma sex steroid levels and urinary excretion of pyridinium cross-link markers of bone turnover. Moreover, in this study a low-boron diet appeared to induce hyperabsorption of calcium since positive calcium balances were found in combination with elevated urinary calcium excretion. The authors concluded that this phenomenon may have inhibited or obscured any effect of boron supplementation.

Arthritis

Boron has been claimed to relieve the symptoms of arthritis, but evidence is very weak. Epidemiological studies suggest that incidence of arthritis is higher in areas of the world where boron intake is low, and subjects with arthritis have been found to have lower bone boron concentrations.[5] One double-blind controlled (but not randomised) trial in 20 patients with osteoarthritis found that boron (6 mg daily) improved symptoms in five out of 10 subjects in the treated group, but only one out of 10 subjects improved in the placebo group. However, statistical analysis was not performed because of the small number of subjects.[6]

Brain function

Three placebo-controlled, double-blind randomised trials in 28 healthy adults showed that low dietary boron (0.25 mg/2000 kcal) was associated with poorer performance of a variety of cognitive and pschychomotor tasks and also depression of mental alertness than higher intake (3.25 mg/2000 kcal).[7]

Precautions/contraindications

No problems have been reported.

Conclusion

There is preliminary evidence that boron has beneficial effects on calcium metabolism in postmenopausal women by preventing calcium loss and bone demineralisation, but no evidence that it can prevent or be of benefit in treating osteoporosis. There is some evidence that diets low in boron impair cognitive function. Evidence that boron can improve symptoms of arthritis is lacking.

Pregnancy and breast-feeding

No problems have been reported, but there have not been sufficient studies to guarantee the safety of boron in pregnancy and breast-feeding. However, supplements are probably best avoided because of possible changes in oestrogen metabolism.

Adverse effects

Boron is relatively non-toxic when administered orally at doses contained in food supplements. High oral doses (>100 mg/day) are associated with disturbances in appetite and digestion, nausea, vomiting, diarrhoea, dermatitis and lethargy.

Toxicity has occurred, especially in children, from the application of boron-containing dusting powders and lotions (in the form of borax or boric acid) to areas of broken skin and mucous membranes. Such preparations are no longer recommended.

Interactions

Nutrients

Riboflavin: large doses of boron may increase excretion of riboflavin.

Dose

Boron is available in the form of tablets and capsules.

The dose is not established. Dietary supplements provide on average, 3 mg per daily dose.

References

1 Nielsen FH, Hunt CD, Mullen LM, Hunt JR. Effect of dietary boron on mineral, estrogen and testosterone metabolism in postmenopausal women. *FASEB J* 1987; 1: 394–397.
2 Nielsen FH, Mullen LM, Gallagher SK. Effect of boron depletion and repletion on blood indicators of calcium status in humans fed a magnesium-low diet. *J Trace Elem Exp Med* 1990; 3: 45–54.
3 Naghii MR, Samman S. The effect of boron supplementation on its urinary excretion and selected cardiovascular risk factors in healthy male subjects. *Biol Trace Elem Res* 1997; 56: 273–286.
4 Beattie JH, Peace HS. The influence of a low-boron diet and boron supplementation on bone, major mineral and sex steroid metabolism in postmenopausal women. *Br J Nutr* 1993; 69: 871–884.
5 Newnham RE. Essentiality of boron for healthy bones and joints. *Environ Health Perspect* 1994; 102 (suppl. 7): 83–85.
6 Travers RL, Rennie GC, Newnham RE. Boron and arthritis: the results of a double-blind, pilot study. *J Nutr Med* 1990; 1: 127–132.
7 Penland JG. Dietary boron, brain function, and cognitive performance. *Environ Health Perspect* 1994; 102 (suppl. 7): 65–72.

Branched-chain amino acids

Description

Branched-chain amino acids (BCAAs) are a group of essential amino acids. They are all found in the muscle, accounting for one-third of all amino acids in muscle protein.

Constituents

L-leucine, L-isoleucine, L-valine.

Action

As with all amino acids, the primary function of BCAAs is as precursors for the synthesis of proteins. In addition, they may be broken down if necessary to serve as an energy source. They may be used directly by skeletal muscle, as opposed to other amino acids which require prior gluconeogenesis in the liver to produce a useful energy source. Muscle tissue appears to demonstrate an increased need for these amino acids during times of intense physical exercise, and there is some evidence that serum BCAA levels fall during exercise.

In addition, because BCAAs are not readily degraded by the liver, they circulate in the blood and compete with the amino acid tryptophan for uptake into the brain. Tryptophan is a precursor of serotonin (5-hydroxytryptamine), which may produce symptoms of fatigue. It appears that exercise increases the ratio of free tryptophan:BCAA, thus raising serotonin levels in the brain. Some researchers consider that supplementation with BCAAs will reduce this ratio and raise serum levels of BCAAs, so improving mental and physical performance.

Possible uses

Exercise performance

Researchers have been interested in the potential role of BCAAs in exercise and whether they can improve performance.

A placebo-controlled (not blinded) study involving 193 experienced runners given 16 g BCAAs or placebo showed that running performance was improved in the slow runners but not the fast runners with BCAAs. A second part of the study showed that 7.5 g BCAAs improved mental performance during exercise compared with placebo, but the study has been criticised for lack of dietary control and poor choice of performance measures.[1]

Another placebo-controlled, but in this case double-blind, study on 16 subjects, participating in a 21-day trek at a mean altitude of 3255 m found that supplementation with BCAAs (11.52 g) improved indices of muscle loss and concluded that BCAAs could prevent muscle loss during chronic hypoxia at high altitude.[2]

In a double-blind, placebo-controlled study, 10 endurance-trained male athletes were studied during cycle exercise while ingesting in random order drinks containing sucrose, sucrose plus tryptophan, sucrose plus BCAAs (6 g) or sucrose plus BCAAs (18 g). There were no differences between the treatment groups in time to exhaustion, suggesting that BCAA did not improve exercise performance. However, BCAAs reduced brain tryptophan uptake and significantly increased plasma ammonia levels compared with the control group.[3]

In a double-blind, placebo-controlled, randomised, cross-over study, nine trained male cyclists performed three laboratory trials consisting of 100 km cycling after ingesting either glucose, glucose plus BCAA or placebo. Neither the glucose nor the BCAAs enhanced performance in these cyclists.[4]

In a further study of seven trained male cyclists, perceived exhaustion was 7% lower and ratings of mental fatigue were 15% lower than when they were given placebo, but there was no difference in physical performance. However, the ratio of tryptophan:BCAAs, which increased during exercise, remained unchanged or decreased when BCAAs were ingested.[5]

In a double-blind, placebo-controlled trial, six men and seven women participated in a cycle trial in the heat. Cycle time to exhaustion increased with BCAAs, indicating that BCAA supplementation prolongs moderate exercise performance in the heat.[6]

In a further double-blind, placebo-controlled trial, eight subjects performed three exercise trials and were given either carbohydrate drinks, carbohydrate plus BCAAs (7 g) or placebo one hour before and then during exercise. Subjects ran longer with both carbohydrate and carbohydrate plus BCAAs, but there were no differences between the carbohydrate and carbohydrate plus BCAA groups, indicating that BCAAs are of no added benefit in exercise.[7]

Other studies have suggested that BCAAs could prevent or decrease the net rate of protein degradation seen in heavy exercise,[8,9] while others have not.[10] One study indicated that BCAAs might have a sparing effect on muscle glycogen degradation during exercise.[11] There is also some evidence that BCAAs can alter mood and cognitive performance during exercise.[12]

Miscellaneous

BCAA can activate glutamate dehydrogenase, an enzyme which is deficient in amyotrophic lateral sclerosis (ALS). In one double-blind, randomised, placebo-controlled trial of BCAA, supplements helped maintenance of muscle strength and continued ability to walk in such patients.[13] However, a larger study was ended early when BCAA not only failed to cause benefit, but also led to excess mortality.[14]

> **Conclusion**
> Evidence from well-controlled trials shows no benefit of BCAAs in exercise performance. Benefit has been shown mainly in poorly controlled trials.

Precautions/contraindications

No problems have been reported, but BCAAs should probably not be used in hepatic and renal impairment without medical supervision. BCAAs are used occasionally in patients with these conditions but in a medical setting.

Pregnancy and breast-feeding

No problems have been reported, but there have not been sufficient studies to guarantee the safety of BCAAs in pregnancy and breast-feeding.

Adverse effects

None reported, but there are no long-term studies assessing the safety of BCAAs. Large doses of BCAAs (>20 g) may increase plasma ammonia levels and may impair water absorption, causing gastrointestinal discomfort.

Interactions

None reported. BCAAs compete with aromatic amino acids (e.g. phenylalanine, tyrosine, tryptophan) for transport into the brain.

Dose

BCAAs are available in tablet and powder form.

The dose is not established. Dietary supplements provide 7–20 g per dose.

References

1 Blomstrand E, Hassmen P, Ekblom B, *et al.* Administration of branched chain amino acids during sustained exercise – effects on performance and plasma concentrations of some amino acids. *Eur J Appl Occup Physiol* 1991; 63: 83–88.

2 Schena F, Guerrini F, Tregnaghi P, Kayser B.

Branched-chain amino acid supplementation during trekking at high altitude. The effects on loss of body mass, body composition and muscle power. *Eur J Appl Physiol Occup Physiol* 1992; 65: 394–398.
3 Van Hall G, Raaymakers J, Saris W, *et al.* Ingestion of branched chain amino acids and tryptophan during sustained exercise in man: failure to affect performance. *J Physiol* 1995; 486: 789–794.
4 Madsen K, MacLean DA, Kiens B, *et al.* Effects of glucose, glucose plus branched chain amino acids or placebo on bike performance over 100 km. *J Appl Physiol* 1996; 81: 2644–2650.
5 Blomstrand E, Hassmen P, Ek S, *et al.* Influence of ingesting a solution of branched chain amino acids on perceived exertion during exercise. *Acta Physiol Scand* 1997; 159: 41–49.
6 Mittleman KD, Ricci MR, Bailey SP. Branched-chain amino acids prolong exercise during heat stress in men and women. *Med Sci Sports Exerc* 1998; 30: 83–91.
7 Davis JM, Welsh RS, De Volve KL, Alderson NA. Effects of branched-chain amino acids and carbohydrate on fatigue during intermittent, high intensity running. *Int J Sports Med* 1999; 20: 309–314.
8 Blomstrand E, Newsholme EA. Effect of branched-chain amino acid supplementation on the exercise induced change in aromatic amino acid concentration in human muscle. *Acta Physiol Scand* 1992; 146: 293–298.
9 MacLean DA, Graham TE, Saltin B. Branched-chain amino acids augment ammonia metabolism while attenuating protein breakdown during exercise. *Am J Physiol* 1994; 267: E1010–E1022.
10 Blomstrand E, Andersson S, Hassmen P, *et al.* Effect of branched-chain amino acid and carbohydrate supplementation on the exercise-induced change in plasma and muscle concentration of amino acids in human subjects. *Acta Physiol Scand* 1995; 153: 87–96.
11 Blomstrand E, Ek S, Newsholme EA. Influence of ingesting a solution of branched-chain amino acids on plasma and muscle concentrations of amino acids during prolonged submaximal exercise. *Nutrition* 1996; 12: 485–490.
12 Hassmen P, Blomstrand E, Ekblom B, Newsholme EA. Branched chain amino acid supplementation during 30-km competitive run: Mood and cognitive performance. *Nutrition* 1994; 10: 405–410.
13 Plaitakis A, Smith J, Mandeli J, Yahr MD. Pilot trial of branched-chain amino acids in amyotrophic lateral sclerosis. *Lancet* 1988; 1: 1015–1018.
14 The Italian ALS Study Group. Branched-chain amino acids and amyotrophic lateral sclerosis: A treatment failure? *Neurology* 1993; 43: 2466–2470.

Brewer's yeast

Description

Brewer's yeast is *Saccharomyces cerevisiae*.

Constituents

The average nutrient composition of dried brewer's yeast is shown in Table 1.

Possible uses

Brewer's yeast is a useful source of B vitamins and several minerals (see Table 1).

Table 1 Average nutrient composition of dried brewer's yeast

Nutrient	Per teaspoon (8 g)	% RNI[1] (approx.)
Vitamin A	Trace	–
Thiamine (mg)	1.2	133
Riboflavin (mg)	0.4	33
Niacin (mg)	2.0	14
Vitamin B_6 (mg)	0.2	16
Folic acid (µg)	320	160
Pantothenic acid (mg)	0.9	–
Biotin (µg)	16	–
Vitamin C	Trace	–
Calcium (mg)	6	0.9
Magnesium (mg)	18	6
Potassium (mg)	160	4.5
Phosphorus (mg)	103	19
Iron (mg)	1.6	13
Zinc (mg)	0.6	7
Copper (mg)	0.4	33

[1]Reference Nutrient Intake for men aged 19–50 years.

Note: Brewer's yeast tablets contain approximately 300 mg brewer's yeast per tablet; extra B vitamins are often added.

Brewer's yeast has been used to treat diarrhoea due to *Clostridium difficile*.[1] Because brewer's yeast contains chromium it has been claimed to help in the control of blood glucose levels. It is also claimed to prevent hypercholesterolaemia. However, there is insufficient evidence to substantiate these claims.

Conclusion

Brewer's yeast has a suggested value in controlling blood glucose levels, preventing hypecholesterolaemia and controlling diarrhoea caused by *Clostridium difficile*. Little evidence is available to support its efficacy in all but the last of these conditions.

Precautions/contraindications

Brewer's yeast should be avoided by patients taking monoamine oxidase inhibitors (see Interactions). It is also best avoided by patients with gout; this is because of high concentrations of nucleic acids which may lead to purine formation.

Pregnancy and breast-feeding

No problems have been reported.

Adverse effects

None reported except flatulence.

Interactions

Drugs

Monoamine oxidase inhibitors: may provoke hypertensive crisis.

Dose

Brewer's yeast is available in the form of tablets and powder.

The dose is not established.

Reference

1 Schellenberg D, Bonington A, Champion CM, *et al.* Treatment of *Clostridium difficile* diarrhoea with brewer's yeast. *Lancet* 1994; 343: 171.

Bromelain

Description

Bromelain is the name for the protease enzymes extracted from the stem and fruit of fresh pineapple. The commercial supplement is usually obtained only from the stem of the pineapple, which contains a higher concentration of the enzymes than the fruit.

Constituents

Bromelains are sulphydryl proteolytic enzymes, including several proteases. In addition, bromelain also contains small amounts of non-proteolytic enzymes (including acid phosphatase, peroxidase and cellulase), polypeptide protease inhibitors and organically bound calcium.

Action

Bromelain is an anti-inflammatory agent and is thought to act through direct or indirect effects on inflammatory mediators. It inhibits the enzyme thromboxane synthetase, which converts prostaglandin H_2 into pro-inflammatory prostaglandins and thromboxanes. Bromelain also stimulates the breakdown of fibrin, which stimulates pro-inflammatory prostaglandins responsible for fluid retention and clot formation. It also appears to promote the conversion of plasminogen to plasmin, causing an increase in fibrinolysis.

Possible uses

Various claims are made for the value of bromelain supplementation, but much of the research underpinning these claims was carried out in the 1960s and 1970s, and there are almost no well-controlled human studies.

Bromelain has been associated with improvement in symptoms of sinusitis, acceleration of wound healing, potentiation of antibiotic action, healing of gastric ulcers, treatment of inflammation and soft tissue injuries, reduction in severity of angina, reduction in sputum production in patients with chronic bronchitis and pneumonia and decrease in symptoms of thrombophlebitis.[1]

Sinusitis

Two double-blind, placebo-controlled studies showed that bromelain 160 mg (400 000 units) could reduce some symptoms of sinusitis.[2,3] However, headache was not improved in either study.

Musculoskeletal injuries

In a double-blind, placebo-controlled trial,[4] 146 boxers with bruises to the face and haematomas to the eyes, lips, ears, arms and chest received either 160 mg bromelain daily or placebo for 14 days. At day 4, 78% of the bromelain treated group were completely cured of their bruises compared with 15% of the placebo group. However, this result was not tested for statistical significance.

Surgical procedures

Bromelain has been reported in at least two studies[5,6] to reduce the degree and duration of swelling and oral pain with oral surgery. However, one study was not controlled and the other had no statistical analysis.

Antibacterial

Bromelain could be useful an antidiarrhoeal

agent. In an *in vitro* study[7] bromelain was shown to prevent intestinal fluid secretion mediated by *Escherichia coli* and *Vibrio cholera*, and in other studies[8,9] to protect piglets from diarrhoea. However, there are no human studies to date.

Cardiovascular disease

Bromelain has been reported to reduce the severity of angina[10] and several *in vitro* studies[11,12] have demonstrated that bromelain reduces platelet aggregation.

Ulcerative colitis

A letter from two US consultants[13] stated that two patients with ulcerative colitis achieved complete clinical and endoscopic remission after initiation of therapy with bromelain.

Cystitis

One double-blind study in humans revealed that bromelain was effective in treating non-infectious cystitis.[14]

> **Conclusion**
> Many claims have been made for bromelain, based largely on studies conducted during the 1960s and 1970s. Many of the published trials are uncontrolled human studies or animal or *in vitro* studies, and well-controlled clinical trials are required to establish the role of bromelain as a potential supplement.

Precautions/contraindications

No problems have been reported, but based on the potential pharmacological activity of bromelain, i.e. that it may inhibit platelet aggregation, bromelain should be used with caution in patients with a history of bleeding or haemostatic disorders.

Pregnancy and breast-feeding

No problems have been reported, but there have been insufficient studies to guarantee the safety of bromelain in pregnancy and breast-feeding.

Adverse effects

None reported, but there are no long-term studies assessing the safety of bromelain.

Interactions

Drugs

None reported, but theoretically, bleeding tendency may be increased with anticoagulants, aspirin and antiplatelet drugs.

Dose

Bromelain is available in the form of tablets, capsules and powders. A variety of designations have been used to indicate the activity of bromelain. These include rorer units (ru), gelatin-dissolving units (gdu) and milk clotting units (mcu). One gram of bromelain standardised to 2000 mcu would be approximately equal to 1 g with 1200 gdu of activity or 8 g with 100 000 ru activity.[1]

The dose is not established. Dietary supplements provide 125–500 mg in a dose.

References

1 Anonymous. Bromelain. *Altern Med Rev* 1998; 3: 302–308.
2 Ryan RE. A double-blind clinical evaluation of bromelains in the treatment of acute sinusitis. *Headache* 1967; 7: 13–17.
3 Seltzer AP. Adjunctive use of bromelains in sinusitis: A controlled study. *Eye Ear Nose Throat Mon* 1967; 46: 1281–1288.
4 Blonstein JL. Control of swelling in boxing injuries. *Practitioner* 1960; 185: 78.
5 Tassman GC, Zafran JN, Zayon GM. Evaluation of a plant proteolytic enzyme for the control of inflammation and pain. *J Dent Med* 1964; 19: 73–77.
6 Tassman GC, Zafran JN, Zayon GM. A double blind crossover study of a plant proteolytic enzyme in oral surgery. *J Dent Med* 1965; 20: 51–54.
7 Mynott TL, Guandalini S, Raimondi F, *et al.* Bromelain prevents secretion caused by *Vibrio cholera* and *Escherichia coli* enterotoxins in rabbit ileum in vitro. *Gastroenterology* 1997; 113: 175–184.
8 Mynott TL, Luke RKJ, Chandler DS. Oral administration of protease inhibits enterotoxigenic *Escherichia coli* (ETEC) activity in piglet small intestine. *Gut* 1996; 38: 28–32.
9 Chandler DS, Mynott TL. Bromelain protects piglets

from diarrhoea caused by oral challenge with K88-positive enterotoxigenic *Escherichia coli*. *Gut* 1998; 43: 196–202.

10 Nieper HA. Effect of bromelain on coronary heart disease and angina pectoris. *Acta Med Empirica* 1978; 5: 274–278.

11 Heinicke RM, Van der Wal M, Yokoyama MM. Effect of bromelain (Ananase) on human platelet aggregation. *Experientia* 1972; 28: 844–845.

12 Metzig C, Grabowska E, Eckert K, *et al*. Bromelain proteases reduce human platelet aggregation in vitro, adhesion to bovine endothelial cells, and thrombus formation in rat vessels in vivo. *In Vivo* 1999; 13: 7–12.

13 Kane S, Goldberg MJ. Use of bromelain for mild ulcerative colitis [letter]. *Ann Intern Med* 2000; 132: 680.

14 Lotti T, Mirone V, Imbimbo C, *et al*. Controlled clinical studies of nimesulide in the treatment of urogenital inflammation. *Drugs* 1993; 46 (suppl. 1): 144–146.

Calcium

Description

Calcium is an essential mineral.

Human requirements

Dietary Reference Values for calcium are shown in Table 1.

Intakes

In the UK, the average daily diet provides: for men, 961 mg; women, 764 mg.

Action

Calcium has a structural role in bones and teeth. Some 90% of calcium is found in the skeleton. Bone density increases during the first three decades of life, reaching its peak at about the age of 30 years. After this age, bone density declines, the decline occurring more rapidly in women after the menopause. However, bone density also declines in older men. Calcium is also essential for cellular structure, blood clotting, muscle contraction, nerve transmission, enzyme activation and hormone function.

Dietary sources

Dietary sources of calcium are shown in Table 2.

Metabolism

Absorption

Calcium is absorbed in the duodenum, jejunum and ileum by an active saturable process which involves vitamin D. At high intakes, some calcium is absorbed by passive diffusion (independent of vitamin D). It can also be absorbed from the colon.

Distribution

More than 99% of the body's calcium is stored in the bones and teeth. The physiologically active form of calcium is the ionised form (in the blood). Blood calcium levels are controlled homeostatically by parathyroid hormone, calcitonin and vitamin D and a range of other hormones.

Elimination

Excretion of calcium occurs in the urine, although a large amount is reabsorbed in the kidney tubules, the amount excreted varying with the quantity of calcium absorbed and the degree of bone loss. Elimination of unabsorbed and endogenously secreted calcium occurs in the faeces. Calcium is also lost in the sweat and is excreted in breast milk.

Bioavailability

Bioavailability is dependent to some extent on vitamin D status. Absorption is reduced by phytates (present in bran and high-fibre cereals), but high-fibre diets at currently recommended levels of intake do not significantly affect calcium absorption in the long term. Absorption is reduced by oxalic acid (present in cauliflower, spinach and rhubarb). High sodium intake may reduce calcium retention.

The efficiency of absorption is increased during periods of high physiological requirement (e.g. in childhood, adolescence, pregnancy and lactation) and impaired in the elderly.

Table 1 Dietary Reference Values for calcium (mg/day)

EU RDA = 800 mg

Age	UK			USA	WHO	Europe
	LNRI	EAR	RNI	AI	RNI	PRI
0–6 months	240	400	525	210	500	–
7–12 months	240	400	525	270	600	400
1–3 years	200	275	350	500	400	400
4–6 years	275	350	450	–	450	450
4–8 years	–	–	–	800	–	–
7–10 years	325	425	550	–	500	550
9–18 years	–	–	–	1300	–	–
Males						
11–14 years	450	750	1000	–	600–700	1000
15–18 years	450	750	1000	–	500–600	1000
19–50 years	400	525	700	1000	400–500	700
50+ years	400	525	700	1200	400–500	700
Females						
11–14 years	480	625	800	–	600–700	800
15–18 years	480	625	800	–	500–600	800
19–50 years	400	525	700	1000	400–500	700
50+ years	400	525	700	1200	400–500	700
Pregnancy	*	*	*	1000[1]	1000–2000	*
Lactation	–	–	+550	1000[1]	1000–2000	+550

*No increment.

AI = Adequate Intake. AI = 1300 mg in women aged ≤18 years (pregnancy and breast-feeding).

PRI = Population Reference Intake.[1]

Note: The National Osteoporosis Society has produced separate guidelines for recommended daily calcium intake as follows: 7–12 years, 800 mg; 13–19 years, 1000 mg; men 20–45 years, 1000 mg; men >45 years, 1500 mg; women 20–45 years, 1000 mg; women >45 years, 1500 mg; women >45 years (using Hormone Replacement Therapy), 1000 mg; pregnant and breast-feeding women, 1200 mg; pregnant and breast-feeding teenagers, 1500 mg.

Deficiency

Simple calcium deficiency is not a recognised clinical disorder. However, low dietary intake during adolescence and young adulthood may reduce peak bone mass and bone mineral content and increase the risk of osteoporosis in later life.

However, requirements may be increased and/or supplements may be necessary in:

- children, adolescents, pre- and post-menopausal women;
- pregnant and breast-feeding women;
- vegans and others who avoid milk and milk products; and
- lactose intolerance (owing to avoidance of milk and milk products).

Possible uses

The role of calcium has been investigated in a number of conditions, including osteoporosis, hypertension, colon cancer, menstrual symptoms and pre-eclampsia.

Table 2 Dietary sources of calcium

Food portion	Calcium content (mg)	Food portion	Calcium content (mg)
Cereal products		*Prawns (80 g)*	*120*
Bread, brown, 2 slices	70	Salmon, canned (115 g)	100
white, 2 slices	70	**Sardines, canned (70 g)**	**350**
wholemeal 2 slices	35	Shrimps (80 g)	100
1 chapati	20	**Whitebait (100 g)**	**860**
Milk and dairy products		**Vegetables**	
½ pint milk (280 ml), whole, semi-skimmed or skimmed	**350**	Broccoli (100 g)	40
½ pint (280 ml) soya milk	50	*Spinach (100 g)*	*150*
1 pot yoghurt, plain (150 g)	*300*	Spring greens (100 g)	75
fruit (150 g)	*250*	1 small can baked beans (200 g)	106
Cheese, Brie (50 g)	*270*	Dahl, chickpea (150 g)	100
Camembert (50 g)	*175*	Lentils, kidney beans or chick peas (105 g)	40–70
Cheddar (50 g)	**360**	Soya beans, cooked (100 g)	85
Cheddar, reduced fat (50 g)	**420**	*Tofu (60 g)*	*300*
Cottage cheese (100 g)	73		
Cream cheese (30 g)	35	**Fruit**	
Edam (50 g)	**350**	1 large orange	70
Feta (50 g)	*180*		
Fromage Frais (100 g)	85	**Nuts**	
White cheese (50 g)	*280*	20 almonds	50
1 egg size 2 (60 g)	35	*1 tablespoon sesame seeds (20 g)*	*140*
		Tahini paste on 1 slice bread (10 g)	70
Fish			
Pilchards, canned (105 g)	*105*	*Milk chocolate (100 g)*	*240*

Excellent sources (**bold**); good sources (*italics*).

Osteoporosis

Calcium supplements may have a role in the prevention of osteoporosis. Most of the available evidence has been obtained from studies looking at three different population groups (i.e. children and adolescents, premenopausal women and postmenopausal women).

Children and adolescents

Adequate intake of calcium is important throughout life, but seems to be particularly important during skeletal growth and development of peak bone mass.[1,2] Data also exist[3,4] to show that high intake of milk and dairy produce increases bone mineralisation and bone growth in adolescence – effects which may not be due entirely to the high calcium content of milk. In addition to other minerals, such as magnesium, phosphorus and zinc (which are themselves important for bone health), milk also provides energy and protein, both of which may stimulate bone growth through their influence on insulin growth factor 1 (IGF-1).

Several controlled intervention studies[5–7] using calcium supplements in children and adolescents have shown that calcium intakes above the current British Reference Nutrient Intake (RNI) are effective in increasing bone mineral accretion, particularly in those youngsters with habitually low calcium intakes. However, more evidence is required to determine whether these effects are translated into a reduced risk of osteoporosis in later life; they may be due merely to short-term effects on bone remodelling.

Premenopausal women

In premenopausal women, results from studies examining the relationship between dietary calcium intake and bone mass and also those from calcium supplementation studies are contradictory. Some show a positive effect of calcium[8,9] on bone mineral density, but others do not.[10–12]

Postmenopausal women

After the menopause, bone loss occurs at an increasing rate, and while calcium may help to slow the loss, it does not prevent it. Moreover, the influence of calcium at this stage of life seems to vary with the length of time that has passed since the menopause occurred. Most studies fail to show a relationship between calcium intake, from either food or supplements, and bone loss during the five years immediately following the menopause. In one study,[13] women who had undergone the menopause within the last five years had rapid bone loss which was not affected by a calcium supplement of 500 mg a day. However, in women who were more than six years after the menopause (and had a calcium intake of less than 400 mg a day), the same supplement significantly reduced bone loss. Another study in women 10 years after the menopause[14] showed that a calcium supplement of 1000 mg a day had a benefit on both total and site-specific bone mass even though their habitual calcium intake was satisfactory, and that this effect of supplementation could last for four years and result in fewer fractures.[15]

Using fracture rather than bone loss as the end-point, some recent studies have demonstrated a benefit of calcium given with vitamin D in older people. A French study[16] showed considerable reduction in fracture rates in a large group of elderly people (mean age 84 ± 6 years) who were living in a nursing home and given 1200 mg calcium with 800 IU of vitamin D. Protection became apparent after 6–12 months, and after three years the probability of hip fractures was reduced by 29%. In a more recent study,[17] also in elderly people, similar results were obtained from calcium supplementation alone, but the subjects were vitamin D replete. Researchers in the USA[18] looked at the effects of 500 mg of calcium plus 700 units of vitamin D for three years in 176 men and 213 women aged 65 years or more who were living at home. The supplemented group had a reduced incidence of non-vertebral fracture and lower bone loss in the femoral neck and the total body than the non-supplemented group.

Hypertension

Epidemiological studies[19,20] support an inverse relationship between the amount of calcium in the diet and blood pressure. However, based on multivariate analyses, the absolute contribution of calcium is very small. Some clinical intervention studies have reported reduction in blood pressure in normotensive and hypertensive subjects[21–23] or no effect.[24] A meta-analysis of 33 randomised, controlled trials concluded that calcium (800–2000 mg daily) may lead to a small reduction in systolic blood pressure.[25] Another meta-analysis of 22 randomised clinical trials showed that calcium supplements (500–1000 mg daily) produced a significant decrease in systolic but not diastolic blood pressure; however, the authors concluded that the effect was too small to support the use of calcium supplementation in hypertension.[26] Calcium may be most effective in patients with hypertension who are Afro-Caribbean[27] or who are responsive to manipulation of dietary sodium.[28]

Cancer

Calcium supplementation may reduce the occurrence of colorectal cancer, but the effects are inconsistent. High calcium intake (1200–1400 mg daily) has been linked with reduced colon cancer risk in epidemiological studies, and high dietary and supplemental calcium have been associated with reduced recurrence of adenomatous polyps.[29–31] Other studies have shown no significant effects of calcium supplementation on colorectal cell proliferation in subjects at high risk for colorectal cancer.[32,33]

Menstrual symptoms

Calcium supplementation (1200 mg daily for three menstrual cycles) was effective in reducing premenstrual pain, but not menstrual pain in a prospective, randomised, double-blind, placebo-controlled trial.[34] In another trial, when given with manganese, calcium (1336 mg daily) reduced menstrual pain and undesirable behavioural symptoms.[35] A further trial showed that calcium (1000 mg daily) reduced both premenstrual and menstrual symptom scores, and there was a significant effect of calcium on menstrual pain.[36]

Pre-eclampsia

Use of calcium supplements during pregnancy may reduce the risk of pre-eclampsia. An analysis of clinical trials which examined the effects of calcium intake on pre-eclampsia and pregnancy outcomes in 2500 women found that those who consumed 1500–2000 mg of calcium daily were 70% less likely to suffer from hypertension in pregnancy.[37] However, a large study, involving 4589 healthy first-time mothers found that calcium supplementation (2000 mg/day) had no effect on the incidence of hypertension, protein excretion or complications of childbirth.[38]

> **Conclusion**
>
> There is evidence that calcium supplementation can improve bone density in adolescents. Calcium may also help to reduce the decline in bone density in older postmenopausal women, particularly when given in conjunction with vitamin D. However, there is little evidence that calcium supplementation attenuates the reduction in bone density around the time of the menopause. Calcium supplementation may lower blood pressure, but the effect is too small to recommend its use in hypertension. Evidence linking calcium to colon cancer is conflicting. There is preliminary evidence that calcium supplementation may help symptoms of premenstrual syndrome, particularly pain.

Precautions/contraindications

Calcium supplements should be avoided in: conditions associated with hypercalcaemia and hypercalcuria; renal impairment (chronic); renal stones or history of renal stones. They should be used with caution and with medical supervision in hypertension because blood pressure control may be altered.

Pregnancy and breast-feeding

No problems have been reported. Calcium supplements may be required during pregnancy and lactation. Some studies have shown that the use of calcium supplements in pregnancy may lower the risk of pre-eclampsia, while another has not (see above).

Adverse effects

Reported adverse effects with supplements include nausea, constipation and flatulence (usually mild). Calcium metabolism is under such tight control that accumulation in blood or tissues from excessive intakes is almost unknown; accumulation is usually due to failure of control mechanisms. Toxic effects and hypercalcaemia are unlikely with oral doses of less than 2000 mg daily. However, in young children, calcium supplements should be used under medical supervision because of a risk of bowel perforation.

Interactions

Drugs

Alcohol: excessive alcohol intake may reduce calcium absorption.

Aluminium-containing antacids: may reduce calcium absorption.

Anticonvulsants: may reduce serum calcium levels.

Bisphosphonates: calcium may reduce absorption of etidronate; give 2 h apart.

Cardiac glycosides: concurrent use with parenteral calcium preparations may increase risk of cardiac arrhythmias (ECG monitoring recommended).

Corticosteroids: may reduce serum calcium levels.

Laxatives: prolonged use of laxatives may reduce calcium absorption.

Loop diuretics: increased excretion of calcium.
4-Quinolones: may reduce absorption of 4-quinolones; give 2 h apart.
Tamoxifen: calcium supplements may increase the risk of hypercalcaemia (a rare side-effect of tamoxifen therapy); calcium supplements are best avoided.
Tetracyclines: may reduce absorption of tetracyclines; give 2 h apart.
Thiazide diuretics: may reduce calcium excretion.

Nutrients
Fluoride: may reduce absorption of fluoride and vice-versa; give 2 h apart.
Iron: calcium carbonate or calcium phosphate may reduce absorption of iron; give two 2 h apart (absorption of iron in multiple formulations containing iron and calcium is not significantly altered).
Vitamin D: increased absorption of calcium and increased risk of hypercalcaemia; may be advantageous in some individuals.
Zinc: may reduce absorption of zinc.

Dose

Calcium is available in the form of tablets and capsules. A review of 35 US calcium supplements showed that four brands contained lower levels of calcium than claimed on the label. However, none of the products failed testing for exceeding contamination levels for lead and other heavy metals.[39] Another survey showed that calcium supplements may contain lead,[40] but levels were not high enough to cause concern.[41]

The dose for potential prevention of osteoporosis, postmenopausal women, 1000–1500 mg (as elemental calcium) daily (not a substitute for hormone replacement therapy).

As a dietary supplement, up to 1000 mg (as elemental calcium) daily.

Note: doses are given in terms of elemental calcium. Patients should be advised that calcium supplements are not identical; they provide different amounts of elemental calcium. The calcium content of various calcium salts commonly used in supplements is shown in Table 3.

Table 3 Calcium content of commonly used calcium salts

Calcium salt	Calcium (mg/g)	Calcium (%)
Calcium amino acid chelate	180	18
Calcium carbonate	400	40
Calcium chloride	272	27.2
Calcium glubionate	65	6.5
Calcium gluconate	90	9
Calcium lactate	130	13
Calcium lactate gluconate	129	13
Calcium orotate	210	21
Calcium phosphate (dibasic)	230	23

Note: Calcium lactate and gluconate are more efficiently absorbed than calcium carbonate (particularly in patients with achlorhydria).

References

1 Matkovik V. Calcium metabolism and calcium requirements during skeletal modelling and consolidation of bone mass. *Am J Clin Nutr* 1991; 54 (suppl.): 245S–259S.
2 Recker RR, Davies MK, Hinders SM, *et al*. Bone gain in young adult women. *JAMA* 1992; 268: 2403–2408.
3 Chan GM, Hoffman K, McMurry M. Effects of dairy produce on bone and body composition in pubertal girls. *J Pediatr* 1995; 126: 551–556.
4 Cadogan J, Eastell R, Jones M, Barker ME. A study of bone growth in adolescents: the effect of an 18-month, milk-based dietary intervention. *Br Med J* 1997; 315: 1255–1260.
5 Johnston CC, Miller JZ, Slemenda CW, *et al*. Calcium supplementation and increases in bone mineral density in children. *N Engl J Med* 1992; 327: 82–87.
6 Lloyd T, Andon MB, Rollings N, *et al*. Calcium supplementation and bone mineral density in adolescent girls. *JAMA* 1993; 270: 841–844.
7 Lee WTK, Leung SSF, Leung DMT, *et al*. A randomised double-blind controlled calcium supplementation trial and bone and height acquisition in children. *Br J Nutr* 1995; 74: 125–139.
8 Ramsdale SJ, Bassy EJ, Pye DJ. Dietary calcium intake relates to bone mineral density in premenopausal women. *Br J Nutr* 1994; 71: 77–84.
9 Rico H, Revilla M, Villa LF, *et al*. Longitudinal study of the effect of calcium pidolate on bone mass in eugonadal women. *Calcif Tissue Int* 1994; 54: 47–80.

10 Valimaki MJ, Karkkainen M, Lamberg-Allardt C, *et al.* Exercise, smoking and calcium intake during adolescence and early adulthood as determinants of peak bone mass. *Br Med J* 1994; 309: 230–235.
11 New SA, Bolton-Smith C, Grubb DA, Reid DM. Nutritional influences on bone mineral density: a cross sectional study in premenopausal women. *Am J Clin Nutr* 1997; 65: 1831–1839.
12 Earnshaw SA, Worley A, Hosking DJ. Current diet does not relate to bone mineral density after the menopause. The Nottingham Early Postmenopausal Intervention Cohort (EPIC) Study Group. *Br J Nutr* 1997; 78: 65–72.
13 Dawson-Hughes B, Dallal GE, Krall EA, *et al.* A controlled trial of the effect of calcium supplementation on bone density in post-menopausal women. *N Engl J Med* 1990; 323: 878–883.
14 Reid IR, Ames RW, Evans MC, *et al.* Effect of calcium supplementation on bone loss in postmenopausal women. *N Engl J Med* 1993; 328: 460–464.
15 Reid IR, Ames RW, Evans MC, *et al.* Long term effects of calcium supplementation on bone loss and fractures in postmenopausal women: a randomised controlled trial. *Am J Med* 1995; 98: 331–335.
16 Chapuy MC, Arlot ME, Duboeuf F, *et al.* Vitamin D and calcium to prevent hip fractures in elderly women. *N Engl J Med* 1992; 327: 1637–1642.
17 Chevalley T, Rizzoli R, Nydegger V, *et al.* The effects of calcium supplements on femoral bone mineral density and vertebral fracture rate in vitamin D-replete elderly patients. *Osteoporosis Int* 1994; 4: 245–252.
18 Dawson-Hughes B, Harris SS, Krall EA, Dallal GE. Effect of calcium and vitamin D supplementation on bone density in men and women 65 years of age or older. *N Engl J Med* 1997; 337: 670–676.
19 Iso H, Terao A, Kitamura A. Calcium intake and blood pressure in seven Japanese populations. *Am J Epidemiol* 1991; 133: 776–783.
20 McCarron DA, Morris CD. The calcium deficiency hypothesis of hypertension. *Ann Intern Med* 1987; 107: 919–922.
21 Grobbee DE, Hofman A. Effect of calcium supplementation on diastolic blood pressure in young people with mild hypertension. *Lancet* 1986; 2: 703–707.
22 McCarron DA, Lipkin M, Rivlin RS, Heaney RP. Dietary calcium and chronic diseases. *Med Hypotheses* 1990; 31: 265–273.
23 Kawano Y, Yoshimi H, Matsuoka H, *et al.* Calcium supplementation in patients with essential hypertension: assessment by office, home and ambulatory blood pressure. *J Hypertens* 1998; 16: 1693–1699.
24 Galloe AM, Graudal N, Moller J, *et al.* Effect of oral calcium supplementation on blood pressure in patients with hypertension: A randomised, double-blind, placebo-controlled, crossover study. *J Hum Hypertens* 1993; 7: 43–45.
25 Bucher HC, Cook RJ, Guyatt GH, *et al.* Effects of dietary calcium supplementation on blood pressure – a meta-analysis of randomized controlled trials. *JAMA* 1996; 275: 1016–1022.
26 Allender PS, Cutler JA, Follman D, *et al.* Dietary calcium and blood pressure: A meta-analysis of randomized controlled trials. *Ann Intern Med* 1996; 124: 825–831.
27 Zemel MB. Dietary calcium, calcitrophic hormones, and hypertension. *Nutr Metab Cardiovasc Dis* 1994; 4: 224–228.
28 Weinberger MH, Wagner UL, Fineberg NS, *et al.* The blood pressure effects of calcium supplementation in humans of known sodium responsiveness. *Am J Hypertens* 1993; 6: 799–805.
29 Hofstad B, Almendigen K, Vatn M, *et al.* Growth and recurrence of colorectal polyps: A double-blind 3-year intervention with calcium and antioxidants. *Digestion* 1998; 59: 148–156.
30 Hyman J, Baron JA, Dain BJ, *et al.* Dietary and supplemental calcium and the recurrence of colorectal adenomas. *Cancer Epidemiol Biomarkers Prev* 1998; 7: 291–295.
31 Bonithon-Kopp C, Kronborg O, Giacosa A, *et al.* Calcium and fibre supplementation in prevention of colorectal adenoma recurrence: Randomised intervention trial. *Lancet* 2000; 356: 1300–1306.
32 Baron JA, Tosteson TD, Wargovich MJ, *et al.* Calcium supplementation and rectal mucosal proliferation: A randomized controlled trial. *J Natl Cancer Inst* 1995; 87: 1303–1307.
33 Weisberger UM, Boeing H, Owen RW, *et al.* Effect of long-term placebo controlled calcium supplementation on sigmoidal cell proliferation in patients with sporadic adenomatous polyps. *Gut* 1996; 38: 396–402.
34 Thys-Jacobs S, Starkey P, Bernstein D, *et al.* Calcium carbonate and the premenstrual syndrome: Effects on premenstrual and menstrual symptoms (Premenstrual Syndrome Study Group). *Am J Obstet Gynecol* 1998; 179: 444–452.
35 Penland JG, Johnson PE. Dietary calcium and manganese effects on menstrual cycle symptoms. *Am J Obstet Gynecol* 1993; 168: 1417–1423.
36 Thys-Jacobs S, Ceccarelli S, Bierman A, *et al.* Calcium supplementation in premenstrual syndrome: A randomized crossover trial. *J Gen Intern Med* 1989; 4: 183–189.
37 Herrara JA, Arevala Herrara M, Herrara S, *et al.* Prevention of preeclampsia by linoleic acid and calcium supplementation: a randomized controlled trial. *Obstet Gynecol* 1998; 91: 585–590.
38 Bucher HC, Guyatt GH, Cook RJ, *et al.* Effect of calcium supplementation on pregnancy induced

hypertension and preeclampsia: A meta-analysis of randomized controlled trials. *JAMA* 1996; 275: 1113–1117.

39 Consumerlab. Product review. Calcium. http://www.consumerlab.com (accessed 5 December 2000).

40 Ross EA, Szabo NJ, Tebbett IR. Lead content of calcium supplements. *JAMA* 2000; 284: 1425–1429.

41 Heaney R. Lead in calcium supplements: Cause for alarm or celebration? *JAMA* 2000; 284: 1263–1270.

Carnitine

Description

Carnitine is an amino acid derivative.

Nomenclature

Carnitine is sometimes known as vitamin B_T; it is not an officially recognised vitamin.

Constituents

Carnitine exists as two distinct isomers, L-carnitine (naturally occurring carnitine) and D-carnitine (synthetic carnitine). Dietary supplements contain L-carnitine or a DL-carnitine mixture.

Human requirements

No proof of a dietary need exists. Carnitine is synthesised in sufficient quantities to meet human requirements.

Intakes

The average omnivorous diet is estimated to provide 100–300 mg of carnitine daily.

Dietary sources

Meat and dairy products are the best sources. Fruit, vegetables and cereals are poor sources of carnitine. Carnitine is added to infant milk formulae.

Action

Carnitine has the following physiological functions:

- Regulation of long-chain fatty acid transport across cell membranes.
- Facilitation of beta-oxidation of long-chain fatty acids and ketoacids.
- Transportation of acyl co-enzyme A compounds.

Metabolism

Dietary carnitine is absorbed rapidly from the intestine by both passive and active transportation mechanisms. Carnitine is synthesised in the liver, brain and kidney from the essential amino acids, lysine and methionine.

Deficiency

Primary carnitine deficiency is caused by impairment in the membrane transportation of carnitine. Symptoms may include: chronic muscle weakness (due to muscle carnitine deficiency), recurrent episodes of coma and hypoglycaemia (usually in infants and children), encephalopathy, and cardiomyopathy.

Secondary carnitine deficiency occurs in several inherited disorders of metabolism (especially organic acidurias and disorders of beta-oxidation).

Despite the fact that plant foods are poor sources of carnitine, there is no evidence that vegetarians are deficient in carnitine. Endogenous synthesis prevents deficiencies.

Possible uses

Carnitine supplementation has been investigated for its potential benefit in cardiovascular disease, exercise performance, chronic fatigue syndrome and Alzheimer's disease.

Cardiovascular disease

Carnitine may be beneficial in patients with ischaemic heart disease, but only those who have low serum carnitine levels.

Orally administered L-carnitine (2 g daily) has been shown to improve symptoms of angina,[1] and to reduce anginal attacks and glyceryl trinitrate consumption.[2] In a dose of 900 mg daily for 12 weeks, it has also been shown to improve exercise tolerance in patients with stable angina.[3]

Carnitine supplementation (4 g daily) has also been reported to improve heart rate, arterial pressures, angina and lipid patterns in a controlled study of patients who had experienced a recent myocardial infarction.[4] Yet another study showed that L-carnitine (1 g twice daily for 45 days) may be beneficial in congestive heart failure, by reducing heart rate, dyspnoea and oedema, and increasing diuresis. Supplementation also allowed for a reduction in daily digoxin dose.[5]

Another study has provided some evidence that L-carnitine (2 g twice daily for three weeks) increases walking distance in patients with intermittent claudication.[6]

Hyperlipidaemia

Preliminary studies have shown that L-carnitine may reduce blood cholesterol levels. Oral administration of L-carnitine (3–4 g daily) significantly reduced serum levels of total cholesterol or triglyceride or both, and increased those of high density lipoprotein (HDL) cholesterol.[7–9]

Exercise performance

There is a potential for carnitine to improve athletic performance by increasing lipid utilisation and conserving glycogen supplies in the muscles.

An increase in maximal aerobic power was observed in subjects who received L-carnitine 2 g daily[10] and 4 g daily.[11,12] Other studies have shown no effect of supplemental carnitine on muscle carnitine.[13,14]

Double blind, placebo-controlled trials have shown no benefit of oral carnitine 2 g,[15] 3 g[16] or 4 g[17] on exercise performance in healthy subjects.

Chronic fatigue syndrome

Patients with chronic fatigue syndrome have been reported to have low carnitine levels. One cross-over (not blinded) parallel design study randomised 30 patients with chronic fatigue syndrome to either 3 g L-carnitine or 100 mg amantadine.[18] At the end of the two-month study, the carnitine group experienced clinical improvement in 12 out of the 18 studied parameters. However, no statistical comparison between carnitine and amantadine was conducted.

Alzheimer's disease

Preliminary evidence from two double-blind, placebo-controlled trials[19,20] suggests that carnitine supplementation could reduce the deterioration in some symptoms of Alzheimer's disease.

Miscellaneous

There is some evidence that carnitine improves insulin resistance in type 2 diabetes.[21] It may support treatment for epilepsy[22] and complement antiretroviral therapy in patients with human immunodeficiency virus (HIV),[23,24] but studies have not assessed the effect of carnitine on morbidity and mortality from AIDS.

> **Conclusion**
>
> Preliminary evidence suggests that carnitine supplementation may be of benefit in several cardiovascular disorders, such as angina, hyperlipidaemia, myocardial infarction, congestive heart failure and intermittent claudication. Evidence also exists that carnitine may be beneficial in Alzheimer's disease and chronic fatigue syndrome. While these results are clearly of interest, further evidence is required before the role of carnitine (if any) in the management of these conditions can be defined. Despite a theoretical rationale, there is as yet no good evidence that carnitine supplementation improves exercise performance.

Precautions/contraindications

The administration of the D-isomer (including a DL-mixture, contained in some supplements) may interfere with the normal function of the L-isomer, and should not be used. Only the L-isomer has been used in studies.

Pregnancy and breast-feeding

No problems have been reported, but there have not been sufficient studies to guarantee the safety of carnitine in pregnancy and breast-feeding.

Adverse effects

Serious toxicity has not been reported. Nausea, vomiting and diarrhoea may occur with high doses. The risk of toxicity is greater with the D-isomer than with L-carnitine (see Precautions); myasthenia has been reported with ingestion of DL-carnitine.

Interactions

Drugs

Anticonvulsants: increased excretion of carnitine.
Pivampicillin: increased excretion of carnitine.
Pivmecillinam: increased excretion of carnitine.

Dose

L-Carnitine supplements are available in the form of tablets and capsules.

The dose is not established. In studies, doses of 1–6 g L-carnitine daily have been used.

References

1 Cherchi A, Lai C, Angelino F, *et al.* Effects of L-carnitine in exercise tolerance in chronic stable angina: A multicenter, double-blind, randomized placebo controlled crossover study. *Int J Clin Pharmacol Ther Toxicol* 1985; 23: 569–572.
2 Garyza G, Amico RM. Comparative study on the activity of racemic and laevorotatory carnitine in stable angina pectoris. *Int J Tissue Reactions* 1980; 2: 175–180.
3 Kamikawa T, Suzuki Y, Kobayashi A, *et al.* Effects of L-carnitine on exercise tolerance in patients with stable angina pectoris. *Jpn Heart J* 1984; 25: 587–597.
4 Davini P, Bigalli A, Lamanna F, *et al.* Controlled study on L-carnitine therapeutic efficacy in post-infarction. *Drugs Exp Clin Res* 1992; 18: 355–365.
5 Ghidini O, Azzurro M, Vita G, *et al.* Evaluation of the therapeutic efficacy of L-carnitine in congestive heart failure. *Int J Clin Pharmacol Ther Toxicol* 1988; 26: 217–220.
6 Brevetti G, Chiariello M, Ferulano G, *et al.* Increases in walking distance in patients with peripheral vascular disease treated with L-carnitine: A double-blind, cross-over study. *Circulation* 1988; 77: 767–773.
7 Pola P, Savi L, Grilli M, *et al.* Carnitine in the therapy of dyslipidemic patients. *Curr Ther Res* 1979; 27: 208–216.
8 Pola P, Tondi P, Dal Lago A, *et al.* Statistical evaluation of long-term L-carnitine therapy in hyperlipoproteinaemias. *Drugs Exp Clin Res* 1983; 12: 925–935.
9 Rossi CS, Silprandi N. Effect of carnitine on serum HDL-cholesterol: Report of two cases. *Johns Hopkins Med J* 1982; 150: 51–54.
10 Swart I, Rossouw J, Loots J, *et al.* The effect of L-carnitine supplementation on plasma carnitine levels and various parameters of male marathon athletes. *Nutr Res* 1997; 17: 405–414.
11 Angelini C, Vergani L, Costa L, *et al.* Clinical study of efficacy of L-carnitine and metabolic observations in exercise physiology. In: Borum D, ed. *Clinical Aspects of Human Carnitine Deficiency*. New York: Pergamon Press, 1986: 36–42.
12 Marconi C, Sassi G, Carpinelli A, Cerretelli P. Effects of L-carnitine loading on the aerobic and aerobic performance of endurance athletes. *Eur J Appl Physiol* 1985; 54: 131–135.
13 Barnett C, Costill D, Vukovitch M, *et al.* Effect of L-carnitine supplementation on muscle and blood carnitine content and lactate accumulation during high-intensity spring cycling. *Int J Sport Nutr* 1994; 4: 280–288.
14 Vukovitch M, Costill D, Fink W, *et al.* Carnitine supplementation: effect on muscle carnitine and glycogen content during exercise. *Med Sci Sports Exerc* 1994; 26: 1122–1129.
15 Colombani P, Wenk C, Kunz I, *et al.* Effects of L-carnitine supplementation on physical performance and energy metabolism of endurance trained athletes: A double-blind crossover filed study. *Eur J Appl Physiol* 1996; 73: 434–439.
16 Trappe SW, Costill DL, Goodpaster P, *et al.* The effects of L-carnitine on performance during interval swimming. *Int J Sports Med* 1994; 15: 181–185.
17 Giamberardino MA, Dragani L, Valente R, *et al.* Effects of prolonged L-carnitine administration on delayed muscle pain and CK release after eccentric effort. *Int J Sports Med* 1996; 17: 320–324.
18 Pliophys A, Pliophys S. Amantadine and L-carnitine treatment of chronic fatigue syndrome. *Neuropsychobiology* 1997; 35: 16–23.
19 Sano M, Bell K, Cote L, *et al.* Double-blind parallel design pilot study of acetyl levocarnitine in patients with Alzheimer's disease. *Arch Neurol* 1992; 49: 1137–1141.

20 Spagnoli A, Lucca U, Menasce G, *et al.* Long term acetyl-L-carnitine treatment in Alzheimer's disease. *Neurology* 1991; 41: 1726–1732.
21 Mingrone G, Greco AV, Capristo E. L-carnitine improves glucose disposal in type 2 diabetic patients. *J Am Coll Nutr* 1999; 18: 77–82.
22 Shuper A, Gutman A, Mimouni M. Intractable epilepsy. *Lancet* 1999; 353: 1238.
23 Moretti S, Alesse E, Di Marzio L. Effect of L-carnitine on human immunodeficiency virus-1 infection-associated apoptosis: A pilot study. *Blood* 1998; 91: 3817–3824.
24 De Simone C, Tzantzoglou S, Famularo G. High dose L-carnitine improves immunologic and metabolic parameters in AIDS patients. *Immunopharmacol Immunotoxicol* 1993; 15: 1–12.

Carotenoids

Description

Carotenoids are natural pigments found in plants, including fruit and vegetables, giving them their bright colour. About 600 carotenoids have been identified of which about six appear to be used in significant ways by the blood or other tissues. About 50 have provitamin A activity, and of these, all-*trans* betacarotene is the most active on a weight basis and makes the most important quantitative contribution to human nutrition. Betacarotene is fat soluble. Apart from betacarotene, other significant carotenoids (according to research conducted so far) are alphacarotene, cryptoxanthin, lycopene, lutein and zeaxanthin.

Units

The bioavailability of those carotenoids with provitamin A activity (e.g. alphacarotene, betacarotene, cryptoxanthin) is less than that of retinol (preformed vitamin A).

Although the absorption and utilisation of carotenoids varies, the generally accepted relationship is that 6 μg betacarotene is equivalent to 1 μg retinol. (Other carotenoids with provitamin A activity are not converted to vitamin to the same extent as is betacarotene.)

The amount of betacarotene in dietary supplements may be expressed in terms of micrograms or International Units. 1 unit of betacarotene is defined as the activity of 0.6 μg betacarotene. Thus:

- 1 unit betacarotene = 0.6 μg betacarotene; and
- 1 μg betacarotene = 1.67 units betacarotene.

Human requirements

There is currently no UK Dietary Reference Value (DRV) for betacarotene (or any other carotenoids). This is because, until recently, its only role has been considered to be as a precursor of vitamin A. Some authorities are starting to make recommendations for betacarotene, e.g. 6 mg daily (Finland); 4 mg daily (France); 2 mg daily (Germany), but the USA has made no recommendations.

Intakes

In the UK, the average adult diet provides 2.28 mg (betacarotene) daily.

Action

Carotenoids have the following functions. They:

- quench singlet oxygen and prevent the formation of free radicals. [Note that natural betacarotene (*cis* form) acts as an antioxidant, while the synthetic (*trans*) form has been suggested to be pro-oxidant[1]];
- react with or scavenge free radicals directly and thus act as an antioxidant; and
- enhance some aspects of immune function.

In addition, alphacarotene, betacarotene and cryptoxanthin can be converted to vitamin A.

Dietary sources

Carotenoids are found in a wide variety of fruits and vegetables, although they may not be the ones commonly consumed. Alphacarotene is found in carrots and pumpkin. Lycopene is concentrated in red fruits, such as tomatoes (particularly cooked and pureéd tomatoes), guava, watermelon and red grapefruit. Lutein and zeaxanthin are found in dark green vegetables, red pepper and pumpkin. Cryptoxanthin is present in mangoes, oranges and peaches. The content of betacarotene in various foods is shown in Table 1.

Metabolism

Although there are a huge number of carotenoids, most research has been conducted on betacarotene, and less is known about the others, particularly in terms of metabolism. Hence, only the metabolism of betacarotene is described here.

Absorption

Betacarotene consists of two molecules of vitamin A which are hydrolysed in the gastrointestinal tract. It is absorbed into the mucosal cell of the small intestine and converted to retinol. The efficiency of absorption is usually 20–50%, but can be as low as 10% when intake is high. The conversion of betacarotene to retinol is regulated by the vitamin A stores of the individual and by the amount ingested; conversion efficiency varies from 2:1 at low intakes to 12:1 at higher intakes. On average, 25% of absorbed betacarotene appears to remain intact and 75% is converted to retinol.

Distribution

Intact betacarotene is transported in very low density lipoprotein (VLDL) or low density lipoprotein (LDL) cholesterol. Blood levels, unlike those of retinol, are not maintained constant but vary roughly in proportion to the amounts ingested. Increased blood levels (hypercarotenaemia) are sometimes associated (as a secondary condition) with hypothyroidism, diabetes mellitus, and hepatic and renal disease. Hypercarotenaemia can also be caused by a rare genetic inability to convert betacarotene to vitamin A.

All carotenoids are deposited in the liver to a lesser extent than is vitamin A. Most is stored in the adipose tissue, epidermal and dermal layers of the skin and the adrenals; there are high levels in the corpus luteum and in colostrum.

Table 1 Dietary sources of betacarotene

Food portion	Betacarotene (μg)[1]
Bread and cereals	Traces
Milk and dairy products	
Milk	Traces
Cheese – average (50 g)	100
Butter on 1 slice bread (10 g)	40
Margarine on 1 slice bread (10 g)	75
2 tablespoons ghee (30 g)	150
Meat and fish	
Liver, ox, cooked (90 g)	**1400**
Liver, lamb's, cooked (90 g)	90
Fish	Traces
Fish oils	Traces
Vegetables	
Peas, boiled (100 g)	400
Broccoli, boiled (100 g)	470
Brussels sprouts, boiled (100 g)	320
Cabbage, raw, (100 g)	385
Cabbage, boiled (100 g)	210
Carrots, boiled (100 g)	**7560**
Kale, boiled (100 g)	**3375**
Lettuce (30 g)	120
Peppers, green, raw (50 g)	130
Peppers, red, raw (50 g)	**1920**
Spinach, boiled (100 g)	**3840**
Sweet potato, boiled (150 g)	**6000**
2 tomatoes, raw (150 g)	960
1 large glass tomato juice	400
Watercress (20 g)	500
Mixed vegetable curry (300 g)	**10 200**
Fruit	
1 apple	20
3 apricots	450
1 banana	30
1 mango	**3600**
½ melon, cantaloupe	**2500**
1 slice melon, honeydew	100
1 slice watermelon	750
1 orange	75
4 passion fruits	**1500**
1 slice paw-paw	**1800**
1 peach	90
1 pear	30
3 plums	300

[1]To convert carotene (μg) to retinol (μg), divide by 6.
Excellent sources (>1000 μg/portion) (**bold**).

Elimination

Betacarotene is eliminated mainly in the faeces.

Bioavailability

Betacarotene is not very stable, and potency is lost if it is exposed to oxygen. Mild cooking processes can improve bioavailability: absorption from raw carrot can be as low as 1%, but this figure increases dramatically when carrots are subjected to short periods of boiling. Overcooking reduces bioavailability, however. Significant losses can also occur in frying, freezing and canning.

Deficiency

No specific symptoms have been defined.

Possible uses

Carotenoids are being investigated in a variety of conditions, particularly cancer, cardiovascular disease and cataract.

Betacarotene

Cancer

More than 50 epidemiological studies have demonstrated that a high intake of foods rich in carotenoids (i.e. fruit and vegetables) and high serum levels of betacarotene are associated with reduced risk of certain cancers, especially lung cancer, but also cancers of the cervix, endometrium, breast, oesophagus, mouth and stomach.[2]

Fruit and vegetables contain several types of carotenoids in addition to betacarotene, and it is incorrect to assume that betacarotene is responsible for all the preventive effects of fruit and vegetables. For example, increased alpha-carotene intakes from diet have been associated with a reduced risk of lung cancer[3,4] with suggestive inverse associations also for other carotenoids.

Serum analysis has shown, however, an association between low serum betacarotene levels and increased cancer risk, possibly indicating a more specific link. Intervention studies published so far have provided little evidence for a beneficial effect of betacarotene supplementation on cancer risk; indeed, some have indicated that there may be an increased risk.

A 12-year US study involving 22 071 male physicians randomly allocated to 50 mg betacarotene or placebo every other day did not demonstrate any statistically significant benefit or harm from supplementation. In the betacarotene group, 1273 subjects developed malignant neoplasms compared with 1293 in the placebo group. No serious adverse effects were noted in the study.[5]

In a double-blind, placebo-controlled Finnish intervention trial, known as the alpha tocopherol, betacarotene cancer prevention (ATBC) study,[6] 29 000 male smokers were randomised to receive either betacarotene 20 mg daily, alpha tocopherol 50 mg daily, both betacarotene and alpha tocopherol, or placebo. Lung cancer incidence increased in all the groups receiving betacarotene, but the effect was stronger in those who smoked heavily, a finding which was consistent with those of the CARET study (see below). However, lung cancer incidence was not correlated with serum betacarotene, suggesting that this was not a direct effect of betacarotene.[7] There was also no significant effect on incidence of or mortality from cancer of the pancreas,[8] nor on the incidence of colorectal adenomas.[9]

Another US study (the betacarotene and retinol efficacy trial – CARET) in 4060 subjects with substantial work-related exposure to asbestos, and also 14 254 heavy smokers, showed that betacarotene 30 mg with vitamin A 25 000 units increased the risk of lung cancer compared with placebo. Mortality was also 17% higher, however, and as a consequence of this the trial was stopped prematurely.[10] Possible explanations for these findings have been given (see Antioxidants, pages 9 and 10).

In patients with documented cervical dysplasia given either betacarotene 30 mg or placebo for nine months, complete remission occurred in 23% of the supplemented group and 47% of the placebo group, showing that betacarotene had no beneficial effect on resolution of cervical dysplasia.[11] However, in another study there was an inverse relationship between breast cancer and betacarotene intake in premenopausal women.[12]

In a further study, betacarotene was neither beneficial nor harmful in reducing the risk of developing skin cancer. A total of 1621 subjects, aged 20 to 69 years, were randomised into four groups: betacarotene and sunscreen; sunscreen and placebo; betacarotene and no sunscreen; and no sunscreen and placebo. Sunscreen was applied daily to all exposed areas of the head, neck, arms and hands, with re-application after swimming or increasing perspiration. No dosing details were given for betacarotene. At the end of the study, there were no statistically significant differences in development of basal or squamous cell carcinoma between the betacarotene and placebo groups.[13]

Cardiovascular disease

Diets rich in fruit and vegetables are generally associated with a lower risk of cardiovascular disease, but evidence for a direct protective effect of betacarotene was reported from the Physician's Health study in America.[14] In an analysis of a subgroup of volunteers who had previously had stable angina or coronary revascularisation, 50 mg betacarotene on alternate days reduced subsequent coronary events by 50% compared with placebo.

However, in a large, placebo-controlled trial, involving men aged between 50 and 69 years who smoked five or more cigarettes a day, supplementation with betacarotene was not helpful in angina pectoris and may even have slightly increased the incidence of the condition.[15] In this study, 5602 patients received betacarotene 20 mg daily, 5570 received alpha tocopherol 50 mg daily, 5548 patients received alpha tocopherol 50 mg and betacarotene 20 mg daily, and 5549 received placebo. Follow-up continued for a maximum of seven years. Patients taking vitamin E alone or in combination with betacarotene showed a minor decrease in angina pectoris, but betacarotene alone was associated with a slight increase in angina incidence.

Incidence of myocardial infarction was not reduced by betacarotene supplementation (50 mg daily) in US male physicians.[5] Betacarotene was not effective in the treatment of increased serum triglycerides or cholesterol levels,[16] and was not shown to reduce the risk of stroke.[17]

Cataract

Betacarotene may protect against cataract formation. In a retrospective study,[18] the group with the lowest serum betacarotene levels had over five times the risk of developing cataract as the group with the highest serum levels.

Diabetes

Serum betacarotene levels may be reduced in diabetic patients, and one case-control study has shown a negative correlation between betacarotene and glycaemic control.[19] However, in the US male physicians' study, betacarotene supplementation (50 mg daily) was ineffective in reducing the risk of developing type 2 diabetes.[20]

Immune function

Data on betacarotene's influence on the immune system are conflicting. One study showed that supplementation (betacarotene 15 mg daily for 26 days) resulted in a significant increase in the proportion of monocytes involved in initiating immune responses.[21] However, in other studies, T-cell immunity was unaffected by betacarotene supplementation.[22]

Lutein

Lutein is a carotenoid which is present in high concentrations in the eye. Within the eye, this pigment filters out blue light, and it may have a protective role in the visual apparatus and its vascular supply. There is evidence that lutein may help to prevent age-related macular degeneration[23] and cataracts.[24] Supplements may also help to improve visual function in patients with retinal degeneration.[25]

Lycopene

Lycopene is a carotenoid pigment, which functions as a free radical scavenger and antioxidant. Supplementation has been reported to protect against macular degeneration,[26] atherosclerosis[27] and cancer (especially of the prostate).[28]

Conclusion
Diets rich in carotenoids are protective against various conditions, particularly cancer and cardiovascular disease. However, evidence that betacarotene supplements are beneficial for this purpose is lacking. Other carotenoids, such as lycopene and lutein are now being studied. Preliminary evidence suggests that lutein may be protective in cataract and macular degeneration, while lycopene may be protective against macular degeneration and prostate cancer.

Precautions/contraindications

No serious problems have been reported. Supplements should be avoided by people with known hypersensitivity to carotenoids.

Pregnancy and breast-feeding

No problems have been reported.

Adverse effects

Unlike retinol, carotenoids are generally non-toxic. Even when ingested in large amounts, they are not known to cause birth defects or to cause hypervitaminosis A, primarily because efficiency of absorption decreases rapidly as the dose increases and because conversion to vitamin A is not sufficiently rapid to induce toxicity.

Intake of >30 mg carotenoids daily (either from commercial supplements or from tomato or carrot juice) may lead to hypercarotenaemia; this is characterised by a yellowish coloration of the skin (including the palms of the hands and soles of feet), and a very high concentration of carotenoids in the plasma. This is harmless and reversible and gradually disappears when excessive intake of carotenoids is corrected.

Hypercarotenaemia is clearly differentiated from jaundice by the appearance of the whites of the eyes (yellow in hypercarotenaemia, but not in jaundice).

Diarrhoea, dizziness and arthralgia may occur occasionally with carotene supplements. Allergic reactions (hay fever and facial swelling), amenorrhoea and leucopenia have been reported rarely.

According to FAO/WHO, intakes up to 5 mg betacarotene/kg body weight are acceptable.

The only serious toxic manifestation of carotenoid intake is canthaxanthin retinopathy which can develop in patients with erythropoietic protoporphyria and related disorders who are treated with large daily doses (50–100 mg) of canthaxanthin (a derivative of betacarotene) for long periods.

Interactions

None specifically established (see also Vitamin A).

Dose

Betacarotene, lutein, lycopene and mixed carotenoids are available in the form of tablets and capsules.

The dose is not established. Dietary supplements provide 6–15 mg (10 000–25 000 units) betacarotene per dose.

References

1 Levin G, Yeshurun M, Mockady S. In vitro antiperoxidative effect of 9-*cis* beta-carotene compared with that of the all-*trans* isomer. *J Nutr Cancer* 1997; 27: 293–297.
2 Gaby SK, Singh VN. Betacarotene. In: Gaby SK, Bendich A, Singh VN, Machlin LJ, eds. *Vitamin Intake and Health: A Scientific Review*. New York: Marcel Dekker, 1991: 89–106.
3 Michaud DS, Feskanich D, Rimm EB, *et al.* Intake of specific carotenoids and risk of lung cancer in 2 prospective US cohorts. *Am J Clin Nutr* 2000; 72: 990–997.
4 Knekt P, Jarvinen R, Tempo A, *et al.* Role of various carotenoids in lung cancer prevention. *J Natl Cancer Inst* 1999; 91: 182–184.
5 Hennekens CH, Buring JE, Manson JE, *et al.* Lack of effect of long-term supplementation with beta-carotene on the incidence of malignant neoplasms and cardiovascular disease. *N Engl J Med* 1996; 334: 1145–1149.
6 The Alpha Tocopherol, Beta-Carotene Cancer Prevention Study Group. The effect of vitamin E and beta carotene on the incidence of lung cancer in male smokers. *N Engl J Med* 1994; 330: 1029–1035.
7 Albanes E, Heinonen OP, Taylor PR, *et al.* Alpha

tocopherol and beta-carotene supplements and lung cancer incidence in the alpha-tocopherol, beta-carotene cancer prevention study: Effects of base-line characteristics and study compliance. *J Natl Cancer Inst* 1996; 88: 1560–1570.

8 Rautalahti MT, Virtamo JRK, Taylor PR, *et al.* The effects of supplementation with alpha-tocopherol and beta-carotene on the incidence and mortality of carcinoma of the pancreas in a randomised, controlled trial. *Cancer* 1999; 86: 37–42.

9 Maliula N, Virtamo J, Virtanen M, *et al.* The effect of alpha-tocopherol and β-carotene supplementation on colorectal adenomas in middle-aged male smokers. *Cancer Epidemiol Biomarkers Prev* 1999; 8: 489–493.

10 Omenn GS, Goodman GE, Thornquist MD, *et al.* Effects of a combination of betacarotene and vitamin A on lung cancer and cardiovascular disease. *N Engl J Med* 1996; 334: 1150–1155.

11 Romney SL, Ho GYF, Palan PR, *et al.* Effects of betacarotene and other factors on outcome of cervical dysplasia and human papillomavirus infection. *Gynecol Oncol* 1997; 65: 483–492.

12 Bohlke K, Spiegelman D, Trichopoulou A, *et al.* Vitamins A, C and E and the risk of breast cancer: Results from a case control study in Greece. *Br J Cancer* 1999; 79: 23–29.

13 Green A, Williams G, Neale R, *et al.* Daily sunscreen application and betacarotene supplementation in prevention of basal cell and squamous cell carcinomas of the skin. *Lancet* 1999; 354: 723–729.

14 Gaziano JM, Manson JE, Ridker PM, *et al.* Beta-carotene supplementation for chronic stable angina. *Circulation* 1990; 82 (Suppl.III): 201 (abstract 0796).

15 Rapola JM, Virtamo J, Haukka JK, *et al.* Effect of vitamin E and betacarotene on the incidence of angina pectoris: a randomized, double-blind, controlled trial. *JAMA* 1996; 275: 693–698.

16 Redlich C, Chung J, Cullen M, *et al.* Effect of long-term betacarotene and vitamin A on serum cholesterol and triglycerides among participants in the carotene and retinol efficacy trial (CARET). *Atherosclerosis* 1999; 145: 425–432.

17 Ascherio A, Rimm E, Hernan MA, *et al.* Relation of consumption of vitamin E, vitamin C and carotenoids to risk for stroke among men in the United States. *Ann Intern Med* 1999; 130: 963–970.

18 Jacques PF, Hartz SC, Chylack LT, *et al.* Nutritional status in persons with and without senile cataract: Blood vitamin and mineral levels. *Am J Clin Nutr* 1988; 48: 152–158.

19 Abahusain MA, Wright J, Dickerson JWT, *et al.* Retinol, alpha-tocopherol and carotenoids in diabetes. *Eur J Clin Nutr* 1999; 53: 630–635.

20 Liu S, Ajanu U, Chae C, *et al.* Long-term β-carotene supplementation and risk of type 2 diabetes mellitus. *JAMA* 1999; 282: 1073–1075.

21 Hughes DA, Wright AJA, Finglas PM, *et al.* The effect of beta-carotene supplementation on the immune function of blood monocytes from healthy male non-smokers. *J Lab Clin Med* 1997; 129: 309–317.

22 Santos MS, Leka LS, Ribaya-Mercado D, *et al.* Short and long-term beta-carotene supplementation do not influence T cell-mediated immunity in healthy elderly persons. *Am J Clin Nutr* 1997; 66: 917–924.

23 Hammond BR Jr, Johnson EJ, Russell RM, *et al.* Dietary modification of human macular pigment density. *Invest Ophthalmol Vis Sci* 1997; 38: 1795–1801.

24 Lyle BJ, Mares-Perlman JA, Klein BE, *et al.* Antioxidant intake and risk of incident age related nuclear cataracts in the Beaver Dam Eye Study. *Am J Epidemiol* 1999; 149: 801–809.

25 Dagnelie G, Zorge IS, McDonald TM. Lutein improves visual function in some patients with retinal degeneration: A pilot study via the Internet. *Optometry* 2000; 7: 147–164.

26 Mares-Perlman JA, Brady WE, Klein R, *et al.* Serum antioxidants and age related macular degeneration in a population-based case-control study. *Arch Ophthalmol* 1995; 113: 1518–1523.

27 Agarwal S, Rao AV. Tomato lycopene and low density lipoprotein oxidation: A human dietary intervention study. *Lipids* 1998; 33: 981–984.

28 Giovanucci E. Tomatoes, tomato-based products, lycopene and cancer: Review of the epidemiologic literature. *J Natl Cancer Inst* 1999; 91: 317–331.

Chitosan

Description

Chitosan is a fibre, extracted from chitin, which is a structural component of crustacean shells, crabs, shrimps and lobsters. Chitin is de-acetylated to produce chitosan.

Constituents

Chitosan is a polysaccharide containing numerous acetyl groups.

Action

Chitosan binds fat molecules due to its ionic nature. When taken orally, chitosan has been reported to bind 8–10 times its own weight in fat from food in the gastrointestinal tract, thus preventing fat from being absorbed. Consequently, the body has to burn stored fat, and this in turn may lead to a reduction in body fat and body weight.

Possible uses

Weight loss

In mice treated with chitosan and given a high-fat diet, chitosan prevented the increase in body weight, hyperlipidaemia and fatty liver induced by a high-fat diet.[1]

In a randomised, placebo-controlled, double-blind study, 34 overweight human volunteers were each given four capsules of chitosan or placebo for 28 consecutive days. Subjects maintained their normal diet and documented their food intake. After four weeks of treatment, body mass index, serum cholesterol, triglycerides, vitamin A, D and E and betacarotene were not significantly different between the two groups. The results suggest that chitosan in the dose given had no effect on body weight in overweight subjects. No serious adverse effects were reported.[2]

In another placebo-controlled, double-blind study, involving 51 healthy obese women, chitosan 1200 mg twice daily was given for eight weeks. No reductions in weight were observed in any treatment group. Low-density lipoprotein (LDL) cholesterol fell to a greater extent in the chitosan group than the placebo group, but there was no significant change in high-density lipoprotein (HDL) cholesterol and triglycerides were slightly increased.[3]

Chitosan reduced blood glucose and cholesterol in an animal model of lean-type non-insulin-dependent diabetes mellitus (NIDDM) with hypoinsulinaemia, but had no effect in an animal model of obese-type NIDDM with hyperinsulinaemia. The authors concluded that chitosan could be a useful treatment for lean-type NIDDM with hypoinsulinaemia.[4]

Conclusion

Chitosan is promoted for weight loss, but there have been few trials, and results have been conflicting.

Precautions/contraindications

Chitosan should be avoided in patients with gastrointestinal malabsorption conditions.

Pregnancy and breast-feeding

No problems have been reported, but weight loss should not be attempted during pregnancy.

Adverse effects

There are no long-term studies assessing the safety of chitosan. However, chitosan may reduce the absorption of fat soluble vitamins (A, D, E and K). This has been shown in animals,[5] but not in humans.[2,3]

Interactions

None reported.

Dose

Chitosan is available in the form of tablets and capsules.

The dose is not established. Dietary supplements provide 1500–3000 mg per daily dose.

References

1 Han LK, Kimura Y, Okuda H. Reduction in fat storage during chitin-chitosan treatment in mice fed a high-fat diet. *Int J Obes Relat Metab Disord* 1999; 23: 174–179.
2 Pittler MH, Abbott NC, Harkness EF, Ernst E. Randomized, double-blind trial of chitosan for body weight reduction. *Eur J Clin Nutr* 1999; 53: 379–381.
3 Wuolijoki E, Hirvela T, Ylitalo P. Decrease in serum LDL cholesterol with microcrystalline chitosan. *Methods Find Exp Clin Pharmacol* 1999; 21: 357–361.
4 Miura T, Usami M, Tsuura Y, *et al.* Hypoglycemic and hypolipidemic effect of chitosan in normal and neonatal streptozotocin-induced diabetic mice. *Biol Pharm Bull* 1995; 18: 1623–1625.
5 Deuchi K, Kanauchi O, Shizukuishi M, *et al.* Continuous and massive intake of chitosan affects soluble vitamin status in rats fed on a high fat diet. *Biosci Biotech Biochem* 1995; 59: 1211–1216.

Chlorella

Description

Chlorella is a single-celled freshwater alga.

Constituents

Chlorella is rich in chlorophyll. Manufacturers claim that it is a source of amino acids, nucleic acids, fatty acids, vitamins and minerals. However, content varies with conditions of growing, harvesting and processing. *Chlorella* is claimed to contain a unique substance called Chlorella Growth Factor. The claimed nutrient content of *Chlorella* is shown in Table 1.

Action

Chlorella may have antitumour and antiviral activities, and it may have the ability to stimulate the immune system. However, these effects have not been clarified in human studies.

Possible uses

Chlorella is promoted as a tonic for general health maintenance; it is a useful source of some nutrients (e.g. betacarotene, riboflavine, vitamin B_{12}, iron and zinc; see Constituents).

In addition, *Chlorella* is claimed to be useful in: accelerating the healing of wounds and ulcers; improving digestion and bowel function; stimulating growth and repair to tissues; retardation of ageing; strengthening the immune system; improving the condition of the hair, skin, teeth and nails; treating colds and respiratory infections; and removing poisonous substances from the body. These claims are based largely on anecdote; *Chlorella* has no proven efficacy for these conditions.

Preliminary evidence from an uncontrolled study in 20 patients over a period of two months showed that *Chlorella* supplementation may help to relieve the symptoms of

Table 1 Claimed[1] nutrient content of *Chlorella*

Nutrient	Per 100 g	Per typical dose (3 g)	% RNI[2]
Protein (g)	66	2	–
Fat (g)	9	0.3	–
Carbohydrate (g)	11	0.3	–
Vitamin A (μg) (as betacarotene)	5500	165	28
Thiamine (mg)	2.0	0.06	8
Riboflavin (mg)	7.0	0.2	24
Niacin (mg)	30.0	0.9	6
Vitamin B_6 (mg)	1.5	0.05	4
Vitamin B_{12} (μg)	134	4	270
Folic acid (μg)	25	0.75	0.4
Pantothenic acid (mg)	3.0	0.09	–
Biotin (μg)	190	6	–
Vitamin C (mg)	60	1.8	5
Vitamin E (mg)	17	0.5	–
Choline (mg)	270	8.1	–
Inositol (mg)	190	5.7	–
Calcium (mg)	500	15	2
Magnesium (mg)	300	9	3
Potassium (mg)	700	21	0.6
Phosphorus (mg)	1200	36	6.5
Iron (mg)	260	8	80
Zinc (mg)	70	2	26
Copper (μg)	80	2.4	0.2
Iodine (μg)	600	18	13

[1]Reported on a product label.
[2]Reference Nutrient Intake for men aged 19–50 years.

fibromyalgia.[1] However, the authors concluded that a larger, more comprehensive double-blind, placebo-controlled trial in patients with fibromyalgia is warranted.

Other preliminary evidence suggests that *Chlorella* could help patients with brain tumours better tolerate chemotherapy and radiotherapy. However, there appears to be no effect on tumour progression or survival.[2]

> **Conclusion**
> There is insufficient reliable information to recommend the use of *Chlorella* for any indication.

Precautions/contraindications

No problems have been reported.

Pregnancy and breast-feeding

No problems have been reported.

Adverse effects

None reported, but *Chlorella* may provoke allergic reactions.

Interactions

None reported, but *Chlorella* may contain significant amounts of vitamin K. This could inhibit the activity of warfarin and other anticoagulants.

Dose

Chlorella is available in the form of tablets, capsules, liquid extracts and powder.

The dose is not established. Dietary supplements provide 500–3000 mg of the intact organism per daily dose.

References

1 Merchant RE, Carmack CA, Wise CM. Nutritional supplementation with *Chlorella pyredinosa* for patients with fibromyalgia syndrome: A pilot study. *Phytother Res* 2000; 14: 167–173.

2 Merchant RE, Rice CD, Young HF. Dietary *Chlorella pyredinosa* for patients with malignant glioma: Effects on immunocompetence, quality of life and survival. *Phytother Res* 1990; 4: 220–231.

Choline

Description

Choline is associated with the vitamin B complex; it is not an officially recognised vitamin. Choline is a component of phosphatidylcholine and an active constituent of dietary lecithin, but the two substances are not synonymous.

Human requirements

Choline is an essential nutrient for several mammalian organisms, but agreement on its essentiality as a vitamin for humans has not been reached. However, the US Food and Nutrition Board of the National Institute of Medicine has established a Dietary Reference Intake for adults of 550 mg a day for men and 425 mg a day for women, with lower amounts for children, together with an upper intake level of 3.5 g daily for adults aged over 18 years.

Intakes

Estimated dietary intake in the UK is 250–500 mg daily. Choline can also be synthesised in the body from phosphatidylethanolamine.

Action

Choline serves as a source of labile methyl groups for transmethylation reactions. It functions as a component of other molecules such as the neurotransmitter acetylcholine, phosphatidylcholine (lecithin) and sphingomyelin, structural constituents of cell membranes and plasma lipoproteins, platelet activating factor and plasmalogen (a phospholipid found in highest concentrations in cardiac muscle membranes).

Lecithin and sphingomyelin participate in signal transduction,[1] an essential process for cell growth, regulation and function. Animal studies suggest that choline or lecithin deficiency may interfere with this critical process and that alterations in signal transduction may lead to abnormalities such as cancer and Alzheimer's disease.

Dietary sources

Choline is widely distributed in foods (mainly in the form of lecithin). The richest sources of choline are brewer's yeast, egg yolk, liver, wheatgerm, soya beans, kidney and brain. Oats, peanuts, beans, and cauliflower also contain significant amounts.

Metabolism

Absorption

Some choline is absorbed intact, probably by a carrier-mediated mechanism; some is metabolised by the gastrointestinal flora to trimethylamine (which produces a fishy odour).

Distribution

Choline is stored in the brain, kidney and liver, primarily as phosphatidylcholine (lecithin) and sphingomyelin.

Elimination

Elimination of choline occurs mainly via the urine.

Deficiency

Dietary choline deficiency occurs in animals, and abnormal liver function, liver cirrhosis and fatty liver may be associated with choline deficiency in humans. Observations in patients on total parenteral nutrition (TPN) have shown a choline-deficient diet to result in fatty infiltration of the liver, hepatocellular damage and liver dysfunction.[2,3]

Possible uses

As a precursor of acetylcholine, choline has been suggested to increase the concentration of acetylcholine in the brain. Choline has therefore been suggested to be beneficial in patients with disease related to impaired cholinergic transmission (e.g. tardive dyskinesia, Huntington's chorea, Alzheimer's disease, Gilles de la Tourette syndrome, mania, memory impairment and ataxia). However, experimental evidence suggests that oral choline has no effect on choline metabolites in the brain.[4]

Comparison of studies involving choline is often complicated by lack of standardisation of doses used. However, clinical trials with tardive dyskinesia patients using choline have met with some success.[4–6]

Choline has also been suggested to improve performance in athletes. This idea arose because of findings that plasma choline concentrations were reduced in trained runners[7] and athletes[8] after sporting events. However, a double-blind, cross-over study in 20 cyclists showed that choline supplementation did not delay fatigue during brief or prolonged exercise.[9]

Claims have been made for the value of choline in the prevention of cardiovascular disease, including angina, atherosclerosis, hypertension, stroke and thrombosis. It has also been claimed to prevent and/or treat Alzheimer's disease, senile dementia and memory loss. Scientific proof for these claims is lacking, however.

Precautions/contraindications

No problems have been reported.

> **Conclusion**
> Research on choline supplementation is limited and studies are generally very poorly controlled. The limited research shows that choline does not appear to improve Alzheimer's disease, memory or athletic performance. Very preliminary evidence suggests that choline might be beneficial in tardive dyskinesia, but the data are not sufficient to recommend supplementation.

Pregnancy and breast-feeding

No problems have been reported.

Adverse effects

Fishy odour due to metabolism by the gut flora; more severe symptoms relate to excessive cholinergic transmission (doses of 10 g daily or more) and include diarrhoea, nausea, dizziness, sweating, salivation, depression and a longer P–R interval in electrocardiograms.

Interactions

None established.

Dose

Choline is available in the form of tablets and capsules.

The dose is not established. Dietary supplements generally provide 250–500 mg per dose (choline chloride provides 80% choline and choline tartrate 50% choline).

References

1 Canty DJ, Zeisel SH. Lecithin and choline in human health and disease. *Nutr Rev* 1994; 52: 327–339.
2 Zeisel SH, DaCosta KA, Franklin PD. Choline, an essential nutrient for humans. *FASEB J* 1991; 5: 2093–2098.
3 Davis KL, Berger PA, Hollister LE. Choline for tardive dyskinesia. *N Engl J Med* 1975; 293: 152–153.
4 Gelenberg AJ, Doller-Wojcik JC, Growdon JH. Choline and lecithin in the treatment of tardive

dyskinesia: preliminary results from a pilot study. *Am J Psychiatr* 1979; 136: 772–776.

5 Growdon JH, Hirsch MJ, Wurtman RJ, Wiener W. Oral choline administration to patients with tardive dyskinesia. *N Engl J Med* 1977; 297: 524–527.

6 Tamminga CA, Smith RC, Erickson SE, *et al.* Cholinergic influences in tardive dyskinesia. *Am J Psychiatr* 1977; 134: 769–774.

7 Conlay LA, Sabounjian LA, Wurtman RJ. Exercise and neuromodulators: Choline and acetylcholine in marathon runners. *Int J Sports Med* 1992; 13: S141–S142.

8 Von Allworden HN, Horn S, Kahl J, *et al.* The influence of lecithin on plasma choline concentrations in triathletes and adolescent runners during exercise. *Eur J Appl Physiol* 1993; 67: 87–91.

9 Spector SA, Jackman MR, Sabounjian LA, *et al.* Effect of choline supplementation on fatigue in trained cyclists. *Med Sci Sports Exerc* 1995; 27: 668–673.

Chondroitin

Description

Chondroitin is a natural physiological compound that is synthesised endogenously and secreted by the chondrocytes. It is found in joint cartilage and connective tissue (including vessel walls).

Description

Chondroitin is a mixture of large molecular weight glycosaminoglycans and disaccharide polymers composed of equimolar amounts of D-glucuronic acid, D-acetylgalactosamine and sulphates in 10–30 disaccharide units. (Glycosaminoglycans are the substances in which collagen fibres are embedded in cartilage.)

Action

Chondroitin absorbs water, adding to the thickness and elasticity of cartilage and its ability to absorb and distribute compressive forces. Chondroitin also appears to control the formation of new cartilage matrix, by stimulating chondrocyte metabolism and synthesis of collagen and proteoglycan. Chondroitin also inhibits degradative enzymes (elastase and hyaluronidase), which break down cartilage matrix and synovial fluid, contributing to cartilage destruction and loss of joint function.

Possible uses

Osteoarthritis

Chondroitin is claimed to be useful as a dietary supplement in combination with glucosamine in osteoarthritis and related disorders. Preliminary evidence suggests that chondroitin reduces the pain of osteoarthritis in the knee compared with placebo.

In a multicentre, randomised, double-blind, controlled study, involving 127 patients with osteoarthritis of the knee, 40 were treated with chondroitin sulphate oral gel 1200 mg daily, capsules 1200 mg daily or placebo for three months. Chondroitin (both formulations) significantly improved subjective symptoms, including joint mobility.[1]

In a randomised, double-blind, placebo-controlled study, 80 patients with knee osteoarthritis participated in a six-month study and received either 2 × 400 mg chondroitin capsules twice a day or placebo. Symptoms of joint pain and time to perform a 20 m walk were significantly reduced in the treated group, and there was a non-significant trend for the placebo group to use more paracetamol.[2]

A one-year, randomised, double-blind, controlled pilot study included 42 patients with symptomatic knee osteoarthritis. Patients were treated orally with 800 mg chondroitin sulphate or placebo. Chondroitin sulphate was well tolerated and significantly reduced pain and increased overall mobility. In addition, bone and joint metabolism stabilised in the treated patients, but not in those on placebo.[3]

A meta-analysis which included seven trials of 372 patients taking chondroitin found that over 120 or more days, chondroitin was significantly superior to placebo with respect to the Lesquesne index and pain rating on a visual analogue scale (VAS). Pooling the data confirmed these results, and showed at least 50% improvement in the treated versus the placebo patients. The authors concluded that further investigations using larger cohorts of patients for longer time periods were needed to prove the usefulness of chondroitin as a symptom-modifying agent in osteoarthritis.[4]

A randomised, double-blind, double-dummy study compared the efficacy of chondroitin with diclofenac in 146 patients with knee osteoarthritis. During the first month, patients received either 3 × 50 mg diclofenac tablets daily plus 3 × 400 mg placebo sachets, or 3 × 400 mg chondroitin sachets daily plus 3 × 50 mg placebo tablets. From months two to three, the diclofenac patients were given placebo sachets alone, and the chondroitin patients were given chondroitin sachets. Both groups were treated with placebo sachets from months four to six. The diclofenac group showed prompt pain reduction, which disappeared after the end of treatment. In the chondroitin group, the therapeutic response appeared later in time, but lasted for up to three months after the end of treatment.[5]

Conclusion
Chondroitin appears to offer some pain relief in osteoarthritis. However, studies conducted so far have involved small numbers of subjects and have been of short duration. Further research is required to establish the place of chondroitin as a supplement for osteoarthritis.

Precautions/contraindications

No problems have been reported.

Pregnancy and breast-feeding

No problems have been reported, but there have not been sufficient studies to guarantee the safety of chondroitin in pregnancy and breast-feeding. Chondroitin is probably best avoided.

Adverse effects

There are no known serious side-effects. However, there are no long-term studies assessing the safety of chondroitin. Rarely, gastrointestinal effects and headache have been reported. However, studies in animals have found significantly decreased haematocrit, haemoglobin, white blood cells and platelet count, and the risk of internal bleeding has been suggested.[6] There are no reports of bleeding as a result of chondroitin use in humans, however.

Interactions

Drugs

Anticoagulants: theoretically, chondroitin could potentiate the effects of anticoagulants.

Dose

Chondroitin is available in the form of capsules, typically containing 250–750 mg, often in combination with glucosamine (see Glucosamine monograph). A review of two US products containing chondroitin showed that both had lower chondroitin levels than declared on the labels; this was also found for six out of 13 glucosamine and chondroitin combination products, all due to low chondroitin levels.[7]

The dose is not established. Manufacturers tend to recommend 400–1200 mg daily.

References

1 Bourgeois P, Chales G, Dehais J, *et al.* Efficacy and tolerability of chondroitin sulfate 1200mg/day vs chondroitin 3 × 400mg/day vs placebo. *Osteoarthritis Cartilage* 1998; 6 (suppl. A): 25–30.
2 Bucsi L, Poor G. Efficacy and tolerability of oral chondroitin sulfate as a symptomatic slow-acting drug for osteoarthritis (SYASDOA) in the treatment of knee osteoarthritis. *Osteoarthritis Cartilage* 1998; 6 (suppl. A): 31–36.
3 Uebelhart D, Thonar EJ, Delmad PD, *et al.* Effects of oral chondroitin sulfate on the progression of knee osteoarthritis: a pilot study. *Osteoarthritis Cartilage* 1998; 6 (suppl. A): 39–46.
4 Leeb BF, Schweitzer H, Montag K, Smolen JS. A meta-analysis of chondroitin sulfate in the treatment of osteoarthritis. *J Rheumatol* 2000; 27: 205–211.
5 Morreale P, Manopulo R, Galati M. Comparison of anti-inflammatory efficacy of chondroitin sulfate and diclofenac sodium in patients with knee osteoarthritis. *J Rheumatol* 1996; 23: 1385–1391.
6 McNamara PS, Barr SC, Erb HN, *et al.* Hematologic, hemostatic and biochemical effects in dogs receiving an oral chondroprotective agent for thirty days. *Am J Vet Res* 1996; 57: 1390–1394.
7 Consumerlab. Product review. Glucosamine and chondroitin. http://www.consumerlab.com (accessed 5 December 2000).

Chromium

Description

Chromium is an essential trace mineral.

Human requirements

In the UK, no Reference Nutrient Intake or Estimated Average Requirements has been set. A safe and adequate intake is, for adults, 50–400 μg daily; children and adolescents, 0.1–1.0 μg/kg daily.

In the USA the daily Adequate Intake (AI) is: for adults aged 51–70+ years, males 30 μg, females 20 μg; 19–50 years, males 35 μg, females 21 μg; pregnancy, 30 μg; lactation, 45 μg; children 9–13 years, males 25 μg, females 21 μg; 4–8 years, 15 μg; 1–3 years, 11 μg; infants aged 0–6 months, 0.2 μg; 7–12 months, 5.5 μg.

Intakes

In the UK, the average adult diet provides 13.6–47.7 μg daily.

Action

Chromium functions as an organic complex known as glucose tolerance factor (GTF), which is thought to be a complex of chromium, nicotinic acid and amino acids. It potentiates the action of insulin, and thus influences carbohydrate, fat and protein metabolism. Chromium also appears to influence nucleic acid synthesis and to play a role in gene expression.

Dietary sources

Wholegrain cereals (including bran cereals), brewer's yeast, broccoli, processed meats and spices are the best sources. Dairy products and most fruits and vegetables are poor sources.

Metabolism

Absorption

Chromium is poorly absorbed (0.5–2% of intake); absorption occurs in the small intestine by mechanisms which have not been clearly elucidated, but which appear to involve processes other than simple diffusion.

Distribution

Chromium is transported in the serum or plasma bound to transferrin and albumin. It is widely distributed in the tissues.

Elimination

Absorbed chromium is excreted mainly by the kidneys, with small amounts lost in hair, sweat and bile.

Bioavailability

Absorption of chromium is increased by oxalate and by iron deficiency, and reduced by phytate. Diets high in simple sugars (glucose, fructose, sucrose) increase urinary chromium losses. Absorption is also increased in patients with diabetes mellitus, and depressed in the elderly. Stress and increased physical activity appear to increase urinary losses.

Deficiency

Gross chromium deficiency is rarely seen in humans, but signs and symptoms of marginal deficiency include: impaired glucose intolerance, fasting hyperglycaemia, raised circulating insulin levels, glycosuria, decreased insulin binding, reduced number of insulin receptors, elevated serum cholesterol, elevated serum triglycerides and central and peripheral neuropathy.

Possible uses

Because of its effects on insulin, chromium has been investigated for a potential role in diabetes mellitus, and it has also been promoted for body-building in athletes. It has also been investigated for a potential role in cholesterol lowering and reducing the risk of cardiovascular disease.

Diabetes mellitus

Chromium deficiency may result in insulin resistance,[1] although other researchers have concluded that low-chromium diets have no effect on either insulin or blood glucose.[2] Chromium supplementation may improve glycaemic control in some patients with type 1 and 2 diabetes and gestational diabetes, but relatively high doses (e.g. 1000 μg daily) may be needed. Serum lipid fractions may also be reduced by chromium in patients with diabetes.

Chromium picolinate (200 μg three times a day) reduced glycosylated haemoglobin in a woman with type 1 diabetes mellitus, and the patient also reported improved blood glucose values.[3] Chromium picolinate (200 μg daily) increased insulin sensitivity in patients with type 1 and type 2 diabetes, allowing for a reduction in dose of insulin or hypoglycaemic drugs without compromising glucose control.[4] Steroid-induced diabetes was improved after supplementation with chromium 200 μg three times a day, and chromium 200 μg daily was sufficient to maintain normal blood glucose thereafter.[5]

In a double-blind, placebo-controlled trial, 180 patients with type 2 diabetes were randomised to receive 250 μg chromium twice a day, 100 μg chromium twice a day, or placebo. After two months, glycosylated haemoglobin levels were significantly lower in the high-dose chromium group and after four months were lower in both chromium groups compared with placebo. Fasting and 2 h insulin levels were significantly lower in both chromium groups at two and four months, but significantly lower glucose values and lower plasma cholesterol were found only in the high-dose chromium group.[6]

In a prospective, double-blind, placebo-controlled, cross-over study in 28 subjects with type 2 diabetes, serum triglycerides were significantly reduced by chromium (200 μg daily for two months).[7] However, there was no change in fasting glucose, plasma low-density lipoprotein (LDL) or high-density lipoprotein (HDL) cholesterol levels.

Supplementation of nicotinic acid together with chromium may increase the effectiveness of chromium. In a study involving 16 healthy elderly volunteers, neither chromium 200 μg daily, nor nicotinic acid 100 mg daily affected fasting glucose nor glucose tolerance. However, chromium administered with nicotinic acid resulted in a 15% decrease in the area under the glucose curve and a 7% decrease in fasting glucose.[8]

Obesity

In some controlled human studies, chromium has been reported to reduce body fat[9,10] and increase fat-free mass.[10] However, other studies showed no such effect.[11,12]

Body-building

Chromium supplements are claimed to influence body composition during body-building programmes, though there is little evidence for this. In a study involving 36 men on a weight-training programme, chromium supplementation had no effect on strength, fat-free mass and muscle mass.[13] Chromium picolinate (200 μg a day) did not alter body fat, lean body mass and skinfold thickness in untrained young men on an exercise programme.[14] Neither body composition nor strength changed as a result of chromium picolinate supplementation (200 μg daily) in football players during a nine-week training programme.[15] Young women in a weight-training programme taking chromium picolinate (200 μg daily for 12 weeks) gained significantly more weight than those taking a placebo, and there was a non-significant increase in lean body mass.[16] However, there were no effects on body composition or strength in young men on the same programme.

Cardiovascular disease

Chromium supplements have been claimed to reduce serum cholesterol levels, and there is some evidence for this.

Two placebo-controlled trials, one in 76 men on beta-blockers (which was double blind),[17] the other in 76 patients with atherosclerosis (not blinded)[18] showed a significant increase in serum HDL cholesterol with chromium (300 μg daily in the first study, 200 μg daily in the second). In a double-blind, placebo-controlled cross-over study in 28 healthy sunjects,[19] chromium supplementation (200 μg daily) resulted in a statistically significant reduction in total and LDL cholesterol. HDL was not raised significantly, although apolipoprotein A-1 (the principal protein in A-1) was increased.

> **Conclusion**
> Preliminary evidence suggests that chromium may improve insulin resistance and glucose control in diabetes, although not all studies have reached this conclusion. Preliminary evidence also suggests that chromium may improve serum lipid levels. However, there is no good evidence that chromium reduces body weight or body fat. Despite claims made for chromium in sports, there is no evidence that it has body-building effects in athletes.

Precautions/contraindications

Chromium supplements containing yeast should be avoided by patients taking monoamine oxidase inhibitors (MAOIs). Patients with diabetes mellitus should not take chromium supplements unless medically supervised (chromium may potentiate the action of insulin).

Pregnancy and breast-feeding

No problems reported at normal intakes.

Adverse effects

Oral chromium, particularly trivalent chromium (the usual form in supplements), is relatively non-toxic and unlikely to induce adverse effects. However, it should be emphasised that there have been no long-term studies assessing the safety of chromium in humans. Industrial exposure to high amounts of chromate dust is associated with an increased incidence of lung cancer, and may cause allergic dermatitis and skin ulcers. The hexavalent form (not found in food or supplements) can cause renal and hepatic necrosis.

Interactions

Drugs

Insulin: may reduce insulin requirements in diabetes mellitus (monitor blood glucose).
Oral hypoglycaemics: may potentiate effects of oral hypoglycaemics.

Dose

Chromium is available in the form of chromium picolinate, chromium nicotinic acid, chromium chloride or as an organic complex in brewer's yeast. It is available in tablet and capsule form, and is present in multivitamin/mineral preparations.

The dose is not established. Studies have been conducted with 200–500 μg elemental chromium daily. Dietary supplements provide, on average, 200 μg in a daily dose.

References

1 Mertz W. Chromium in human nutrition: A review. *J Nutr* 1993; 123: 626–633.
2 Anderson RA. Nutritional factors influencing the glucose/insulin system: Chromium. *J Am Coll Nutr* 1997; 16: 404–410.
3 Fox GN, Sabovic Z. Chromium picolinate supplementation for diabetes mellitus. *J Fam Pract* 1998; 46: 83–86.
4 Ravina A, Slezak L, Rubal A. Clinical use of the trace element chromium (III) in the treatment of diabetes mellitus. *J Trace Elem Exp Med* 1995; 8: 183–190.
5 Ravina A, Slezak L, Mirsky N. Reversal of corticosteroid-induced diabetes mellitus with supplemental chromium. *Diabetes Med* 1999; 16: 164–167.

6 Anderson RA, Cheng N, Bryden NA. Elevated intakes of supplemental chromium improve glucose and insulin variables in individuals with type 2 diabetes. *Diabetes* 1997; 46: 1786–1791.
7 Lee NA, Reasner CA. Beneficial effect of chromium supplementation on serum triglyceride levels in NIDDM. *Diabetes Care* 1994; 17: 1449–1452.
8 Urberg M, Zemel MB. Evidence for synergism between chromium and nicotinic acid in the control of glucose tolerance in elderly humans. *Metabolism* 1987; 36: 896–899.
9 Kaats GR, Blum K, Fisher JA. Effects of chromium picolinate supplementation on body composition: A randomized, double-masked, placebo-controlled study. *Curr Ther Res* 1996; 57: 747–756.
10 Kaats GR, Blum K, Pullin D. A randomized double-masked, placebo-controlled study of the effects of chromium picolinate supplementation on body composition: A replication and extension of a previous study. *Curr Ther Res* 1998; 59: 379–388.
11 Cefalu WT, Bell-Farrow AD, Wang ZQ. The effect of chromium supplementation on carbohydrate metabolism and body fat distribution. *Diabetes* 1997; 46 (suppl. 1): 55A.
12 Trent LK, Thieding-Cancel D. Effects of chromium picolinate on body composition. *J Sports Med Phys Fitness* 1995; 35: 273–280.
13 Lukaski HC, Bolonchuk WW, Siders WA. Chromium supplementation and resistance training: Effects on body composition, strength and trace element status of men. *Am J Clin Nutr* 1982; 35: 661–667.
14 Hallmark MA, Reynolds TH, DeSouza TA. Effects of chromium and resistive training on muscle strength and body composition. *Med Sci Sports Exerc* 1996; 28: 139–144.
15 Clancy SP, Clarkson PM, DeCheke ME. Effects of chromium picolinate supplementation on body composition, strength and urinary chromium loss in football players. *Int J Sports Nutr* 1994; 4: 142–153.
16 Hasten DL, Rome EP, Franks BD. Effects of chromium picolinate on beginning weight training students. *Int J Sports Nutr* 1992; 2: 343–350.
17 Roeback JR, Hla KM, Chambless LE, *et al.* Effects of chromium supplementation on serum high density lipoprotein cholesterol in men taking beta-blockers: A randomized, controlled trial. *Ann Intern Med* 1991; 115: 917–924.
18 Abraham AS, Brooks BA, Eylath U. The effect of chromium supplementation on serum glucose and lipids in patients with and without non-insulin dependent diabetes. *Metabolism* 1992; 41: 768–771.
19 Press RI, Geller J, Evans GW. The effect of chromium picolinate on serum cholesterol and apolipoprotein fractions in human subjects. *West J Med* 1990; 152: 41–45.

Co-enzyme Q

Description

Co-enzyme Q is a naturally occurring enzyme (found in the mitochondria of body cells).

Nomenclature

Alternative names include co-enzyme Q_{10} and ubiquinone.

Action

Co-enzyme Q is involved in electron transport in the mitochondrial membrane. It is important for energy production in cells, is thought to be a free radical scavenger, an antioxidant and to have membrane-stabilising properties.

Dietary sources

The co-enzyme Q content of different types of food has been evaluated.[1] Co-enzyme Q is found in fatty fish, such as sardines and mackerel, wholegrain cereals, soya beans, nuts, meat and poultry, and vegetables, especially spinach and broccoli. Milk and cheese have a lower content of co-enzyme Q.

Endogenous synthesis is also important, and the relative significance of biosynthesis and dietary intake to co-enzyme Q status has not been clarified.

Metabolism

Co-enzyme Q is synthesised endogenously using tyrosine, methionine and acetyl co-enzyme A as starting materials. The acetyl co-enzyme A pathway proceeds to both cholesterol and co-enzyme Q synthesis, so co-enzyme Q_{10} and cholesterol share, to some extent, the same biosynthetic pathway.

The ability to synthesise co-enzyme Q may decrease with age. Evidence for a reduction in co-enzyme Q_{10} concentrations with age in various human tissues has been demonstrated.[2,3]

Possible uses

Co-enzyme Q has been investigated for possible effects in cardiovascular disease, cancer, exercise performance, periodontal disease, acquired immunodeficiency syndrome (AIDS) and Parkinson's disease.

Cardiovascular disease

Co-enzyme Q has been suggested to have a role in the management of cardiovascular disease.

Several small studies have suggested that co-enzyme Q_{10} has the ability to protect the ischaemic myocardium in patients with stable angina.[4–6] With doses of 150–600 mg daily, co-enzyme Q_{10}, in comparison with placebo, significantly prolonged exercise duration, but at least in one study, angina symptoms and nitrate use were not reduced.[6]

In another study, in patients with acute myocardial infarction given co-enzyme Q_{10} there was no prolongation of the QT interval, while 40% of the patients on placebo had a prolonged QT interval. After one year, six patients in the placebo group died of re-infarction, while there was one non-cardiac death in the co-enzyme Q_{10} group.[7] Therapy with co-enzyme Q_{10} (60 mg daily) has also been shown effective in treating ventricular arrhythmias.[5]

Several studies have reported clinical benefits of therapy with co-enzyme Q_{10} (50–100 mg daily) in congestive heart failure when added to conventional therapy, including digoxin, diuretics and angiotensin-converting enzyme inhibitors.[4,5,8–13] However, one study failed to show improvement of ventricular function with co-enzyme Q_{10}.[14]

A meta-analysis of eight clinical trials concluded that addition of co-enzyme Q_{10} to standard therapy for congestive heart failure was associated with significant improvements in ejection fraction, stroke volume and cardiac output.[15] Two case reports suggest that in non-responders to co-enzyme Q_{10}, increasing the dose to 300 mg daily may result in improved left ventricular function and improved quality of life.[16]

Co-enzyme Q_{10} therapy (30–90 mg daily) has been reported to reduce both systolic and diastolic blood pressure in uncontrolled studies involving small numbers of patients.[5,17,18] A large multicentre trial is needed to further assess the efficacy of co-enzyme Q_{10} in hypertension.

Cancer

Co-enzyme Q is claimed to have a protective effect against cancer, but data are limited. Folkers *et al.*[19] reported that co-enzyme Q has shown macrophage-potentiating activity in cancer patients with some evidence of increased survival. In a Danish trial,[20,21] 32 women were given routine chemotherapy, radiotherapy, surgery, vitamins, minerals and co-enzyme Q. Six of the women showed partial or complete cancer regression. The authors concluded that, statistically, six women would normally have died, but during the two years of the trial there were no deaths. However, the multiplicity of nutritional supplements used in the study prevents identification of co-enzyme Q as the dominant factor. In two patients with metastatic breast cancer whose co-enzyme Q_{10} dose was increased from 90 to 360 mg daily, liver metastases and pleural cavity metastases apparently disappeared.[22]

Exercise performance

Controlled studies investigating the effects of co-enzyme Q supplementation in exercise performance have not generally shown positive results. A dose of 1 mg co-enzyme Q/kg/day had no effect on exercise performance in trained cyclists and athletes.[23] Co-enzyme Q did not improve performance in either aerobic exercise[24] or cyclists.[25]

Miscellaneous

Case reports and small trials have shown beneficial effects of co-enzyme Q in periodontal disease,[26–28] AIDS[29,30] and Parkinson's disease.[31] Several other claims have been made for co-enzyme Q, including improved energy levels, reduced menopausal symptoms, improved immunity and as an aid to slimming, though there is limited evidence for these claims.

Conclusion

Results from preliminary studies with co-enzyme Q suggest that it may help to improve symptoms of congestive heart failure, and may also help to protect against myocardial infarction. Studies in angina and hypertension are inconclusive. It is likely that co-enzyme Q is beneficial mainly in people who are deficient. Studies conducted so far do not justify the use of co-enzyme Q in cancer, athletes and sports people and AIDS. However, some of the preliminary research justifies more rigorous trials to investigate potential benefits. At present, there is insufficient evidence to make definite recommendations for co-enzyme Q as a dietary supplement.

Precautions/contraindications

Co-enzyme Q should not be used to treat cardiovascular disorders without medical supervision.

Pregnancy and breast-feeding

No problems reported, but probably best avoided.

Adverse effects

No adverse effects have been reported except for occasional, mild nausea. Withdrawal of co-enzyme Q could cause relapse in patients with cardiovascular disorders.

Interactions

Drugs

Warfarin: may reduce the effect of warfarin; decreases in international normalised ratio (INR) have been reported.[32]

Dose

Co-enzyme Q is available in the form of tablets and capsules. A review of 29 US products showed that only one product failed to contain the amount of co-enzyme Q stated on the label.[33]

The dose is not established; as an adjunct to conventional treatment in cardiovascular disorders (with medical supervision only), doses of 150–300 mg daily have been used; dietary supplements generally provide 15–60 mg per dose.

References

1 Kamei M, Fujita T, Ranke T, *et al.* The distribution and content of ubiquinone in foods. *Int J Vit Nutr Res* 1986; 56: 57–64.

2 Kalen A, Appelkvist EL, Dallner G. Age related changes in the lipid composition of rat and human tissue. *Lipids* 1989; 24: 579–584.

3 Soderberg M, Edlund C, Kristensson K, Dallner G. Lipid composition of different regions of the brain during aging. *J Neurochem* 1990; 54: 415–423.

4 Mortensen SA, Vadhanavikit S, Baandrup U. Long term co-enzyme Q_{10} therapy: A major advance in the management of resistant myocardial failure. *Drugs Exp Clin Res* 1985; 11: 581–593.

5 Greenberg S, Frishman WH. Co-enzyme Q10: A new drug for cardiovascular disease. *J Clin Pharmacol* 1990; 30: 596–608.

6 Kamikawa T, Kobayashi A, Tamashita T. Effects of co-enzyme Q10 on exercise tolerance in chronic stable angina pectoris. *Am J Cardiol* 1985; 56: 247–251.

7 Kuklinski B, Weissenbacher E, Fahnrich A. Co-enzyme Q10 and antioxidant in acute myocardial infarction. *Mol Aspects Med* 1994; 15 (suppl.): S143–S147.

8 Lampertico M, Comis S. Italian multicenter study on the efficacy and safety of co-enzyme Q10 as adjuvant therapy in heart failure. *Clin Invest* 1993; 71: 129–133.

9 Mortensen SA. Perspectives on therapy of cardiovascular disease with co-enzyme Q10 (Ubiquinone). *Clin Invest* 1993; 71: 116–123.

10 Baggio E, Gandini R, Plancher AC. Italian multicenter study on the safety and efficacy of co-enzyme Q10 as adjunctive therapy in heart failure (interim analysis). *Clin Invest* 1993; 71: 145–149.

11 Langsjoen PH, Langsjoen PH, Folkers K. Long-term efficacy and safety of co-enzyme Q10 therapy for idiopathic dilated cardiomyopathy. *Am J Cardiol* 1990; 65: 521–523.

12 Langsjoen PH, Folkers K, Lyson K. Effective and safe therapy with co-enzyme Q10 for cardiomyopathy. *Klin Wochenschr* 1988; 66: 583–590.

13 Ishiyama T, Morita Y, Toyama S. A clinical study of the effect of co-enzyme Q on congestive heart failure. *Jpn Heart J* 1976; 17: 32–42.

14 Khatta M, Alexander BS, Kritchen CM, *et al.* The effect of co-enzyme Q_{10} in patients with congestive heart failure. *Ann Intern Med* 2000; 132: 636–640.

15 Soja AM, Mortensen SA. Treatment of congestive heart failure with co-enzyme Q10 illuminated by meta-analyses of clinical trials. *Mol Aspects Med* 1997; 18 (suppl.): S159–S168.

16 Sinatra ST. Refractory congestive heart failure successfully managed with high dose co-enzyme Q10 administration. *Mol Aspects Med* 1997; 18 (suppl.): S299–S305.

17 Folkers K, Drzewoski J, Richardson PC. Bioenergetics in clinical medicine, XVI: Reduction of hypertension in patients by therapy with co-enzyme Q10. *Res Commun Chem Pathol Pharmacol* 1981; 31: 129–140.

18 Yamaagami T, Shibata N, Folkers K. Bioenergetics in clinical medicine, XVIII: Administration of co-enzyme Q10 to patients with essential hypertension. *Res Commun Chem Pathol Pharmacol* 1976; 14: 721–727.

19 Folkers K, Brown R, Judy WV, Morita M. Survival of cancer patients on therapy with co-enzyme Q10. *Biochem Biophys Res Commun* 1993; 192: 241–245.

20 Lockwood K, Moesgaard S, Folkers K. Partial and complete regression of breast cancer in patients in relation to DOSE of co-enzyme Q10. *Biochem Biophys Res Commun* 1994; 199: 1504–1508.

21 Lockwood K, Moesgaard S, Hanioka T. Apparent partial remission of breast cancer in 'high risk' patients supplemented with nutritional antioxidants, essential fatty acids and co-enzyme Q10. *Mol Aspects Med* 1994; 10 (suppl.): S231–S240.

22 Lockwood K, Moesgaard S, Hanioka T. Progress on therapy of breast cancer with vitamin Q10 and the regression of metastases. *Biochem Biophys Res Commun* 1995; 212: 172–177.

23 Weston SB, Zhou S, Weatherby RP, *et al.* Does exogenous co-enzyme Q_{10} affect aerobic capacity in

endurance athletes? *Int J Sports Nutr* 1997; 7: 197–206.

24 Malm C, Svensson M, Ekblom B, *et al*. Effects of ubiquinone-10 supplementation and high intensity training on physical performance in humans. *Acta Physiol Scand* 1997; 161: 379–384.

25 Braun B, Clarkson PM, Freedson PS, Kohl RL. Effects of co-enzyme Q_{10} supplementation on exercise performance, VO_{2max} and lipid peroxidation in trained cyclists. *Int J Sport Nutr* 1991; 1: 353–365.

26 Iwamoto Y, Nakamura R, Folkers K. Study of periodontal disease and co-enzyme Q. *Res Commun Chem Pathol Pharmacol* 1975; 11: 265–271.

27 Wilkinson EG, Arnold RM, Folkers K. Bioenergetics in clinical medicine, VI: Adjunctive treatment for periodontal disease with co-enzyme Q10. *Res Commun Chem Pathol Pharmacol* 1976; 14: 715–719.

28 Wilkinson EG, Arnold RM, Folkers K. Bioenergetics in clinical medicine, II: Adjunctive treatment for periodontal disease with co-enzyme Q10. *Res Commun Chem Pathol Pharmacol* 1975; 12: 111–124.

29 Folkers K, Shizukuishi S, Takemura K. Increase in levels of IgG in serum of patients treated with co-enzyme Q10. *Res Commun Chem Pathol Pharmacol* 1982; 38: 335–338.

30 Folkers K, Langsjoen P, Nara Y. Biochemical deficiencies of co-enzyme Q10 on HIV-infection and exploratory treatment. *Biochem Biophys Res Commun* 1988; 2: 88–96.

31 Shultz CW, Beel MF, Fontaine D, *et al*. Absorption, tolerability and effects on mitochondrial activity of oral co-enzyme Q_{10} in parkinsonian patients. *Neurology* 1998; 50: 793–795.

32 Spigset O. Reduced effect of warfarin caused by ubidecarone. *Lancet* 1994; 344: 1372–1373.

33 Consumerlab. Product review. Co-enzyme Q_{10}. http://www.consumerlab.com (accessed 5 December 2000).

Conjugated linoleic acid

Description

Conjugated linoleic acid (CLA) is a naturally occurring polyunsaturated fatty acid. Nine different isomers of CLA have been identified, and their double bonds are conjugated at carbons 9 and 11 or 10 and 12 in the *cis* and *trans* configurations. CLA is found in low concentrations in blood and tissues, although the body does not synthesise CLA endogenously. It is readily absorbed from food and supplements.

Dietary sources

CLA is present in small quantities in many foods, especially beef and dairy produce. Cooking has been shown to increase the CLA content of meat. Changes in the way that beef and dairy animals have been reared during the past decades have reduced the amount of CLA in the diet.

Action

CLA is essential for the delivery of dietary fat into cells. It transports glucose into cells, and helps glucose to be used to provide energy and build muscle rather than being converted to fat. It is this effect which lies behind the claims that CLA is useful for promoting weight loss. CLA is also an antioxidant and enhances the immune system.

Possible uses

CLA is being marketed for loss of body weight, and is also being investigated for prevention of cancer.

Body weight and energy expenditure

In mice, CLA has been shown to reduce fat accumulation and increase protein accumulation without any change in food intake,[1] to reduce energy intake, increase metabolism and reduce body fat,[2] to reduce body fat and increase lean body mass without affecting body weight,[3] and to reduce body fat and increase energy expenditure.[4] A human study showed that 5.6–7.2 g of CLA daily produced non-significant gains in muscle size and strength in both experienced and inexperienced training men.[5]

Cancer

Preliminary evidence from *in vitro* studies and animal models suggests that CLA may reduce the risk of cancer,[6–8] but other studies have not confirmed this.[9] Linoleic acid itself has been shown to promote tumorigenesis in some studies.

Miscellaneous

Animal research suggests an effect of CLA supplementation on preventing atherosclerosis,[10–12] but one study has shown that CLA does not produce beneficial lipid profiles.[13] Another animal study has shown that CLA may reduce the risk of rheumatoid arthritis,[14] and another that it inhibits the development of impaired glucose tolerance and hyperinsulinaemia, while reducing levels of triglyceride and free fatty acids.[15]

Conclusion

CLA is being promoted for control of body weight. As yet, however, evidence for this – as for other possible indications – comes mainly from animal studies.

Precautions/contraindications

None known.

Pregnancy and breast-feeding

No problems have been reported, but there have not been sufficient studies to guarantee the safety of CLA in pregnancy and breast-feeding.

Adverse effects

No known toxicity or side-effects, apart from one report of gastrointestinal problems. However, there are no long-term studies assessing the safety of CLA.

Interactions

None reported.

Dose

CLA is produced for supplements from sunflower oil and is available in the form of capsules.

The dose is not established. Animal research has used large doses, equivalent to several grams a day for humans. However, dietary supplements tend to provide a dose of 1–4 g daily.

References

1 DeLany JP, Blohm F, Truett AA, *et al.* Conjugated linoleic acid rapidly reduces body fat content in mice without affecting energy intake. *Am J Physiol* 1999; 276 (part 2): R1172–R1179.
2 West DB, DeLany JP, Camet PM, *et al.* Effects of conjugated linoleic acid on body fat and energy metabolism in the mouse. *Am J Physiol* 1998 (part 2); 275: R667–R672.
3 Park Y, Allbright KJ, Liu W, *et al.* Effect of conjugated linoleic acid on body composition in mice. *Lipids* 1997; 32: 853–858.
4 West DB, Blohm FY, Truett AA, DeLany JP. Conjugated linoleic acid persistently increases total energy expenditure in AKR/J mice without uncoupling protein gene expression. *J Nutr* 2000; 130: 2471–2477.
5 Ferreira M, Krieder R, Wilson M. Effects of CLA supplementation during resistance training on body muscle and strength. *J Strength Conditioning Res* 1998; 11: 280.
6 Cesano A, Visonneau S, Scimeca JA, *et al.* Opposite effects of linoleic acid and conjugated linolenic acid on human prostatic cancer in SCID mice. *Anticancer Res* 1998; 18 (3A): 1429–1434.
7 Thompson H, Zhu Z, Banni S, *et al.* Morphological and biochemical status of the mammary gland influenced by conjugated linoleic acid: Implication for a reduction in mammary cancer risk. *Cancer Res* 1997: 57: 5067–5072.
8 Parodi PW. Cow's milk fat components as potential carcinogenic agents. *J Nutr* 1997; 127: 1055–1060.
9 Petrik MB, McEntee MF, Johnson BT, *et al.* Highly unsaturated (n-3) fatty acids, but not alpha linolenic, conjugated linoleic or gamma-linolenic acids, reduce tumorigenesis in Apc(Min/+) mice. *J Nutr* 2000; 130: 2434–2443.
10 Lee KN, Kritchevsky D, Pariza MW. Conjugated linoleic acid and atherosclerosis in rabbits. *Atherosclerosis* 1994; 108: 19–25.
11 Nicolosi RJ, Rogers EJ, Kritchevsky D, *et al.* Dietary conjugated linoleic acid reduces plasma lipoproteins and early aortic atherosclerosis in hypercholesterolemic hamsters. *Artery* 1997; 22: 266–277.
12 Kritchevsky D, Tepper SA, Wright S, *et al.* Influence of conjugated linoleic acid (CLA) on establishment and progression of atherosclerosis in rabbits. *J Am Coll Nutr* 2000; 19: 472S–477S.
13 Stangl GI, Muller H, Kirchgessner M. Conjugated linoleic acid effects on circulating hormones, metabolites and lipoproteins, and its proportions in fasting serum and erythrocyte membranes in swine. *Eur J Nutr* 1999; 38: 271–277.
14 Watkins BA, Seifert MF. Conjugated linoleic acid and bone biology. *J Am Coll Nutr* 2000; 19: 478S–486S.
15 Houseknecht KL, Vanden Heuvel JP, Moya-Camarena SY, *et al.* Dietary conjugated linoleic acid normalises impaired glucose tolerance in the Zucker diabetic fatty fa/fa rat. *Biochem Biophys Res Commun* 1998; 244: 678–682.

Copper

Description

Copper is an essential trace mineral.

Human requirements

See Table 1 for Dietary Reference Values for copper.

Table 1 Dietary Reference Values for copper (mg/day)

		EU RDA (for labelling purposes)			
Age	RNI	USA safe intake		WHO	Europe PRI
		RDA	UL		
0–3 months	0.3	0.2[1]	–	0.33–0.55	–
4–6 months	0.3	0.2[1]	–	0.37–0.62	–
7–12 months	0.3	0.22[1]	–	0.6	0.3
1–3 years	0.4	0.34	1.0	0.56	0.4
4–6 years	0.6	–	–	0.57	0.6
4–8 years	–	0.44	3.0	–	–
7–10 years	0.7	–	–	0.75	0.7
9–13 years	–	0.7	5.0	–	–
14–18 years	–	0.89	8.0	–	–
Males					
11–14 years	0.8	–	–	1.00	0.8
15–18 years	1.0	–	–	1.33	1.0
19–50+ years	1.2	0.9	10.0	1.15	1.1
Females					
11–14 years	0.8	–	–	1.0	0.8
15–18 years	1.0	–	–	1.15	1.0
19–50+ years	1.2	0.9	10.0	1.15	1.1
Pregnancy	*	1.0	8.0	*	*
Lactation	+0.3	1.3	10.0[2]	1.25	+0.3

*No increment.
[1]Adequate Intakes (AIs).
[2]aged <18 years, 8.0 mg daily.
UL = Tolerable Upper Intake Level.
Note: No EAR or LRNI have been derived for copper.

Intakes

In the UK, the average adult daily diet provides: for men, 1.82 mg; for women, 1.31 mg.

Action

Copper functions as an essential component of several enzymes (e.g. superoxide dismutase) and other proteins. It plays a role in bone formation and mineralisation, and in the integrity of the connective tissue of the cardiovascular system. Copper promotes iron absorption and is required for the synthesis of haemoglobin. It is involved in melanin pigment formation, cholesterol metabolism and glucose metabolism. In the central nervous system, it is required for the formation of myelin and is important for normal neurotransmission. Copper has pro-oxidant effects *in vitro*, but antioxidant effects *in vivo*; there is also accumulating evidence that adequate copper is required to maintain antioxidant effects within the body.[1]

Dietary sources

See Table 2 for dietary sources of copper.

Table 2 Dietary sources of copper

Food portion	Copper content (mg)
Breakfast cereals	
1 bowl All–Bran (45 g)	*0.2*
1 bowl Bran Flakes (45 g)	0.1
1 bowl Muesli (95 g)	*0.3*
2 pieces Shredded Wheat	*0.2*
2 Weetabix	*0.2*
Cereal products	
Bread, brown, 2 slices	0.1
white, 2 slices	0.1
wholemeal 2 slices	*0.2*
1 chapati	0.1
Pasta, brown, boiled (150 g)	*0.3*
white, boiled (150 g)	0.1
Rice, brown, boiled (165 g)	*0.5*
white, boiled (165 g)	*0.2*
Meat	
Meat, average, cooked (100 g)	*0.2*
Liver, lambs, cooked (90 g)	9.0
calf, cooked (90 g)	11.0
Kidney, lambs, cooked (75 g)	*0.4*
Vegetables	
Chick peas, lentils, or red kidney beans, cooked (105 g)	*0.2*
Potatoes, boiled (150 g)	0.1
Mushrooms, cooked (100 g)	**0.4**
Green vegetables (100 g)	0.02
Fruit	
1 banana	*0.3*
1 orange	0.1
2 handfuls raisins	0.1
8 dried apricots	*0.2*
Nuts	
20 almonds	*0.2*
10 Brazil nuts	*0.4*
30 hazelnuts	*0.4*
30 peanuts	*0.3*
Chocolate	
Milk chocolate (100 g)	*0.3*
Plain chocolate (100 g)	**0.7**

Excellent sources (**bold**); good sources (*italic*).

Metabolism

Absorption

Copper is absorbed mainly in the small intestine, with a small amount absorbed in the stomach; absorption is probably by a saturable carrier-mediated mechanism at low levels of intake, and by passive diffusion at high levels of intake.

Distribution

Copper is rapidly taken up by the liver and incorporated into caeruloplasmin. It is stored primarily in the liver. Copper is transported bound to caeruloplasmin.

Elimination

Elimination is mainly via bile into the faeces; small amounts are excreted in the urine, sweat and via epidermal shedding.

Bioavailability

Absorption may be reduced by phytate (present in bran and high-fibre foods) and non-starch polysaccharides (dietary fibre), but recommended intakes of fibre-containing foods are unlikely to compromise copper status.

Deficiency

Deficiency of copper is rare, but may lead to hypochromic and microcytic anaemias, leucopenia, neutropenia, impaired immunity and bone demineralisation. Deficiency may also be caused by Menke's syndrome (an X-linked genetic disorder in which copper absorption is defective); this disease is characterised by a reduced level of copper in the blood, liver and hair, progressive mental deterioration, defective keratinisation of the hair and hypothermia.

Marginal deficiency may result in elevated cholesterol levels, impaired glucose tolerance, defects in pigmentation and structure of the hair, and demyelination and degeneration of the nervous system. In infants and children, copper deficiency can lead to skeletal fragility and increased susceptibility to infections, especially those of the respiratory tract.

Copper deficiency has been linked to many of the processes, including atherosclerosis and thrombosis, associated with ischaemic heart disease. Whether this relationship is important in humans remains unanswered. More information is required concerning possible mild copper deficiency in human populations.

Possible uses

Copper has been claimed to be protective against hypercholesterolaemia. In various animal species, it has been demonstrated that feeding a copper-deficient diet results in increased serum cholesterol levels,[1] but studies in humans have shown inconsistent results.[1–3]

Claims for the value of copper supplements in rheumatoid arthritis and psoriasis have not been proved.

Conclusion
There are no proven benefits in taking copper supplements unless there is a proven deficiency, which should be treated under medical supervision.

Precautions/contraindications

Copper should not be used in Wilson's disease (the disorder may be exacerbated), or in hepatic and biliary diseases.

Pregnancy and breast-feeding

No problems reported with normal intakes.

Adverse effects

With excessive doses (unlikely from supplements): epigastric pain, anorexia, nausea, vomiting and diarrhoea; hepatic toxicity and jaundice; hypotension; haematuria (blood in urine, pain on urination, lower back pain); metallic taste; convulsions and coma.

Copper toxicity may also occur in patients with Wilson's disease (an inherited disorder in which patients exhibit a deficiency of plasma caeruloplasmin and an excess of copper in the liver and bloodstream). There is a theoretical possibility of copper toxicity in women who use copper-containing intrauterine contraceptive devices (further studies required).

Interactions

Drugs

Penicillamine: reduces absorption of copper and vice-versa; give 2 h apart.
Trientine: reduces absorption of copper and vice-versa; give 2 h apart.

Nutrients

Iron: large doses of iron may reduce copper status and vice-versa; give 2 h apart.
Vitamin C: large doses of vitamin C (>1 g daily) may reduce copper status.
Zinc: large doses of zinc may reduce absorption of copper and vice-versa; give 2 h apart.

Dose

Copper supplements are available in the form of tablets and capsules, but mostly they are found in multivitamin and mineral supplements. The copper content of various commonly used salts is: copper amino acid chelate (20 mg/g); copper gluconate (140 mg/g); copper sulphate (254 mg/g).

There is no established use or dose for copper as an isolated supplement. Dietary supplements tend to provide 3 mg (elemental copper) daily.

References

1 Klevay LM, Inman L, Johnson LK, *et al*. Increased cholesterol in plasma in a young man during experimental copper depletion. *Metabolism* 1984; 33: 1112–1118.
2 Medeiros D, Pellum L, Brown B. Serum lipids and glucose as associated with haemoglobin levels and copper and zinc intake in young adults. *Life Sci* 1983; 32: 1897–1904.
3 Shapcott D, Vobecky JS, Vobecky J, Demers PP. Plasma cholesterol and the plasma copper/zinc ratio in young children. *Sci Total Environ* 1985; 42: 197–200.

Creatine

Description

Creatine is an amino acid synthesised from the amino acid precursors, arginine, glycine and methionine. The kidneys use arginine and glycine to make guanidinoacetate, which the liver methylates to form creatine. The highest concentrations of creatine are found in skeletal muscle, but high concentrations are also found in heart and smooth muscle, as well as brain, kidney and spermatozoa.

Action

Creatine combines readily with phosphate to form creatine phosphate, which is a source of high-energy phosphate that is released during the anaerobic phase of muscle contraction. The phosphorus from creatine phosphate is transferred to adenosine diphosphate (ADP), creating adenosine triphosphate (ATP) and releasing creatine. Stored creatine phosphate can fuel the first 4–5 s of a sprint, but another fuel must provide the energy to sustain the activity.

Creatine supplements increase the storage of creatine phosphate, thus making more ATP available for the working muscles and enabling them to work harder before becoming fatigued. There appears to be an upper limit for creatine storage in muscle, and supplementation increases levels most in athletes with low stores of creatine, rather than those with high levels.

Dietary sources

Creatine is found in food, and the average omnivorous diet supplies about 1–2 g creatinine daily, although vegetarians consume less. This is because creatine is found principally in animal foods, such as fish and meat. Only trace amounts are found in plant foods. If the dietary supply is limited, creatine can be synthesised endogenously.

Possible uses

Creatine has been investigated for a possible role in sports and athletics.

Exercise performance

Supplementation increases levels of creatine in plasma and sketelal muscle, and it is used to enhance exercise performance. A study in 1992 was the first to show that creatine supplementation (5 g four to six times a day) for several consecutive days increased the creatine concentration of skeletal muscle; the authors concluded that creatine supplementation might enhance exercise performance in humans.[1]

The first published investigation into the effect of oral creatine supplementation on exercise performance in humans showed that ingestion of creatine (20 g daily for five days) was found to improve performance during repeated bouts of maximal isokinetic knee-extensor exercise, reducing fatigue by 6%.[2]

In a subsequent more invasive study, subjects performed two bouts of maximal isokinetic cycling exercise before and after creatine ingestion (20 g daily for five days). Each exercise bout lasted 30 s, and the recovery period between bouts was 4 min. Total work performance increased during both bouts of exercise after creatine supplementation and was related to muscle creatine uptake.[3]

A randomised, placebo-controlled trial involving 16 male subjects investigated the effects of creatine supplementation (20 g daily for five days) on the ability to perform kayak ergometer performances of different durations. The results indicated that creatine could significantly increase the amount of work accomplished at durations ranging from 90–300 s.[4]

In a double-blind, cross-over study 12 subjects were either creatine loaded (25 g daily for five days), or were creatine-loaded and took extra creatine (5 g/h) during an exercise test or placebo on three occasions followed by a five-week wash-out period. Each subject underwent a 2.5 h endurance test on their own bicycle followed by five maximal 10 s sprints separated by 2 min recovery intervals. Creatine loading for five days, but not creatine loading plus acute ingestion, significantly increased peak and mean sprint power for all five sprints, but endurance time to exhaustion was not affected by either creatine regimen.[5]

Ten physically active untrained college-age males received creatine (5 g four times daily) or placebo for five days in a double-blind, randomised, balanced, cross-over design and were assessed during maximal and three repeated submaximal bouts of isometric knee extension and handgrip exercises. Creatine significantly increased maximal isometric strength during knee extension, but not during handgrip exercise, and increased time to fatigue during all bouts of exercise. The authors concluded that improvements in maximal isometric strength following creatine supplementation were restricted to movements performed with a large muscle mass.[6]

Further studies have confirmed the ability of creatine supplements to improve performance during heavy resistance training,[7] ice hockey,[8] bicycle exercise[9] and soccer.[10]

However, several studies reported no effects of creatine supplementation on exercise performance. There was no effect on power output during two bouts of 15 s maximal exercise separated by a recovery of 20 min, but this finding may reflect the design in that several bouts of exercise and a shorter recovery time may have been needed to show an effect of creatine supplementation.[11] However, in another study where subjects were assigned to recovery intervals of 30, 60, 90 or 120 s, creatine 20 g daily for five days still had no effect on the subjects' ability to reproduce or maintain a high percentage of peak power during the second of two bouts of high-intensity cycling.[12] This was also the case in a study that showed no effect of creatine supplementation on performance during a single 20 s bout of maximal exercise.[13]

Another study showed no effect of creatine supplementation on performance during single bouts of maximal exercise lasting 15 s, 30 s and 60 s in elite swimmers,[14] and in a further study, no effect was seen of creatine supplementation on performance during a single 30 s bout of maximal exercise,[15] though this may also have reflected the short supplementation period of three days. In a further study, no changes in performance were found after a small dose of creatine (2 g daily) was taken over several weeks.[16]

Conclusion

Despite a large number of clinical trials, there remains a dearth of high-quality research on creatine supplementation. Investigations of the effect of creatine on performance, strength and endurance in laboratory studies have yielded approximately equal numbers of studies showing positive effects and no effect. Field studies (i.e. of individuals participating in normal sports activities) have shown less impressive results than laboratory studies.

Creatine supplementation improves performance during exercise of high to maximal intensity, and its use could potentially benefit sports involving either single bouts of high-intensity exercise (e.g. sprint running, swimming, rowing, cycling) or multiple bouts (e.g. soccer, rugby, hockey). It also has the potential to benefit an athlete involved in training that involves repetitive bouts of high-intensity exercise. However, there is no evidence that creatine can benefit prolonged, submaximal exercise (e.g. middle- or long-distance running), and it may impair endurance exercise by contributing to weight gain.

Miscellaneous

There is preliminary evidence that creatine may improve strength in people with congestive heart failure[17] and in those with neuromuscular diseases.[18]

Precautions/contraindications

Use with caution in renal or hepatic disease. However, the increase in urinary excretion of creatinine observed with creatine supplementation does not indicate renal impairment. Rather, it correlates with the increase in muscle creatine storage and the increased rate of muscle creatine degradation to creatinine.

Creatine is not on the International Olympic Committee Drug List, but some consider it to be in the 'grey zone' between doping and substances allowed to enhance performance.

Pregnancy and breast-feeding

No problems have been reported. However, there have not been sufficient studies to guarantee the safety of creatine in pregnancy and breast-feeding. Creatine is best avoided.

Adverse effects

No serious toxic effects have been documented. However, there are no studies lasting longer than eight weeks assessing the safety of creatine. In a survey of 52 college athletes supplementing with creatine, 16 reported diarrhoea, 13 reported muscle cramps and seven dehydration.[19] Another survey, which involved 28 male baseball players and 24 male football players, aged 18–23 years, found that 16 (31%) experienced diarrhoea, 13 (25%) experienced muscle cramps, seven (13%) reported unwanted weight gain, seven (13%) reported dehydration and 12 reported various other side-effects.[20] In the same survey, 39 (75%) exceeded the maintenance dose of 2–5 g daily.

A report by the US Food and Drug Administration[21] lists 32 creatine-associated events that have been reported to the FDA. These include seizure, vomiting, diarrhoea, anxiety, myopathy, atrial fibrillation, cardiac arrhythmia, shortness of breath, deep-vein thromboses and death. However, the FDA states that there is no certainty that a reported adverse event can be attributed to a particular product.

In another report a patient with nephrotic syndrome who had been supplementing with creatine experienced deterioration in renal function,[22] and a previously healthy 20-year-old man developed interstitial nephritis after taking creatine (20 g daily) for four weeks.[23]

Chronic administration of a large quantity of creatine can increase the production of formaldehyde; this is well known to cross-link proteins and DNA, and may cause potentially serious side-effects.[24]

Creatine supplementation often causes weight gain, which can be mistaken for increase in muscle mass. Increasing intracellular creatine may cause an osmotic influx of water into the cell because creatine is an osmotically active substance. It is therefore possible that the weight gained is due to water retention, and not increased muscle.

The safety of prolonged use of creatine is of concern. Individuals should be advised not to take the loading dose of 20 g daily for more than five days and not to supplement for a total period of longer than 30 days until effects are better known.

Interactions

No known drug interactions. Caffeine may reduce or abolish the ergogenic effects of creatine.

Dose

Creatine is available mainly in the form of powder. A review of 13 US products showed that 11 contained the claimed weight of creatine. One of the products was found to contain less than the claimed amount, and one failed to meet its claim of being free from the impurity dicyandiamide.[25]

The usual dose regimen used in studies is 5 g creatine monohydrate four times daily for the first five days as a loading dose, then 2–5 g daily as maintenance. These doses should not be exceeded because of the risk of adverse effects (see above).

References

1 Harris RC, Soderlund K, Hultman E. Elevation of creatine in resting and exercised muscle of normal subjects by creatine supplementation. *Clin Sci* 1992; 83: 367–374.

2 Greenhaff PL, Casey A, Short AH, *et al.* Influence of oral creatine supplementation on muscle torque during repeated bouts of maximal voluntary exercise in man. *Clin Sci* 1993; 84: 565–571.

3 Casey A, Constantin-Teodosiu D, Howell S, *et al.* Creatine ingestion favorably influences exercise performance and muscle metabolism during maximal exercise in humans. *Am J Physiol* 1996; 27: E31–E37.

4 McNaughton LR, Dalton B, Tarr J. The effects of creatine supplementation on high-intensity exercise performance in elite performers. *Eur J Appl Physiol Occup Physiol* 1998; 78: 236–240.

5 Vandebuerie F, Vanden Eynde B, Vandenberghe K, Hespel P. Effect of creatine loading on endurance capacity and sprint power in cyclists. *Int J Sports Med* 1998; 19: 490–495.

6 Urbanski RL, Vincent WJ, Yaspelkis BB, III. Creatine supplementation differentially affects maximal isometric strength and time to fatigue in large and small muscle groups. *Int J Sports Nutr* 1999; 9: 136–145.

7 Volek JS, Duncan ND, Mazzetti SA, *et al.* Performance and muscle fiber adaptation to creatine supplementation and heavy resistance training. *Med Sci Sports Exerc* 1999; 31: 1147–1156.

8 Jones AM, Atter T, Georg TP. Oral creatine supplementation improves multiple sprint performance in elite ice-hockey players. *J Sports Med Phys Fitness* 1999; 39: 189–196.

9 Rici-Sanz J, Mendez Marco MT. Creatine enhances oxygen uptake and performance during alternating intensity exercise. *Med Sci Sports Exerc* 2000; 32: 379–385.

10 Mujika I, Padilla S, Ibanez J, *et al.* Creatine supplementation and sprint performance in soccer players. *Med Sci Sports Exerc* 2000; 32: 518–525.

11 Cooke WH, Grandjean PW, Barnes WS. Effect of oral creatine supplementation on power output and fatigue during bicycle ergometry. *J Appl Physiol* 1995; 78: 670–673.

12 Cooke WH, Barnes WS. The influence of recovery duration on high intensity exercise performance after oral creatine supplementation. *Can J Appl Physiol* 1997; 22: 454–467.

13 Snow RJ, McKenna MJ, Selig SE, *et al.* Effect of creatine supplementation on sprint exercise performance and muscle metabolism. *J Appl Physiol* 1998; 84: 1667–1673.

14 Mukija I, Chatard JC, Lacoste L, *et al.* Creatine supplementation does not improve sprint performance in competitive swimmers. *Med Sci Sports Exerc* 1996; 28: 1435–1441.

15 Odland LM, MacDougall JD, Tarnopolsky MA, *et al.* Effect of oral creatine supplementation on muscle (PCr) and short-term maximum power output. *Med Sci Sports Exerc* 1997; 29: 216–219.

16 Thompson CH, Kemp GJ, Sanderson AL, *et al.* Effect of creatine on aerobic and anaerobic metabolism in skeletal muscle in swimmers. *Br J Sports Med* 1996; 30: 222–225.

17 Andrews R, Greenhaff P, Curtis S, *et al.* The effect of dietary creatine supplementation on skeletal muscle metabolism in congestive heart failure. *Eur Heart J* 1998; 19: 617–622.

18 Tarnopolsky M, Martin J. Creatine monohydrate increases strength in patients with neuromuscular disease. *Neurology* 1999; 52: 854–857.

19 Juhn MS, Tarnopolsky M. Potential side effects of oral creatine supplementation: A critical review. *J Am Diet Assoc* 1998; 98: 298–304.

20 Juhn MS, O'Kane JW, Vinci DM. Oral creatine supplementation in male college athletes: A survey of dosing habits and side effects. *J Am Diet Assoc* 1999; 99: 593–595.

21 US Food and Drug Administration. Special nutritionals adverse event monitoring system. http://vm.cfscan.fda.gov/cgi-bin/aems.cgi (accessed 1 November 2000).

22 Pritchard NR, Kalra PA. Renal dysfunction accompanying oral creatine supplements. *Lancet* 1998; 351: 1252–1253.

23 Koshy KM, Griswold E, Schneeberger EE. Interstitial nephritis in a patient taking creatine. *N Engl J Med* 1999; 340: 814–815.

24 Yu PH, Deng Y. Potential cytotoxic effect of chronic administration of creatine, a nutrition supplement to augment athletic performance. *Med Hypoth* 2000; 54: 726–728.

25 Consumerlab. Product review. Creatine. http://www.consumerlab.com (accessed 5 December 2000).

Dehydroepiandrosterone

Description

Dehydroepiandrosterone (DHEA) is the most abundant hormone secreted by the adrenal glands. It is a steroid hormone and is secreted by the zona reticularis of the adrenals. DHEA circulates in the blood as dehydroepiandrosterone-3-sulphate (DHEAS), which is converted as required to DHEA. Production of DHEA in humans normally peaks between the ages of 20 and 30 years, and then begins a steady, progressive decline.[1]

Action

DHEA and DHEAS are the precursors for other hormones, including oestrogens and androgens. The degree of androgenic versus oestrogenic effect of DHEA may depend on the individual's hormonal status. For example, there is some evidence that DHEA has different effects in premenopausal and postmenopausal women.[2]

DHEA has also been shown to stimulate insulin growth factor-1 (IGF-1),[3] a hormone which stimulates anabolic metabolism, enhances insulin sensitivity, accelerates muscle growth and enhances energy production.

Possible uses

Supplementation with DHEA has been claimed to produce several health benefits including enhancement of immune function, increased muscle mass, improvements in memory and mood, improvement in symptoms of autoimmune disorders such as lupus erythematosus, and to have a general anti-ageing effect. However, evidence for a beneficial effect of DHEA supplements in all these conditions is inconclusive.

Immunity

The first *in vivo* evidence of an immunomodulatory effect of DHEA came from a prospective, randomised, double-blind, cross-over study involving 11 postmenopausal women with three-week treatment arms. Results showed that DHEA supplementation reduced T helper cell populations and increased natural killer cell populations.[4]

In a single-blind, placebo-controlled study, nine healthy men (mean age 63 years) were supplemented with a placebo for two weeks, followed by DHEA 50 mg daily for 20 weeks.[5] DHEA stimulated immune function by significantly increasing the number of monocyte and B cells, stimulating B- and T-cell mitogenic response, interleukin-2 secretion and the number and cytotoxicity of natural killer cells. The authors acknowledged that the results of this study had limited application because post-treatment immune response was not measured.

However, in two other studies,[6,7] DHEA produced no significant effects on antibody response to influenza vaccine.

Body composition

In a double-blind, placebo-controlled study, 10 healthy men were randomised to receive either 1600 mg DHEA or placebo daily for 28 days. Compared with placebo, body fat was reduced significantly by 31% in the supplemented group, but there was no change in body weight. There was also a 7.5% reduction in low density lipoprotein (LDL) cholesterol.[8] Furthermore, in another randomised, double-blind, placebo-controlled study in morbidly obese adolescents,[9] 40 mg DHEA twice a day had no effect on body weight. In two other studies,[10,11] DHEA 1600 mg daily for four weeks had no significant effect on either body weight or lean body mass.

Memory, mood and depression

In a double-blind, placebo-controlled, cross-over study, 30 healthy subjects aged 40–70 years were randomised to receive in random order either 50 mg DHEA or placebo daily for three months each. During DHEA supplementation there was a significant increase in perceived physical and psychological well-being, but no effect on insulin sensitivity, body fat or libido.[12]

In a double-blind, placebo-controlled, cross-over study, 17 healthy, elderly, male subjects received 50 mg DHEA daily or a placebo for two weeks. There was no change in memory or mood in the supplemented group.[13]

A Cochrane systematic review[14] investigated the effect of DHEA supplementation on cognition and well-being. Five studies matched the reviewers' criteria, four of which were short term (DHEA administered for two weeks or less) and one where DHEA was given for three months. There was no significant change in ability to perform cognitive tests, or mood or well-being (as assessed by standard scales) in the short-term studies. In the longer-term study, the results of an open-ended questionnaire showed that 67% of men and 82% of women reported enhanced well-being with DHEA compared with placebo. The reviewers concluded that present data offer limited support for a beneficial effect of DHEA on well-being, but not on memory or cognitive function.

In a double-blind, placebo-controlled study,[15] 32 patients with severe depression, either medication-free or stabilised on antidepressants, received either DHEA (maximum dose = 90 mg daily) or placebo for six weeks. DHEA was associated with a significantly greater decrease in the Hamilton depression rating scale than placebo, and five of the 11 patients treated with DHEA compared with none of the 11 subjects in the placebo group showed a 50% or greater reduction in symptoms of depression.

Systemic lupus erythematosus

In a double-blind, placebo-controlled study,[16] 28 women with mild to moderate systemic lupus erythematosus (SLE) were randomised to receive 200 mg DHEA or placebo daily for three months. In the supplemented group, there were insignificant improvements in SLE Disease Activity Index scores, physicians' assessment of disease activity and a reduction in the dose of prednisone used. There was also a significant improvement in patients' assessment of disease activity with DHEA compared with placebo.

In an open study, 50 women with mild to moderate SLE were treated with 50–200 mg of DHEA daily for 6–12 months. Supplementation was associated with a significant reduction in disease activity and significant improvement in patient and physician assessment compared with baseline.[17]

Miscellaneous

There is no evidence that DHEA supplements prevent ageing in humans, though some reports have suggested that it might reduce the risk of heart disease. Epidemiological studies have been conflicting, and although some animal and human studies have shown that DHEA may reduce LDL cholesterol and platelet aggregation, controlled trials are needed to assess the effects of DHEA supplementation on cardiovascular risk. DHEA has also been reported to improve insulin sensitivity and reduce blood glucose levels, but again results from studies have been conflicting.

Conclusion

The role of DHEA supplements in all conditions studied is inconclusive. Some studies have shown that DHEA improves the immune response, while others have not. There is no good evidence that DHEA helps to reduce body weight. There is limited evidence that it may improve well-being and reduce symptoms of depression, but it seems to have no effect on memory or cognition. Preliminary evidence suggests that DHEA could improve symptoms of SLE.

Precautions/contraindications

DHEA is contraindicated in individuals who have (or have a history of) prostate cancer or oestrogen-dependent tumours (e.g. breast or uterine cancer). It should be used with caution in patients with diabetes mellitus (because it may alter blood glucose regulation). Blood glucose and doses of insulin and oral hypoglycaemic agents should be monitored in patients with diabetes.

Pregnancy and breast-feeding

The effects of DHEA in pregnancy and breast-feeding are unknown. Because of its potential oestrogenic effect, it is probably best avoided.

Adverse effects

There is no known toxicity or serious side-effects. However, the safety of long-term administration is unknown. DHEA alters the levels of other hormones, and has both oestrogenic and androgenic activity. Potential side-effects in women are therefore increased facial hair and increased loss of head hair, menstrual irregularities and deepening of the voice. The risk of breast cancer may also be increased, but results from studies are conflicting, with some showing that DHEA may reduce risk while others show that it may increase risk. A review[18] concluded that prolonged intake of DHEA may promote breast cancer in postmenopausal women. Potential side-effects in men include an increased risk of prostate cancer.

A study in 22 healthy men[19] suggested that DHEA doses up to 200 mg daily for four weeks were safe and well tolerated. Results of another study[20] in 24 healthy elderly men and women (67.8 ± 4.3 years) suggested that daily doses of 25 or 50 mg DHEA are safe in elderly subjects. There were no large increases in blood levels of androgens and oestrogens in this study.

Interactions

None reported, but theoretically DHEA could interact with insulin, oral hypoglycaemic agents, oestrogens (including hormone replacement therapy) and androgens.

Dose

DHEA is available in the form of tablets and capsules.

The dose is not established. Dietary supplements tend to provide 5–50 mg daily.

References

1 Nafziger AN, Bowlin SJ, Jenkins PL, *et al.* Longitudinal changes in dehydroepiandrosterone sulfate and concentrations in men and women. *J Lab Clin Med* 1998; 131: 316–323.
2 Ebeling P, Koivisto VA. Physiological importance of dehydroepiandrosterone. *Lancet* 1994; 343: 1479–1481.
3 Casson PR, Santoro N, Elkind-Hirsch K, *et al.* Postmenopausal dehydroepiandrosterone administration increases free insulin-like growth factor-1 and decreases high density lipoprotein: A six-month trial. *Fertil Steril* 1998; 70: 107–110.
4 Casson PR, Andersen RN, Herrod HG, *et al.* Oral dehydroepiandrosterone in physiologic doses modulates immune function in postmenopausal women. *Am J Obstet Gynecol* 1993; 169: 1536–1539.
5 Khorram O, Vu L, Yen SS. Activation of immune function by dehydroepiandrosterone (DHEA) in age-advanced men. *J Gerontol A Biol Sci Med Sci* 1997; 52: M1–M7.
6 Degelau J, Guay D, Hallgren H. The effect of DHEAS on influenza vaccine in aging adults. *J Am Geriatr Soc* 1997; 45: 747–751.
7 Ben-Yehuda A, Daneberg HD, Zakay-Rones Z, *et al.* The influence of sequential annual vaccination and of DHEA administration on the efficacy of the immune response to influenza vaccine in the elderly. *Mech Ageing Dev* 1998; 102: 299–306.
8 Nestler JE, Barlascini CO, Clore JN, *et al.* Dehydroepiandrosterone reduces serum low density lipoprotein levels and body fat but does not alter insulin sensitivity in normal men. *J Clin Endocrinol Metab* 1988; 66: 57–61.
9 Vogiatzi MG, Boeck MA, Vlachopapadopoulou E, *et al.* Dehydroepiandrosterone in morbidly obese adolescents: Effects on weight, body composition, lipids and insulin resistance. *Metabolism* 1996; 45: 1011–1015.
10 Welle S, Jozefowicz R, Statt M. Failure of dehydroepiandrosterone to influence energy and protein metabolism in humans. *J Clin Endocrinol Metab* 1990; 71: 1259–1264.
11 Usiskin KS, Butterworth S, Clore JN, *et al.* Lack of effect of dehydroepiandrosterone in obese men. *Int J Obesity* 1990; 14: 457–463.
12 Morales AJ, Nolan JJ, Nelson JC, *et al.* Effects of replacement dose of DHEA in men and women of advancing age. *J Clin Endocrinol Metab* 1994; 78: 1360–1367.
13 Wolf OT, Naumann E, Helhammer DH, *et al.* Effects of dehydroepiandrosterone replacement in elderly men on event-related potentials, memory and well

being. *J Gerontol A Biol Sci Med Sci* 1998; 53: M385–M390.

14 Huppert FA, Van Nickerk JK, Herbert J. Dehydroepiandrosterone (DHEA) supplementation for cognition and well being. *Cochrane Database Syst Rev* 2000; (2): CD000304.

15 Wolkowitz OM, Reus VI, Keebler A, *et al.* Double-blind treatment of major depression with dehydroepiandrosterone. *Am J Psychiatry* 1999; 156: 646–649.

16 Van Vollenhoven RF, Engleman EG, McGuire GL, *et al.* Dehydroepiandrosterone systemic lupus erythematosus: Results of a double-blind, placebo-controlled, randomised clinical trial. *Arthritis Rheum* 1995; 38: 1826–1831.

17 Van Vollenhoven RF, Morabito LM, Engleman EG, *et al.* Treatment of systemic lupus erythematosus with dehydroepiandrosterone: 50 patients treated up to 12 months. *J Rheumatol* 1998; 25: 285–289.

18 Stoll BA. Dietary supplements of dehydroepiandrosterone in relation to breast cancer risk. *Eur J Clin Nutr* 1999; 53: 771–775.

19 Davidson M, Marwah A, Sawchuk RJ, *et al.* Safety and pharmacokinetic study with escalating doses of 3-acetyl-7-oxo-dehydroepiandrosterone in healthy male volunteers. *Clin Invest Med* 2000; 23: 300–310.

20 Legrain S, Massien C, Lahlou N, *et al.* Dehydroepiandrosterone replacement administration: Pharmacokinetic and pharmacodynamic studies in healthy elderly subjects. *J Clin Endocrinol Metab* 2000; 85: 3208–3217.

Evening primrose oil

Description

Evening primrose oil is derived from the seeds of *Oenothera biennis* and other species.

Constituents

Evening primrose oil contains gamma-linolenic acid (GLA) and linoleic acid. Starflower oil (borage oil) and blackcurrant oil are also used as sources of GLA in dietary supplements. Evening primrose oil contains 8–11% GLA. Starflower oil contains 20–25% GLA, but the biological activity of starflower oil may be no greater than that of evening primrose oil, i.e. on a weight-for-weight basis, starflower oil has not been proved to be twice as active as evening primrose oil. Blackcurrant oil contains 15–25% GLA.

Action

GLA is not an essential dietary component. It is normally synthesised in the body by the action of delta-6-desaturase on linoleic acid (obtained in the diet from vegetable and seed oils, e.g. sunflower oil).

GLA is a precursor of dihomogamma-linolenic acid (DGLA) and the series 1 prostaglandins (PG), and also of arachidonic acid (see Figure 1). Most of the DGLA formed from GLA is metabolised to PG1s; conversion of DGLA to arachidonic acid is very slow. Arachidonic acid is normally obtained from meat in the diet.

Supplementation with GLA increases the ratio of DGLA to arachidonic acid. DGLA levels are elevated to a greater extent by the administration of GLA than by the administration of linoleic acid (the reasons for this are not entirely clear).

Prostaglandin PGE_1 (produced from DGLA) inhibits platelet aggregation and is also a vasodilator; it has less potent inflammatory effects than prostaglandins of the PG2 series, thromboxane A_2 and series 4 leukotrienes (produced from arachidonic acid).

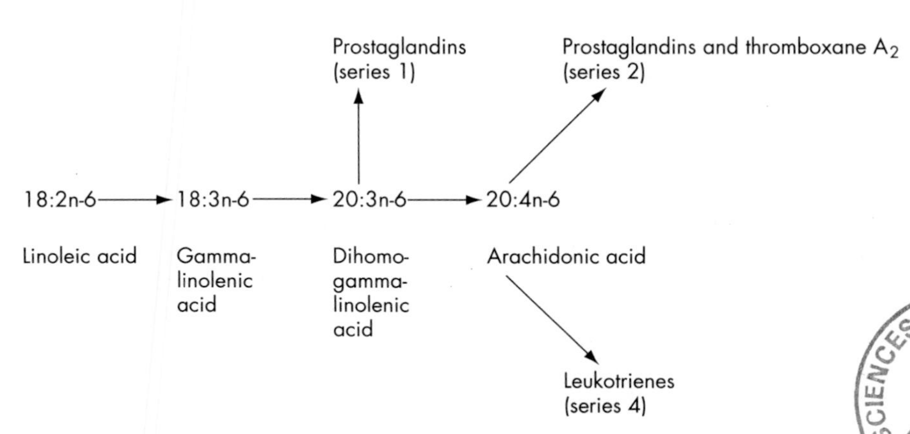

Figure 1 Metabolism of gamma-linolenic acid.

The efficacy of GLA is thus thought to be due, in part, to the increased production of PG1 series prostaglandins at the expense of PG2 series prostaglandins, thromboxane A_2 and series 4 leukotrienes.

Deficiency

Patients with diabetes mellitus or eczema may be at risk of GLA deficiency. Despite some claims, however, there is little evidence that foods rich in saturated fat and sugar, drinking alcohol, stress, pollution, high blood cholesterol, ageing, viral infections and hormone imbalances lead to deficiency of GLA.

Possible uses

Evening primrose oil is used widely as a dietary supplement for various disorders, including the premenstrual syndrome, hypertension, asthma and angina. It is also claimed to reduce blood cholesterol levels, and to act as a slimming aid.

Disorders for which evening primrose oil has been tested in controlled clinical trials include atopic dermatitis, diabetic neuropathy, mastalgia and breast cysts, menopausal flushing, Raynaud's phenomenon, rheumatoid arthritis, schizophrenia, Sjogren's syndrome, ulcerative colitis and various cancers. Evening primrose oil is being investigated in a range of other disorders including multiple sclerosis and hyperactivity in children.

Skin conditions

The efficacy of evening primrose oil in inflammatory skin conditions such as eczema is difficult to judge because several trials have shown improvements in both the treatment and placebo groups. However, results indicate that for efficacy, high doses and long-term treatment are necessary. Evening primrose oil may work in these conditions not only by supplying precursors of prostaglandins but also by supplying the essential fatty acids to maintain cell membranes. One GLA product is available on the National Health Service for alleviation of symptoms of eczema; any benefit is thought to be modest.

A double-blind, cross-over study involving 99 patients showed improvement in symptoms of eczema with doses of 4–6 g daily of evening primrose oil in adults and 2 g daily in children.[1] Another trial involving 25 patients showed that evening primrose oil (45 mg GLA per capsule) improved symptoms of eczema. Although there was also an improvement in the placebo group, this was not as great as in the evening primrose oil group.[2] A further double-blind, cross-over study showed no clinical benefit with the use of evening primrose oil for atopic eczema in a mixed group of adults and children.[3] Adult doses in this study were 12 or 16 × 500 mg capsules each day. Another study in patients with chronic dermatitis of the hands[3] showed no difference between the effects of evening primrose oil (12 × 500 mg capsules each day) or placebo (sunflower oil capsules). Similarly conflicting results have been found in studies in children.[4,5]

Premenstrual syndrome and the menopause

Evening primrose oil may be effective in relieving the physical and psychological symptoms of premenstrual syndrome (PMS) in some women. However, few good studies have been carried out. A review of four studies[6] concluded that evening primrose oil is effective for the treatment of PMS. However, another study in 38 women[7] showed no differences between the effect of placebo and evening primrose oil on symptoms such as fluid retention, breast pain or swelling or mood changes.

Some trials with evening primrose oil in cyclical mastalgia and breast tenderness have shown positive results.[8,9] However, since the response can be slow, treatment should be continued for several months before it is decided whether or not treatment is successful.

Trial data on the effects of evening primrose oil during the menopause are conflicting. In one of the most recent studies,[10] involving 56 postmenopausal women suffering hot flushes, GLA offered no benefit over placebo.

Rheumatoid arthritis

Results from trials with evening primrose oil in rheumatoid arthritis have been mixed. In one study of 20 patients, treatment with non-steroidal anti-inflammatory drugs was stopped and administration of evening primrose oil resulted in no significant changes in symptoms of arthritis.[11] In an another study involving 49 patients,[12] treatment with evening primrose oil (equivalent to 540 mg GLA daily) or a combination of evening primrose oil and fish oil (450 mg GLA plus 240 mg eicosapentaenoic acid) allowed for a significant reduction in the dose of non-steroidal anti-inflammatory drugs. However, another study in 20 patients[13] who received either evening primrose oil or olive oil twice daily for 12 weeks, showed no significant differences in terms of prostaglandin levels, therapeutic response or laboratory parameters. However, those individuals whose pro-inflammatory prostaglandin and thromboxane levels were reduced tended to have better therapeutic responses.

Miscellaneous

Encouraging findings have been reported with trials of evening primrose oil in diabetic neuropathy,[14,15] but not in asthma,[16,17] hypercholesterolaemia.[18,19] or in obesity.[20]

> **Conclusion**
> Results of clinical studies with gamma-linolenic acid (GLA) in skin conditions, including atopic dermatitis, as well as premenstrual syndrome and rheumatoid arthritis have produced conflicting results. However, some individuals with these conditions do appear to benefit. Preliminary research indicates that GLA may be beneficial in diabetic neuropathy.

Precautions/contraindications

Avoid in patients with epilepsy and in those taking epileptogenic drugs, e.g. phenothiazines. There is some evidence that GLA may increase the risk of seizures in these patients.[21]

Pregnancy and breast-feeding

Caution in pregnancy (possible hormonal effects). No problems have been reported in breast-feeding.

Adverse effects

Toxicity appears to be low. The only adverse effects reported are nausea, diarrhoea and headache. However, one report[22] has warned of a potential risk of inflammation, thrombosis and immunosuppression due to slow accumulation of tissue arachidonic acid after prolonged use of GLA for more than one year.

Interactions

Drugs

Phenothiazines: increased risk (small) of epileptic fits.

Dose

Evening primrose oil and other supplements containing GLA are generally available in the form of capsules.

Symptomatic relief of eczema, 320–480 mg (as GLA) daily; child 1–12 years, 160–320 mg daily.

Symptomatic relief of cyclical and non-cyclical mastalgia, 240–320 mg (as GLA) daily for 12 weeks (then stopped if no improvement).

Dietary supplements provide 40–300 mg (as GLA) per daily dose.

Note: doses are given in terms of GLA; evening primrose oil supplements are not identical; they provide different amounts of GLA.

References

1. Wright S, Burton JL. Oral evening primrose seed oil improves atopic eczema. *Lancet* 1982; 2: 1120–1122.
2. Schalin-Karrila M, Mattila L, Jansen CT. Evening primrose oil in the treatment of atopic eczema: Effect on clinical status, plasma phospholipid fatty acids and circulating blood prostaglandins. *Br J Dermatol* 1987; 117: 11–19.
3. Bamford JT, Gibson RW, Renier CM. Atopic eczema unresponsive to evening primrose oil. *J Am Acad Dermatol* 1985; 13: 959–965.
4. Biagi PL, Bordoni A, Masi M. A long-term study on the use of evening primrose oil (Efamol) in atopic children. *Drugs Exp Clin Res* 1988; 14: 285–290.
5. Hederos CA, Berg A. Epogam evening primrose oil treatment in atopic dermatitis and asthma. *Arch Dis Child* 1996; 75: 494–497.

6 Horrobin DF. The role of essential fatty acids and prostaglandins in the premenstrual syndrome. *J Reprod Med* 1983; 28: 465–468.
7 Khoo SK, Munro C, Battistutta D. Evening primrose oil and treatment of pre-menstrual syndrome. *Med J Austr* 1990; 153: 189–192.
8 McFayden IJ, Forrest AP, Chetty U. Cyclical breast pain – some observations and the difficulties in treatment. *Br J Gen Pract* 1992; 46: 161–164.
9 Steinbrunn BS, Zera RT, Rodriguez JL. Mastalgia – tailoring treatment to type of breast pain. *Postgrad Med J* 1997; 102: 183–188.
10 Chenoy S, Hussain S, Tayob Y, *et al.* Effect of oral gamolenic acid from evening primrose oil on menopausal flushing. *Br Med J* 1994; 308: 501–503.
11 Belch JJ, Ansell D, Madhock R, *et al.* The effects of altering dietary essential fatty acids on requirements for non-steroidal anti-inflammatory drugs in patients with rheumatoid arthritis. *Ann Rheum Dis* 1988; 47: 96–104.
12 Hansen TM, Lerche A, Kassis V, *et al.* Treatment of rheumatoid arthritis with prostaglandin E1 precursors cis-linoleic acid and gamma-linolenic acid. *Scand J Rheumatol* 1983; 12: 85–88.
13 Janntti J, Seppala E, Vapaatalo H. Evening primrose oil and olive oil in the treatment of rheumatoid arthritis. *Clin Rheumatol* 1989; 8: 238–244.
14 Gamma-Linolenic Acid Multicenter Trial Group. Treatment of diabetic neuropathy with gamma-linolenic acid. *Diabetes Care* 1993; 16: 8–15.
15 Jamal GA, Carmichael H. The effect of gamma-linolenic acid on human diabetic peripheral neuropathy: A double-blind placebo-controlled trial. *Diabetic Med* 1990; 7: 319–323.
16 Ebden P, Bevan C, Banks J. A study of evening primrose seed oil in atopic asthma. *Prostaglandins Leukot Essent Fatty Acids* 1989; 35: 69–72.
17 Stenius-Aarniala B, Aro A, Hakulinen A. Evening primrose and fish oil are ineffective as supplementary treatment of bronchial asthma. *Ann Allergy* 1989; 62: 534–537.
18 Viikari J, Lehtonen A. Effect of evening primrose oil on serum lipids and blood pressure in hyperlipidemic subjects. *Int J Clin Pharmacol Ther Toxicol* 1986; 24: 668–670.
19 Boberg M, Vessby B, Selenius I. Effects of dietary supplementation with n-6 and n-3 long-chain polyunsaturated fatty acids on serum lipoproteins and platelet function in hypertriglyceridaemic patients. *Acta Med Scand* 1986; 220: 153–160.
20 Haslett C, Douglas JG, Chalmers SR. A double-blind evaluation of evening primrose oil as an anti-obesity agent. *Int J Obesity* 1983; 7: 549–553.
21 Miller LG. Herbal medicines: Selected clinical considerations focusing on known or potential drug-herb interactions. *Arch Intern Med* 1998; 158: 2200–2211.
22 Phinney S. Potential risk of prolonged gamma-linolenic acid use. *Ann Intern Med* 1994; 120: 692.

Fish oils

Description

In the UK, there are two types of fish oil supplements:

- Fish liver oil; this is generally obtained from the liver of the cod, halibut or shark.
- Fish body oil; this is normally derived from the flesh of the herring, sardine or anchovy.

Constituents

Fish liver oil is a rich source of vitamins A and D; concentrations in cod liver oil liquids normally range between 750 and 1200 μg (2500–4000 units) vitamin A per 10 ml and 2.5–10 μg (100–400 units) vitamin D per 10 ml; halibut and shark liver oils are more concentrated sources of these vitamins. Fish body oil is low in vitamins A and D. Vitamin E is also present in both types of fish oil and extra vitamin E is normally added to supplements.

Both fish liver oil and fish body oil are sources of polyunsaturated fatty acids (PUFAs) of the omega-3 series (eicosapentaenoic acid (EPA) and docosahexanoic acid (DHA)).

Human requirements

EPA and DHA can be synthesised in the body (in small amounts) from alpha-linolenic acid (contained in vegetable oils, e.g. soyabean, linseed and rapeseed oils). However, there may, in addition, be a small dietary requirement (more evidence is required).

Intakes

Various recommendations, both in the UK and elsewhere, have been made for the intake of very-long-chain n-3 fatty acids (EPA/DHA) as follows:

UK Department of Heath:[1]	200 mg daily
British Nutrition Foundation:[2]	1250 mg daily
International Society for the Study of Fatty Acids and Lipids:[3]	650 mg daily
The Danish Ministry of Health	300 mg daily
Deutsche Gesellschaft für Ernährung (DGE)	1500 mg daily

Action

Fish oils have several effects. These include:

- Alteration of lipoprotein metabolism. Fish oils reduce both fasting and postprandial plasma triacylglycerols and very-low-density lipoproteins (VLDL). With moderate intakes of fish oils both high-density lipoprotein (HDL) cholesterol and low-density lipoprotein (LDL) cholesterol tend to increase. High intakes reduce HDL cholesterol and may increase LDL cholesterol in some patients. A meta-analysis of published human trials (that each provided 7 g daily of fish oils for at least two weeks) showed that serum cholesterol was unaffected by long-chain n-3 fatty acid consumption. However, triacylglycerols fell by 25–30%, LDL rose by 5–10% and HDL fell by 1–3%.[4]
- Inhibition of atherosclerosis. Fish oils reduce the plasma concentrations of several atherogenic lipoproteins (see above), but other mechanisms may be important. Thus, these effects may be associated with reduced synthesis of cytokines and interleukin 1α and through

stimulation of the endothelial production of nitric oxide.[5]

- Prevention of thrombosis. Thrombosis is a major complication of coronary atherosclerosis, which can lead to myocardial infarction. The n-3 fatty acids have antithrombotic actions through inhibiting the synthesis of thromboxane A_2 from arachidonic acids in platelets.[6] Thromboxane A_2 causes platelet aggregation and vasoconstriction, and as a result fish oil increases bleeding time and reduces the 'stickiness' of the platelets. Fish oil also enhances the production of prostacyclin, which leads to vasodilation and less-sticky platelets. These effects help to reduce the risk of thrombosis.

- Inhibition of inflammation. Diets rich in omega-3 fatty acids appear to reduce the inflammatory response.[7]

- Inhibition of the immune response. Immune reactivity is generally reduced by omega-3 fatty acids.[8,9]

Mechanism of action

Fish oils appear to act by:

- modulation of pro-inflammatory and prothrombotic eicosanoid (prostaglandin, thromboxane and leukotriene) production; and
- reduction in interleukin-1 and other cytokines.

Eicosanoid production

The effects of omega-3 fatty acids are thought to be due to the partial replacement of arachidonic acid with EPA in cell membrane lipids. This leads to increased production of PG3 series prostaglandins, thromboxane A_3 and series 5 leukotrienes at the expense of PG2 series prostaglandins, thromboxane A_2 and series 4 leukotrienes (see Figure 1).

Thromboxane A_3 (produced from EPA) is weaker at stimulating platelet aggregation than thromboxane A_2 (produced from arachidonic acid). Prostaglandins of the PG3 series have less potent inflammatory effects than prostaglandins of the PG2 series. In addition, DHA inhibits the formation of the more inflammatory prostaglandins of the PG2 series, while EPA acts as a substrate for the synthesis of the less inflammatory prostaglandins of the PG3 series.

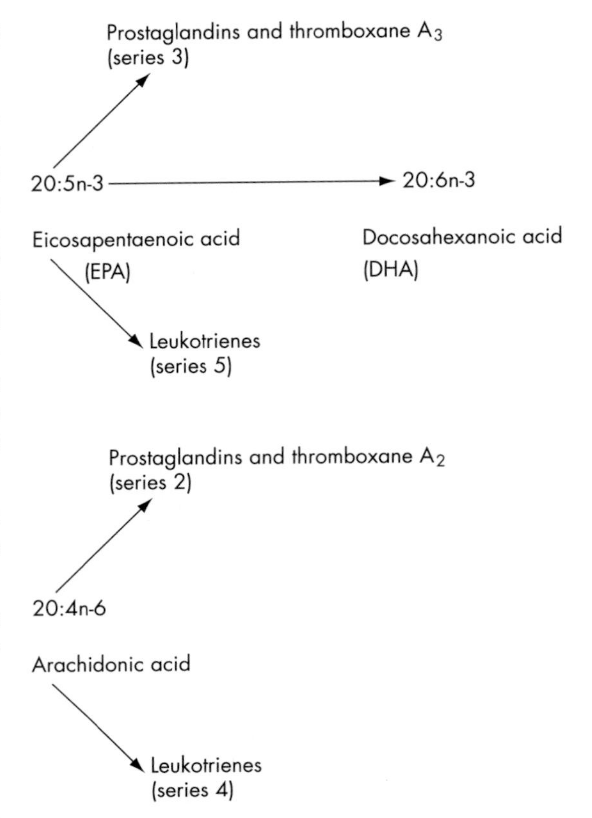

Figure 1 Metabolism of eicosapentaenoic acid and arachidonic acid.

Series 5 leukotrienes (produced by EPA) have weaker inflammatory effects than series 4 leukotrienes (produced by arachidonic acid).

Dietary sources

Oily fish is the best source, but some so-called 'functional foods' including eggs, bread, margarines and milk are fortified with EPA/DHA (Table 1).

Possible uses

Fish liver oils are used as a source of vitamins A and D. Both fish liver oils and fish body oils are used as a source of EPA and DHA.

Table 1 Typical very-long-chain n-3 fatty acid (EPA and DHA) content of fish and fish oils

Food	Average serving (g)	Total EPA/DHA per serving[1] (g)
Cod	120	0.30
Haddock	120	0.19
Plaice	130	0.39
Herring	119	1.56
Kippers	130	3.37
Mackerel	160	3.09
Sardines (canned in tomato sauce)	100	1.67
Pilchards (canned in tomato sauce)	110	2.86
Tuna (canned in brine, drained)	45	0.08
Tuna (canned in oil, drained)	45	0.17
Crab (canned)	85	0.85
Salmon	100	2.2
Salmon (canned in brine, drained)	100	1.55
Trout	230	2.65
Prawns	60	0.06
Mussels	40	0.24
Cod liver oil liquid[2]	10 ml	1.5–3.0
Cod liver oil capsules[2]	Varies	0.1–0.4
Fish oil capsules[2]	Varies	0.1–0.4

[1]Source (except 2): Holland B, Brown J, Buss DH. Fish and fish products; the third supplement to *McCance & Widdowson's The Composition of Food* (5th edition). London: HMSO, 1993.

[2]Source: product labels. Doses and amounts of EPA/DHA vary between products.

In addition, fish oils appear to have a role in the prevention and management of certain conditions such as coronary heart disease (CHD) and stroke, rheumatoid arthritis, inflammatory bowel disease, psoriasis and asthma, mental disorders such as depression, schizophrenia and Alzheimer's disease, nephropathy, various cancers and diabetes mellitus.

Cardiovascular disease

The consumption of fish is associated with lower rates of CHD in many epidemiological studies. Seminal findings in Eskimos have been confirmed and extended to western populations, and in most studies there is an inverse relationship between the intake of fish or n-3 fatty acids and total mortality or cardiovascular mortality.[10–14] However, some studies[15,16] have not shown any benefit, possibly because fish intake was higher in the studied population as a whole.

Intervention studies, in which the intake of fish or fish oil was increased, have also shown beneficial effects. A classic study[17] investigated 2000 Welsh men who had just recovered from their first heart attack. The men were randomised to a 'fish advice group' in which they were asked to eat at least two portions of oily fish a week, or failing this fish oil in capsule form, or a 'no fish advice group'. After two years, there was a 29% reduction in mortality in the fish/fish oil group, which was attributable to a reduction in CHD deaths. However, although there were fewer fatal heart attacks in the fish group, the total number of heart attacks did not decrease.

The GISSI Prevenzione trial[18] investigated the effects of n-3 PUFAs (1 g daily), vitamin E (300 mg daily) or both as supplements in a study involving 11 324 patients surviving recent myocardial infarction. Treatment with n-3 PUFAs, but not vitamin E, reduced total deaths and cardiovascular deaths, and the effect of the combined treatment was similar to that for n-3 PUFAs alone.

In a double-blind, placebo-controlled study in India,[19] 360 patients with suspected myocardial infarction were randomised to receive fish oil (1.09 g daily EPA/DHA), mustard oil (2.9 g daily alpha-linolenic acid) or placebo for one year. Total cardiac events, including cardiac arrhythmias, and also angina pectoris and left ventricular enlargement were significantly reduced in both the fish oil and mustard oil groups compared with placebo. Fish oil, but not mustard oil, was significantly correlated with fewer cardiac deaths than placebo.

Rheumatoid arthritis

Fish oils appear to alleviate the symptoms of rheumatoid arthritis, and this is commensurate with the role of n-3 fatty acids in suppression of the production of inflammatory eicosanoids. Several studies have shown that very-long-chain n-3 fatty acids reduce pain and morning stiffness[20] and decrease the need for non-steroidal anti-inflammatory drugs (NSAIDs).[21,22] Moreover, a meta-analysis of 10 double-blind, placebo-controlled, randomised trials in 395 patients showed that fish oil taken for three months was associated with a statistically significant reduction in joint tenderness and morning stiffness, but no significant improvements in joint swelling, grip strength or erythrocyte sedimentation rate (a marker of inflammation).[23]

Inflammatory bowel disease

Fish oil has been found to have some benefits in patients with Crohn's disease or ulcerative colitis, but no real conclusions can be drawn. A review of five studies[24] investigating the effect of n-3 fatty acids in Crohn's disease was inconclusive, but a later study[25] showed that an enteric coated preparation of very-long-chain n-3 fatty acids significantly reduced the rate of relapse in patients with Crohn's disease in remission.

In patients with ulcerative colitis, fish oil supplements have been found to reduce corticosteroid requirements,[26] improve gastrointestinal histology,[27] and reduce disease activity index.[28]

Psoriasis

Fish oils have been found to be beneficial in some individuals with psoriasis, leading to reduced itching and erythema. However, two double-blind, placebo-controlled studies[29,30] showed that fish oil did not produce any clinical benefit in the treatment of psoriasis.

Asthma

Because asthma is an inflammatory condition, which appears to involve eicosanoids, it is biologically plausible that fish oil could be of benefit. However, results of studies have been discouraging and there is no clear evidence that fish oils are beneficial in asthma.

There is also growing interest in the role of n-3 fatty acids in other conditions affecting respiration, including hay fever, chronic obstructive pulmonary disease (COPD) and cystic fibrosis.

Mental disorders

The potential role of fish oil in mental disorders is now being investigated. A number of studies have found low levels of n-3 fatty acids in cell membranes of patients with depression, schizophrenia and Alzheimer's disease, and it has been suggested that low dietary intakes of n-3 fatty acids or an imbalance in the n-6:n-3 ratio might be associated with these conditions. However, it remains to be seen whether the observed low levels of cell membrane n-3 fatty acids are the cause or the effect of the illnesses.

Nephropathy

Nephropathy is a form of kidney disease that occurs particularly in older men with impaired kidney function and high blood pressure. In a placebo-controlled, multicentre trial, 106 patients were randomised to receive either 12 g of fish oil or placebo daily over a period of two years.[31] The rate of loss of kidney function was retarded in the supplemented group and the beneficial effect was suggested to be due to the impact of n-3 fatty acids on eicosanoid production and other factors. However, other studies have shown no such benefits, and further investigation is needed in this respect.

Cancers

In animal studies, fish oils have been shown to reduce cell proliferation and pre-cancerous cell changes, and some epidemiological studies in humans have suggested that fish oils might be protective against cancer. However, there is no consistent evidence that fish oil decreases cancer risk in humans.

Diabetes

Although fish oil has been linked with deterioration in glucose and insulin control in patients with diabetes mellitus, results of studies with fish oil in diabetic patients have been inconsistent. Treatment with n-3 fatty acids led to a small increase in blood glucose levels in diabetes in one study,[32] but not in another.[33] However, a meta-analysis concluded that fish oil has no adverse effects on glucose or insulin metabolism in patients with diabetes, and lowers triacylglycerols levels effectively by 30%.[34]

Conclusion

Fish oil appears to reduce the risk of CHD. It may help to: reduce the risk of thrombosis by increasing bleeding tendency; reduce blood levels of triacylglycerols; prevent atherosclerosis and arrhythmias; and reduce blood pressure. Fish oil could have beneficial effects in inflammatory conditions such as rheumatoid arthritis, Crohn's disease and ulcerative colitis, but evidence of benefit in asthma and psoriasis is poor. Fish oil may have a role in various mental disorders, such as depression, schizophrenia and Alzheimer's disease, but research in this area is in its infancy.

Precautions/contraindications

Patients with blood clotting disorders or those taking anticoagulants should be monitored while taking fish oils.

Pregnancy and breast-feeding

Use in pregnancy should be supervised (because of the potential for vitamin A toxicity with excessive intakes of fish liver oil).

Adverse effects

Vitamin A and D toxicity (fish liver oil only). The unpleasant taste of fish liver oil liquids may be masked by mixing with fruit juice or milk.

Fish oil supplements are generally safe, and in one prospective study, involving 295 people aged 18 to 76 years,[35] 10–20 ml of fish oil providing 1.8–3.6 g EPA/DHA daily for seven years was not associated with any serious adverse effects. The safety of n-3 fatty acids from fish oil (derived from menhaden oil) was reviewed by the US Food and Drug Administration (FDA) in 1997. After reviewing more than 2600 articles, the FDA concluded that dietary intakes of up to 3 g daily of EPA/DHA from menhaden oil were generally regarded as safe (GRAS).[36] The FDA came to this conclusion after considering three main issues related to the safety of fish oils: first, the risk of deteriorating glycaemic control in type 2 diabetes; second, prolonged bleeding times; third, the risk of increasing LDL cholesterol levels in patients with hypertriglyceridaemia.

Many fish oil supplements (e.g. cod liver oil, halibut liver oil) contain vitamin A and vitamin D – fat-soluble vitamins that can be toxic in excessive amounts. However, the amount of these vitamins contained, for example, in an average multivitamin supplement containing no more than 100% of the RDAs together with the amounts in a recommended dose of, say, ordinary cod liver oil are unlikely to be harmful. However, care should be taken in pregnancy not to take excessive amounts of vitamin A (see Vitamin A monograph), and product labels should be checked.

Other safety concerns expressed in relation to fish oils include the potential to increase bleeding time (a beneficial effect in relation to prevention of CHD) and the possibility of altering glycaemic control in diabetes. However, it is unlikely that any of these effects are a problem, particularly with intakes of less than 3 g EPA/DHA daily. Nevertheless, patients taking anticoagulant medication or those with blood clotting disorders should be monitored while taking fish oils. This does not mean that such patients have to avoid fish oils – just that their doctor should be aware of any intake.

Interactions

Drugs

Anticoagulants: may increase the risk of bleeding; use of fish oils should be medically supervised.
Aspirin: may increase the risk of bleeding; use of fish oils in patients on long-term treatment with aspirin should be medically supervised.
Dipyridamole: may increase the risk of bleeding; use of fish oils should be medically supervised.

Nutrients

Vitamin E: fish oils increase the requirement for vitamin E (absolute additional requirements not established, but 3–4 mg vitamin E per gram of total EPA/DHA appears to be adequate; sufficient amounts of vitamin E are added to most fish oil supplements; there is unlikely to be a need for any extra). In addition, vitamin E may be synergistic in increasing the bleeding tendency with fish oil, although there is no evidence for this.

Supplements

Gingko biloba: gingko biloba may increase the bleeding tendency with fish oils. However, there is no evidence for this.

Ginseng: ginseng may increase the bleeding tendency with fish oils. However, there is no evidence for this.

Dose

Fish oil supplements are available in the form of capsules and liquids.

The dose is not established. Dietary supplements provide 100–1500 mg combined EPA/DHA per dose; clinical trials of fish oil supplements showing beneficial effects have often used 3–4 g daily (combined EPA/DHA), but doses of 1–2 g daily may be adequate.

Note 1: Intake of cod liver oil should not be increased above the doses recommended on the product label to achieve higher intakes of EPA/DHA (risk of vitamin A and D toxicity). Several capsules of cod liver oil could be required to provide the same amount of EPA/DHA as a single dose of cod liver oil liquid. There is no risk of vitamin toxicity with one dose of cod liver oil liquid, but toxicity is likely if several capsules are ingested (the vitamin concentration is usually higher in capsules).

Note 2: fish oil supplements are not identical; they provide different amounts of EPA/DHA.

References

1 Department of Health. *Report on health and social subjects, no 46. Nutritional aspects of cardiovascular disease.* Report of the Cardiovascular Review Group Committee on Medical Aspects of Food Policy. London: HMSO, 1994.

2 British Nutrition Foundation. *Unsaturated Fatty Acids: Nutritional and Physiological Significance.* Task Force Report. London: HMSO, 1992.

3 International Society for the Study of Fatty Acids and Lipids. The full text of its statement can be seen at http://www.issfal.org.uk (accessed 12 December 2000).

4 Harris WS. n-3 fatty acids and serum lipoproteins: Human studies. *Am J Clin Nutr* 1997; 65 (suppl.): 1645S–1654S.

5 Shimokawa H, Vanhoutte PM. Dietary omega-3 fatty acids and endothelium-dependent relaxations in porcine coronary arteries. *Am J Physiol* 1989; 256: H968–H973.

6 Goodnight Jr, SH, Harris WS, Connor WE, Illingworth DR. Polyunsaturated fatty acids, hyperlipidaemia and thrombosis. *Arteriosclerosis* 1982; 2: 87–113.

7 Terano T, Salmon JA, Higg GA, Moncada S. Eicosapentaenoic acid as a modulator of inflammation: Effect on prostaglandin and leukotriene synthesis. *Biochem Pharmacol* 1986; 35: 779–785.

8 Endres S, Ghorbani R, Kelley VE. The effect of dietary supplementation with n-3 polyunsaturated fatty acids on the synthesis of interleukin-1 and tumour necrosis factor by mononuclear cells. *N Engl J Med* 1989; 320: 265–271.

9 Meydani SN, Lichtenstein AH, Colwell S. Immunologic effects of national cholesterol education panel step-2 diets with and without fish-derived n-3 fatty acid enrichment. *J Clin Invest* 1993; 92: 105–113.

10 Dolecek TA. Epidemiological evidence of relationships between dietary polyunsaturated fatty acids and mortality in the multiple risk factor intervention trial. *Proc Soc Exp Biol Med* 1992; 200: 177–182.

11 Ascherio A, Rimm RB, Stampfer MJ, *et al.* Dietary intake of marine n-3 fatty acids, fish intake and the risk of coronary disease among men. *N Engl J Med* 1995; 332: 977–982.

12 Siscovick DS, Raghunathan TE, King I, *et al.* Dietary intake and cell membrane levels of long chain fatty acids and the risk of primary cardiac arrest. *JAMA* 1995; 274: 1363–1367.

13 Daviglus ML, Stamler J, Orencia AJ, *et al.* Fish consumption and the 30-year risk of fatal myocardial infarction. *N Engl J Med* 1997; 336: 1046–1052.

14 Albert CM, Hennekens CH, O'Donnell CJ, *et al.* Fish consumption and risk of sudden cardiac death. *JAMA* 1998; 279: 23–28.

15 Lapidus L, Andersson H, Bengtsson C, Bosaeus I. Dietary habits in relation to incidence of cardiovascular disease and death in women: A 12-year follow-up of participants in the population study of women in Gothenburg, Sweden. *Am J Clin Nutr* 1986; 44: 444–448.

16 Morris MC, Mason JE, Rosner B, *et al.* Fish consumption and cardiovascular disease in the Physicians' Health Study: A prospective study. *Am J Epidemiol* 1995; 142: 166–175.

17 Burr ML, Fehily AM, Gilbert JF, *et al.* Effects of changes in fat, fish and fibre intakes on death and myocardial infarction: Diet and reinfarction trial (DART). *Lancet* 1989; 2: 757–761.

18 Dietary supplementation with n-3 polyunsaturated

fatty acids and vitamin E after myocardial infarction: Results of the GISSI-Prevenzione trial. Gruppo Italiano per lo Studio della Sopravvivenza nell'Infarto Miocardico. *Lancet* 1999; 354: 447–455.
19 Singh RB, Niaz MA, Sharma JP, *et al.* Randomized, double-blind, placebo-controlled trial of fish oil and mustard oil in patients with suspected acute myocardial infarction: The Indian experiment of infarct survival – 4. *Cardiovasc Drugs Ther* 1997; 11: 485–491.
20 Kremer JM. Effects of modulation of inflammatory and immune parameters in patients with rheumatic and inflammatory disease receiving dietary supplements of n-3 and n-6 fatty acids. *Lipids* 1996; 31: S243–S247.
21 Lau CS, Morely KD, Belch JJ. Effects of fish oil supplementation on non-steroidal anti-inflammatory drug requirements in patients with mild rheumatoid arthritis – a double blind placebo-controlled study. *Br J Rheumatol* 1993; 32: 982–989.
22 Geusens P, Wouters C, Nijs J, *et al.* Long term effect of omega-3 fatty acid supplementation in active rheumatoid arthritis. *Arthritis Rheum* 1994; 37: 824–829.
23 Fortin PR, Lew RA, Liang MH, *et al.* Validation of a meta-analysis: The effects of fish oil on rheumatoid arthritis. *J Clin Epidemiol* 1995; 48: 1379–1390.
24 Young-In K. Can fish oil maintain Crohn's disease in remission? *Nutr Rev* 1996; 54: 248–257.
25 Belluzzi A, Brignola C, Campieri M, *et al.* Effect of enteric-coated fish oil preparation on relapses in Crohn's disease. *N Engl J Med* 1996; 334: 1557–1560.
26 Hawthorne AB, Daneshmend TK, Hawkey CJ, *et al.* Treatment of ulcerative colitis with fish oil supplementation: A prospective 12-month randomized controlled trial. *Gut* 1992; 33: 922–928.
27 Stenson WF, Cort D, Rodgers J, *et al.* Dietary supplementation with fish oil in ulcerative colitis. *Ann Intern Med* 1992; 116: 609–614.
28 Aslan A, Triadafilopoulos G. Fish oil fatty acid supplementation in active ulcerative colitis: A double-blind, placebo-controlled, crossover study. *Am J Gastroenterol* 1992; 87: 432–437.
29 Veale DJ, Torley HI, Richards IM, *et al.* A double-blind placebo controlled trial of Efamol Marine on skin and joint symptoms of psoriatic arthritis. *Br J Rheumatol* 1994; 33: 954–958.
30 Soyland E, Funk J, Rajka G, *et al.* Effect of dietary supplementation with very long chain fatty acids in patients with psoriasis. *N Engl J Med* 1993; 328: 1812–1816.
31 Donadio JV, Bergstralh EJ, Offord KP, *et al.* A controlled trial of fish oil in IgA nephropathy. Mayo Nephrology Collaborative Group. *N Engl J Med* 1994; 331: 1194–1199.
32 Vessby B, Karlstrom B, Boberg M, *et al.* Polyunsaturated fatty acids may impair blood glucose control in type 2 diabetic patients. *Diabetic Med* 1992; 9: 126–133.
33 Toft I, Bonaa KH, Ingebretsen OC, *et al.* Effects of n-3 polyunsaturated fatty acids on glucose homeostasis and blood pressure in essential hypertension: A randomized, controlled trial. *Ann Intern Med* 1995; 123: 911–918.
34 Friedberg CE, Janssen MJ, Heine RJ, Grobbee DE. Fish oil and glycaemic control in diabetes. *Diabetes Care* 1998; 21: 494–500.
35 Saynor R, Gillott T. Changes in blood lipids and fibrinogen with a note on safety in a long term study on the effects of n-3 fatty acids in subjects receiving fish oil supplements and followed for seven years. *Lipids* 1992; 27: 533–538.
36 Food and Drug Administration Final Rule. Substances affirmed as generally recognized as safe: Menhaden oil. *Fed Reg* 1997; 62: 30750–30757.

Flavonoids

Description and nomenclature

Flavonoids (or bioflavonoids) are a large group of polyphenolic compounds, which are ubiquitously present in foods of plant origin. Some flavonoids (e.g. quercetin, rutin) are available as dietary supplements.

Constituents

Bioflavonoids are a group of polyphenolic antioxidants, which often occur as glycosides. Flavonoids can be further subdivided into five main groups: flavones (apigenin and luteolin), flavonols (e.g. kaempferol, quercetin and myricetin), proanthocyanidins (abundant in grape seed extract – see Grape seed extract monograph), anthocyanins (the red pigments in e.g. red wine, blackberries, raspberries, elderberries, redcurrants), and C-glycosylflavones. Other flavonoid groups include aurones, biflavonyls, chalcones, dihydrochalcones, flavanones, dihydroflavonols, flavans and isoflavones. (Isoflavones are detailed in a separate monograph.)

More than 4000 flavonoids have been identified and, though many have been studied in the laboratory and in animals, few (apart from quercetin) have been studied in humans. Most flavonoids are colourless, but some are responsible for the bright colours of many fruit and vegetables. Flavonoids are distinguished from the carotenoids (see Carotenoids monograph), which are the red, yellow and orange pigments found in fruit and vegetables. Unlike carotenoids, flavonoids are water-soluble.

Action

Flavonoids appear to display several effects.[1] They:

- act as scavengers of free radicals, including superoxide anions, singlet oxygen, and lipid peroxyl radicals (they have antioxidant properties);
- sequester metal ions;
- inhibit *in vitro* oxidation of low-density lipoproteins (LDL);
- inhibit cyclo-oxygenase, leading to lower platelet aggregation, decreased thrombotic tendency and reduced anti-inflammatory activity;
- inhibit histamine release;
- improve capillary function by reducing fragility of capillary walls and thus preventing abnormal leakage; and
- inhibit various stages of tumour development (animal studies only).

The activities of flavonoids are dependent on their chemical structure.

Human requirements

No proof of any dietary need exists.

Intakes

Estimates of dietary flavonoid intake vary from 10 to 100 mg daily, depending on the population studied, the technique used, and the number and identity of flavonoids measured. If all flavonoids are included, intake may be several hundreds of milligrams a day, particularly if red wine is consumed in large amounts.

Dietary sources

Flavonoids are found in the white segment or ring of fruit (especially citrus fruit) and vegetables, and also in tea and red wine. In the UK, tea, apples and onions seem to be major sources. Flavonoid content of foods varies widely. Cherry tomatoes contain higher concentrations than normal-sized tomatoes, and Lollo Rosso lettuce more than iceberg lettuce.[1] The flavonoid content of red wine may also vary widely, depending on the source, growing conditions and harvesting of the grapes.[2]

Possible uses

Flavonoids have been investigated for a potential role in cardiovascular disease, cancer and cataracts.

Cardiovascular disease

Epidemiological studies have suggested that consumption of fruit and vegetables may protect against cardiovascular disease. That such a benefit could occur as a result of dietary antioxidants is well known, but the presence of flavonoids in these foods may also account for these findings.

Flavonoids may help to reduce the risk of heart disease (possibly by helping to dilate the coronary arteries and by preventing atherosclerosis). The Zutphen study from the Netherlands[3] demonstrated a reduced risk of coronary heart disease (CHD) and a reduced incidence of myocardial infarction in men aged 65–84 years associated with increased ingestion of dietary flavonoids. The major dietary sources of flavonoids in this study were tea (61%), onions (13%) and apples (10%). Flavonoid intake was inversely associated with CHD mortality, with a 68% reduction in risk for intake >19 mg daily. There was, however, no correlation between flavonoid intake and CHD incidence among those with no history of myocardial infarction. The researchers later updated their results,[4] extending follow-up to 10 years. Similar results for CHD mortality were found, but a smaller risk reduction and a borderline significant trend ($P = 0.08$) for the incidence of CHD existed.

Another part of the Zutphen study[5] investigated a cohort of men aged 50–69 years, following them up for 15 years. Dietary flavonoids (mainly quercetin) were inversely associated with stroke incidence after adjustment for potential confounders, including antioxidant vitamins. The relative risk of stroke for the highest versus the lowest quartile of flavonoid intake was 0.27. A lower stroke risk was also observed for the highest quartile of betacarotene intake, but vitamin C and E were not associated with stroke risk. Black tea contributed about 70% to flavonoid intake. The relative risk for daily consumption of 4.7 cups more of tea versus less than 2.6 cups of tea was 0.31 (95% CI, 0.12–0.84).

However, the Caerphilly study in Wales showed no reduced risk of heart disease with increasing flavonoid consumption.[6] This investigation involved 1900 men aged 45–59 years who were studied for up to 14 years. Tea provided 82% of the flavonoid intake, and was strongly and positively associated with the risk of CHD.

Baseline flavonoid intake was estimated in 16 cohorts of the Seven Countries Study,[7] and mortality from CHD, cancer and all causes was investigated after 25 years of follow-up. Average intake of flavonoids was inversely associated with mortality from CHD and explained about 25% of the variance in CHD rates in the 16 cohorts. Flavonoid intake was not independently associated with mortality from other causes, including cancer.

Two studies used data from American cohorts of men and women. The relationship between flavonoid intake and CHD risk was investigated in 34 789 men aged 40–75 years in 1986 with a follow-up of six years.[8] The main sources of flavonoids were tea and onions. Flavonoid intake >40 mg daily was not associated with reduced CHD risk. The Iowa Womens' Health Study[9] investigated 34 492 postmenopausal women aged 55–69 years for subsequent risk of CHD over a 10-year follow-up period. Compared to women in the lowest quintile (<5.8 mg daily) of flavonoid intake, those in the highest quintile (18.7 mg daily) had a significant 32% reduced risk of CHD death.

The association of tea intake with aortic atherosclerosis has also been investigated in a

Dutch study.[10] In a prospective study of 3454 men and women aged 55 years and older, who were free of cardiovascular disease at baseline, tea intake was inversely correlated with severe (but not mild or moderate) aortic atherosclerosis.

Cancer

Activity of flavonoids against malignant cells has been demonstrated *in vitro*,[11–13] and there is much current interest in the potential use of flavonoids in the prevention and treatment of cancer.

In a Finnish study involving 9959 men and women (initially cancer free) aged from 15 to 99 years, high dietary flavonoid intake was shown to reduce the risk of cancer.[14] Researchers involved in the Iowa Women's Health Study showed that of 35 000 post-menopausal women, those who drank more than two cups of tea a day were 32% less likely to have cancers of the mouth, oesophagus, stomach, colon and rectum. Risk of urinary tract cancer was reduced by 60%. In those who drank more than four cups of tea a day, the risk of cancer was lowered by 63%.[15] Onions contain large amounts of flavonoids, which might explain the reduced risk of stomach cancer among those with a high intake of onions in a study involving a group of 120 852 men and women aged 55 to 69 years.[16]

Cataract

There may be a role for flavonoids in preventing diabetes-related cataract formation. In diabetes mellitus, excess sorbitol or dulcitol is produced by the conversion of glucose by aldose reductase. The dulcitol cannot be further metabolised and therefore forms a hard crystalline layer in the lens, which forms the cataract. Flavonoids are potent inhibitors of the enzyme,[17] but further studies are required before they could be recommended for cataract prevention.

Miscellaneous

Experimental studies have demonstrated that some flavonoids prevent ulcer formation,[18] and that they may be useful in treating ulcers.

Flavonoids have been investigated for potential anti-viral activity. *In vitro* tests have shown some activity against rhinovirus (responsible for 50% of common colds), but little activity against herpes simplex and influenza virus.[19]

Many claims have been made for the usefulness of flavonoids in a range of disorders, including haemorrhoids, allergy, asthma, menopausal symptoms and the prevention of habitual abortion, but scientific studies are required to investigate these claims.

Quercetin

As a dietary supplement, quercetin is promoted for prevention and treatment of atherosclerosis and hyperlipidaemia, diabetes, cataracts, hayfever, peptic ulcer, inflammation, prevention of cancer and for treating prostatitis. A preliminary, double-blind, placebo-controlled trial in chronic non-bacterial prostatitis showed that quercetin reduced pain and improved quality of life, but had no effect on voiding dysfunction.[20] However, there is insufficient reliable information about the effectiveness of quercetin for other indications.

Rutin

As a dietary supplement, rutin is used for reducing capillary permeability and treating symptoms of varicose veins. In combination with bromelain and trypsin, rutin is used for the treatment of osteoarthritis. In one double-blind trial, 73 patients with osteoarthritis of the knee were randomly assigned to a combination enzyme product (containing rutin, bromelain, trypsin) or diclofenac. The enzyme product had a similar effect on reducing pain and mobility of the knee to diclofenac.[21] However, there is insufficient reliable information about the effectiveness of rutin for other indications.

Conclusion

High dietary intakes of flavonoids have been linked with a reduced risk of CHD, cancer and cataracts. However, although a number of supplements (e.g. quercetin, rutin) are now available, there is currently only limited evidence that these supplements are beneficial in any condition.

Pregnancy and breast-feeding

No problems have been reported.

Adverse effects

None reported. However, there are no long-term studies assessing the safety of flavonoid supplements.

Interactions

None reported.

Dose

Flavonoids (e.g. quercetin, rutin) are available in the form of tablets and capsules.

The dose is not established; dietary supplements of quercetin and rutin provide around 500 mg in a single dose.

References

1 Crozier A, McDonald MS, Lean MEJ, Black C. Quantitative analysis of the flavonoid content of tomatoes, onions, lettuce and celery. *J Agric Food Chem* 1997; 45: 590–595.

2 McDonald MS, Hughes M, Burns J, *et al.* A survey of the free and conjugated flavonol content of sixty five red wines of different geographical origin. *J Agric Food Chem* 1998; 46: 368–375.

3 Hertog MGL, Feskens EJM, Hollman PCH, *et al.* Dietary antioxidant flavonoids and risk of coronary heart disease: The Zutphen elderly study. *Lancet* 1993; 342: 1007–1011.

4 Hertog MG, Feskens EJ, Hollman PC, *et al.* Antioxidant flavonols and coronary heart disease risk [letter]. *Lancet* 1997; 349: 699.

5 Keli SO, Hertog MG, Feskens EJ. Dietary flavonoids, antioxidant vitamins and the incidence of stroke; the Zutphen study. *Arch Intern Med* 1996; 156: 637–642.

6 Hertog MG, Sweetman PM, Fehily AM, *et al.* Antioxidant flavonols and ischaemic heart disease in a Welsh population of men: The Caerphilly Study. *Am J Clin Nutr* 1997; 65: 1489–1494.

7 Hertog MG, Kromhout D, Aravanis C, *et al.* Flavonoid intake and long-term risk of coronary heart disease and cancer in the seven countries study. *Arch Intern Med* 1995; 155: 381–386.

8 Rimm EB, Katam MB, Ascherio A, *et al.* Relation between intakes of flavonoids and risk for coronary heart disease in male health professionals. *Ann Intern Med* 1996; 125: 384–389.

9 Yochum L, Kushi LH, Meyer K, Folsom AR. Dietary flavonoid intake and risk of cardiovascular disease in postmenopausal women. *Am J Epidemiol* 1999; 149: 943–949.

10 Geleijinse JM, Launer LJ, Hofman A, *et al.* Tea flavonoids may protect against atherosclerosis. *Arch Intern Med* 1999; 159: 2170–2174.

11 Havsteen B. Flavonoids. A class of natural products of high pharmacological potency. *Biochem Pharmacol* 1983; 32: 1141.

12 Tripathi VD, Rastogi RP. Flavonoids in biology and medicine. *J Sci Ind Res* 1981; 40: 116.

13 Kandaswami C, Perkins E, Soloniuk DS, *et al.* Antiproliferative effects of citrus flavonoids on a human squamous cell carcinoma in vitro. *Cancer Lett* 1991; 56: 147–152.

14 Knekt P, Jarvinen R, Seppanen R, *et al.* Dietary flavonoids and the risk of lung cancer and other malignant neoplasms. *Am J Epidemiol* 1997; 146: 223–230.

15 Zheng W, Doyle TJ, Kushi LH. Tea consumption and cancer incidence in a prospective cohort study of postmenopausal women. *Am J Epidemiol* 1996; 144: 175–182.

16 Dorant E, van den Brandt PA, Goldbohm RA. Consumption of onions and a reduced risk of stomach carcinoma. *Gastroenterology* 1996; 110: 12–20.

17 Wagner H. Phenolic compounds of pharmaceutical interest. In: *Recent Advances in Phytochemistry, Vol. 12, Biochemistry of Plant Phenolics*, 1977: 589.

18 Farkas L, Gabor M, Kallay F, Wagner H. Flavonoids and bioflavonoids. Proceedings, International Bioflavonoid Symposium, Munich. Amsterdam: Elsevier, 1977.

19 Tshuiya Y, Shimuzu M, Hiyama Y, *et al.* Antiviral activity of naturally occurring flavonoids in vitro. *Chem Pharm Bull* 1985; 33: 3881.

20 Shoskes DA, Zeitlin SI, Shahed A, Rajfer A. Quercetin in men with category III chronic prostatitis: A preliminary prospective, double-blind, placebo-controlled trial. *Urology* 1999; 54: 960–963.

21 Klein G, Kullich W. Short-term treatment of painful osteoarthritis of the knee with oral enzymes. *Clin Drug Invest* 2000; 19: 15–23.

Flaxseed oil

Description

Flaxseed is the soluble fibre mucilage obtained from the fully developed seed of *Linus usitatissimum*.

Constituents

Flaxseed is a rich source of alpha-linolenic acid and lignans. Alpha-linolenic acid is an essential fatty acid of the n-3 (omega-3) series, which must be supplied by the diet. It can be converted into longer chain fatty acids of the n-3 series, such as eicosapentaenoic acid (EPA) and docosahexanoic acid (DHA), the fatty acids found in fish oils (see Fish oils monograph).

Action

Fatty acids of the n-3 series (like those of the n-6 series) are precursors to a range of prostaglandins, thromboxanes and leukotrienes, and those formed from the n-3 series are generally less pro-inflammatory and atherogenic than those formed from the n-6 series. In addition, there is competition between the fatty acids of both series for the enzyme systems which effect chain elongation, suggesting that a balance between the two types of fatty acids is important; it is estimated that an optimal ratio between n-3 and n-6 fatty acid is 1:4. However, changes in food production and advice to consume polyunsaturated fats has led to an increase in the n-6 fatty acids at the expense of the n-3 fats, and the ratio of n-3 to n-6 fats is between 1:10 to 1:30. Flaxseed oil, which contains approximately three times more n-3 than n-6 fatty acids, may help to reverse the imbalance between n-3 and n-6 fats.

Lignans are a type of phyto-oestrogen. They are digested in the colon to produce enterodiol and enterolactone – lignans which are thought to be protective against cancer.

Possible uses

Traditionally, flaxseed has been used for constipation and other bowel disorders such as diverticulitis and irritable bowel syndrome (IBS). In theory, it may also be useful as a source of n-3 fatty acids for the same conditions (e.g. cardiovascular disease and other inflammatory disorders) where fish oil has benefit.

Cardiovascular disease

In a small trial, 11 healthy male subjects were randomly assigned to receive 40 g flaxseed oil or sunflower seed oil for 23 days.[1] A statistically significant reduction in platelet aggregation response to collagen was found in subjects supplemented with flaxseed but not with sunflower seed. The authors noted that the higher percentage of energy from fat in the sunflower oil might have skewed the results. In spite of this limitation, the conclusion was that oils rich in alpha-linolenic acid may offer increased protection in cardiovascular disease (via reduction in platelet aggregation) in comparison with oils rich in linoleic acid.

In a randomised, double-blind study, 32 healthy subjects received either 35 mg flaxseed oil or 35 mg fish oil for three months.[2] In contrast to fish oil, flaxseed had no effect on serum triglyceride or cholesterol levels, but the authors concluded that the dose may have been insufficient, or that conversion of alpha-linolenic acid to EPA was inadequate.

In a double-blind, cross-over study, 29

subjects with hyperlipidaemia were given in random order muffins containing either 50 g partially defatted flaxseed or wheat bran (control) each day for three weeks. Flaxseed significantly reduced total serum cholesterol by 4.6% and low-density lipoprotein (LDL) cholesterol by 7.6%, but there were no effects on high-density lipoprotein (HDL) cholesterol.[3]

In a double-blind, placebo-controlled study, 11 patients with well-controlled type 2 diabetes were given flaxseed oil or fish oil capsules for three months each in random order. Fish oil, but not flaxseed oil reduced serum triglycerides, but there were no significant differences between the two oils in relation to total, LDL and HDL cholesterol levels.[4]

Cancer

There is some evidence from animal studies that flaxseed inhibits tumour growth, particularly mammary tumours,[5,6] but clinical trials are needed to assess whether flaxseed has anti-cancer properties in humans.

Autoimmune disorders

In a double-blind, placebo-controlled study involving 22 patients with rheumatoid arthritis, 30 g flaxseed powder daily for three months had no effect on clinical subjective parameters of the disorder compared with sunflower oil.[7]

A small study in eight patients with systemic lupus erythematosus (SLE), present as lupus nephritis, found that flaxseed in a dose of 30 g daily improved renal function and inflammatory mediators, and was well tolerated.[8]

Conclusion

Theoretically, flaxseed as a source of n-3 fatty acids could benefit the same conditions as those indicated for fish oil. However, research data are currently insufficient to make recommendations for supplements for reduction in risk of heart disease and cancer or management of rheumatoid arthritis and other inflammatory conditions.

Precautions/contraindications

No problems have been reported.

Pregnancy and breast-feeding

No problems have been reported, but there have not been sufficient studies to guarantee the safety of flaxseed in pregnancy and breast-feeding.

Adverse effects

There are no known toxicity or serious side-effects, but no long-term studies have assessed the safety of flaxseed. Flaxseed contains cyanogenic glycosides, which are naturally occurring toxicants. The long-term effects of these compounds are unknown, but high doses could increase plasma thiocyanate levels.

Interactions

None reported.

Dose

Flaxseed oil is available in the form of a liquid.

The dose is not established. Manufacturers suggest one tablespoon of flaxseed oil daily.

References

1 Allman MA, Pena NM, Pang D. Supplementation with flaxseed oil versus sunflower oil in healthy young men consuming a low fat diet: Effects on platelet composition and function. *Eur J Clin Nutr* 1995; 49:169–178.
2 Layne KS, Goh YK, Jumpsen JA, *et al.* Normal subjects consuming physiological levels of 18:3(n-3) and 20:5(n-3) from flaxseed or fish oils have characteristic differences in plasma lipid and lipoprotein fatty acid levels. *J Nutr* 1996; 126: 2130–2140.
3 Jenkins DJA, Kendall CWC, Vidgen E, *et al.* Health aspects of partially defatted flaxseed, including effects on serum lipids, oxidative measures, and ex vivo androgen and progestin activity: A controlled crossover trial. *Am J Clin Nutr* 1999; 69: 395–402.
4 McManus RM, Jumpson J, Finegood DT. A comparison of the effects of n-3 fatty acids from linseed oil and fish oil in well-controlled type II diabetes. *Diabetes Care* 1996; 19: 463–467.

5 Serraino M, Thompson LU. The effect of flaxseed supplementation on the initiation and promotional stages of mammary tumorigenesis. *Nutr Cancer* 1992; 17: 153–159.
6 Thompson LU, Rickard SE, Orcheson LJ, *et al.* Flaxseed and its lignan and oil components reduce mammary tumour growth at a late stage of carcinogenesis. *Carcinogenesis* 1996; 17: 1373–1376.
7 Nordstrom DC, Honkanen VE, Nasu Y, *et al.* Alpha-linolenic acid in the treatment of rheumatoid arthritis: A double-blind placebo controlled and randomized study; flaxseed versus safflower seed. *Rheumatol Int* 1995; 14: 231–234.
8 Clark WF, Parbtani A, Huff MW, *et al.* Flaxseed: A potential treatment for lupus nephritis. *Kidney Int* 1995; 48: 475–480.

Fluoride

Description

Fluoride is a trace element.

Human requirements

There does not appear to be a physiological requirement for fluoride and, in the UK, no Reference Nutrient Intake has been set, but a safe and adequate intake, for infants only, is 0.05 mg/kg daily.

Action

Fluoride has a marked affinity for hard tissues, and forms calcium fluorapatite in teeth and bone. It protects against dental caries and may have a role in bone mineralisation. It helps remineralisation of bone in pathological conditions of demineralisation.

Dietary sources

Foods high in fluoride include seafoods and tea. Cereals and milk are poorer sources. An important source of fluoride is fluoridated drinking water. In the UK, tea provides 70% of the total intake; if the water is fluoridated, consumption of large volumes of tea can result in fluoride intakes of 4–12 mg daily.

Metabolism

Absorption

Oral fluoride is rapidly absorbed by passive transport from the gastrointestinal tract; some is absorbed from the stomach, and some from the small intestine.

Distribution

Fluoride is found principally in bones and teeth.

Elimination

Elimination is mainly via the urine, with small amounts lost in sweat (especially in warm climates) and bile.

Deficiency

No essential function has been clearly established; low levels of fluoride in drinking water are associated with dental caries, while high levels (provided they are not too high) prevent caries.

Possible uses

Dental caries

Fluoride is recommended for the prophylaxis of dental caries in infants and children (see Dose, below).

Osteoporosis

Evidence for a role of fluoride in osteoporosis and prevention of fracture is conflicting. In one study[1] there was a higher incidence of fractures in an area of Italy with a lower concentration of fluoride in the water than another area. In another study[2] women with continuous exposure to fluoridated water for 20 years were compared with those with no exposure. In those with exposure, bone mineral density was 2.6% higher at the femoral neck, 2.5% higher at the lumbar spine and 1.9% lower at the distal radius. In addition, the risk of hip fracture was slightly reduced, as was the risk of vertebral

Table 1 Daily doses[1] of fluoride (expressed as fluoride ion) in infants and children

Fluoride content of water (μg)	Under 6 months	6 months–3 years	3–6 years	Over 6 years
<300	None	250 μg	500 μg	1 mg
300–700	None	None	250 μg	500 μg
>700	None	None	None	None

[1]Recommended by the British Dental Association, the British Society of Paediatric Dentistry and the British Association for the Study of Community Dentistry (*Br Dent J* 1997; 182: 6–7).

fracture. However, there was no difference in the risk of humerus fracture and a non-significant trend towards an increased risk of wrist fracture.

In an intervention study[3], sodium fluoride (75 mg daily) was no more effective than placebo in retarding the progression of spinal osteoporosis. Another study in 202 post-menopausal women[4] with vertebral fractures showed that sodium fluoride 75 mg daily was not an effective treatment. Yet another intervention study[5] showed that fluoride (as sodium fluoride 50 mg daily or monofluorophosphate 200 mg daily or 150 mg daily) was no more effective than calcium and vitamin D in preventing new vertebral fractures in women with postmenopausal osteoporosis. A trial comparing etidronate with fluoride[6] in the treatment of postmenopausal osteoporosis showed that, although fluoride was more effective at increasing lumbar bone mass, there were no differences in fracture incidence.

Precautions/contraindications

The British Association for Community Dentistry advises that fluoride is unnecessary for infants aged under six months and that fluoride should not be given in areas where the drinking water contains fluoride levels which exceed 700 μg/l.

Adverse effects

Chalky white patches on the surface of the teeth (may occur with recommended doses); yellow-brown staining of teeth, stiffness and aching of bones (with chronic excessive intake). Symptoms of acute overdose include diarrhoea, nausea, gastrointestinal cramp, bloody vomit, black stools, drowsiness, weakness, faintness, shallow breathing, tremors and increased watering of mouth and eyes.

Dose

Systemic fluoride supplements should not be prescribed without reference to the fluoride content of the local water supply (information available from the local Water Board). See Table 1 for daily fluoride doses in infants and children.

References

1 Fabiani L, Leoni V, Vitali M. Bone-fracture incidence rate in two Italian regions with different fluoride concentration levels in drinking water. *J Trace Elem Med Biol* 1999; 13: 232–237.
2 Phipps KR, Orwoll ES, Mason JD, Cauley JA. Community water fluoridation, bone mineral density, and fractures: Prospective study of effects in older women. *Br Med J* 2000; 321: 860–864.
3 Kleerekoper M, Peterson EL, Nelson DA, *et al.* A randomized trial of sodium fluoride as a treatment for osteoporosis. *Osteoporosis Int* 1991; 1: 155–161.
4 Riggs BL, Hodgson SF, O'Fallon M, *et al.* Effect of fluoride treatment on the fracture rate in postmenopausal women with osteoporosis. *N Engl J Med* 1990; 322: 802–809.
5 Meunier PJ, Sebert JL, Reginster JY, *et al.* Fluoride

salts are no better at preventing new vertebral fractures than calcium-vitamin D in postmenopausal osteoporosis; the FAVO study. *Osteoporosis Int* 1998; 8: 4–12.

6 Guanabens N, Farrerons J, Perez-Edo L, *et al*. Cyclical etidronate versus sodium fluoride in established postmenopausal osteoporosis: A randomized 3 year trial. *Bone* 2000; 27: 123–128.

Folic acid

Description

Folic acid is a water-soluble vitamin of the vitamin B complex.

Nomenclature

Folic acid (pteroylglutamic acid) is the parent compound for a large number of derivatives collectively known as folates. Folate is the generic term used to describe the compounds that exhibit the biological activity of folic acid; it is the preferred term for the vitamin present in foods which represents a mixture of related compounds (folates).

Human requirements

See Table 1 for Dietary Reference Values for folic acid.

Table 1 Dietary Reference Values for folic acid (μg/day)

EU RDA = 200 μg

Age	UK			USA	WHO	Europe PRI
	LRNI	EAR	RNI	RDA		
0–3 months	30	40	50	65	16	50
4–6 months	30	40	50	65	24	50
7–12 months	30	40	50	80	32	50
1–3 years	35	50	70	150	32	50
4–6 years	50	75	100	200	50	130
7–10 years	75	110	150	200	102	150
Males						
11–14 years	100	150	200	300	170	180
15–50+ years	100	150	200	400	200	200
Females						
11–14 years	100	150	200	300	170	180
15–50+ years	100	150	200	400	170	200
Pregnancy	–	–	+100	600	370–400	400
Lactation	–	–	+60	500	270	350

Note: The Department of Health recommends that all women who are pregnant or planning a pregnancy should take a folic acid supplement (see Dose).
US Tolerable Upper Intake Level = 1 mg for adults aged >19 years.

Intakes

In the UK, the average adult daily diet provides: for men, 322 μg; for women, 224 μg.

Action

Folates are involved in a number of single carbon transfer reactions, especially in the synthesis of purines and pyrimidines (and hence the synthesis of DNA), glycine and methionine. They are also involved in some amino acid conversions and the formation and utilisation of formate. Deficiency leads to impaired cell division (effects most noticeable in rapidly regenerating tissues).

Dietary sources

See Table 2 for dietary sources of folic acid.

Table 2 Dietary sources of folic acid

Food portion	Folate content (μg)
Breakfast cereals	
1 bowl All–Bran (45 g)	*80*
1 bowl Bran Flakes (45 g)	**110**
1 bowl Corn Flakes (30 g)	*70*
1 bowl Muesli (95 g)	**130**
1 bowl Start (40 g)	**140**
Cereal products	
Bread, brown, 2 slices	*30*
white, 2 slices	25
wholemeal, 2 slices	*30*
fortified, 2 slices	**70**
1 chapati	10
Milk and dairy products	
½ pint (280 ml) milk, whole, semi–skimmed, or skimmed	15
½ pint (280 ml) soya milk	*50*
1 pot yoghurt (150 g)	25
Cheese, average (50 g)	15
Camembert (50 g)	*50*
Meat	
Liver, lambs, cooked (90 g)	**220**
Kidney, lambs, cooked (75 g)	*60*
Vegetables	
Broccoli, boiled (100 g)	*65*
Brussels sprouts, boiled (100 g)	**110**
Cabbage, boiled (100 g)	*30*
Cauliflower, boiled (100 g)	*50*
Kale, boiled (100 g)	*90*
Lettuce (30 g)	20
Peas, boiled (100 g)	*50*
Potatoes, boiled (150 g)	**145**
Spinach, boiled (100 g)	**100**
1 small can baked beans (200 g)	*45*
Chickpeas, cooked (105 g)	**110**
Red kidney beans (105 g)	*90*
Fruit	
1 orange	*45*
1 large glass orange juice	*40*
Half a grapefruit	20
Yeast	
Brewer's yeast (10 g)	**400**
Marmite, spread on 1 slice bread	*50*

Excellent sources (**bold**); good sources (*italics*).

Metabolism

Absorption

Absorption of folate takes place mainly in the jejunum.

Distribution

Folate is stored mainly in the liver. Enterohepatic recycling is important for maintaining serum levels.

Elimination

Excretion of folate is largely renal, but folates may also be eliminated in the faeces (mainly as a result of folate synthesis by the gut microflora). Folates are also found in breast milk.

Bioavailability

Folates leach into cooking water and are destroyed by cooking or food processing at high temperatures.

Deficiency

Folate deficiency results in reduction of DNA synthesis and hence in reduction of cell division. While DNA synthesis occurs in all dividing cells, deficiency is most easily seen in tissues with high rates of cell turnover such as erythrocytes (red blood cells). The main clinical observation associated with folate deficiency is, therefore, megaloblastic anaemia.

The main causes of folate deficiency are as follows:

- Decreased dietary intake. This occurs in people eating inadequate diets, such as some elderly people, those on low incomes, and alcoholics who substitute alcoholic drinks for good sources of nutrition.
- Decreased intestinal absorption. Patients with disorders of malabsorption (e.g. coeliac disease) may suffer folate deficiency.
- Increased requirements. Increased requirement for folate, and hence an increased risk of deficiency, can occur in pregnancy, during lactation, in haemolytic anaemia and leukaemia.
- Alcoholism. Chronic alcoholism is a common cause of folate deficiency. This may occur as a result of poor dietary intake, reduced absorption or increased excretion by the kidney. The presence of alcoholic liver disease increases the likelihood of folate deficiency.
- Drugs. Long-term use of certain drugs (e.g. phenytoin, sulfasalazine) is associated with folate deficiency.

Signs and symptoms include megaloblastic, macrocytic anaemia; weakness, tiredness, irritability, forgetfulness, dyspnoea, anorexia, diarrhoea, weight loss, headache, syncope, palpitations and glossitis. In babies and young children, growth may be affected.

Possible uses

Pregnancy and pre-pregnancy

The risk of neural tube defects (NTDs) can be reduced by increased folic acid intake during the periconceptual period.[1–5] Such studies have given rise to recommendations in several countries that women intending to become pregnant should consume additional folic acid. The reason for the beneficial effect of folic acid is unclear. Although it may be a result of deficiency, a genetic defect in the methylene tetrahydrofolate reductase (MTHFR) gene, estimated to occur in about 5 to 15% of white populations, appears to result in an increased requirement for folates and an increased risk of recurrent early pregnancy loss and NTDs.[6,7] In addition, elevated levels of plasma homocysteine have been observed in mothers producing offspring with NTDs,[8] and the possibility that this factor could have toxic effects on the fetus at the time of neural tube closure is currently under further investigation.

Cardiovascular disease

Marginal folate status is also associated with elevated plasma homocysteine levels, an emerging risk factor for cardiovascular disease mortality.[9–11] Mechanisms by which plasma homocysteine may be associated with increased risk of cardiovascular disease have not been clearly established, but possibilities include:[12]

- oxidative damage to the vascular endothelium;
- inhibition of endothelial anticoagulant factors, resulting in increased clot formation;
- increased platelet aggregation; and
- proliferation of smooth muscle cells, resulting in increased vulnerability of the arteries to obstruction.

Homocysteine is derived from dietary methionine, and it is removed by conversion to cystathionine, cysteine and pyruvate, or by remethylation to methionine. Rare inborn errors of metabolism can cause severe elevations in plasma homocysteine levels. One example is homocystinuria, which occurs as a result of a genetic defect in the enzyme cystathione beta synthase. Genetic changes in the enzymes involved in the remethylation pathway, including MTHFR and methionine synthase, are also associated with increase in plasma homocysteine concentrations. All such cases are associated with premature vascular disease, thrombosis and early death.

Such genetic disorders are, however, rare and cannot account for the raised homocysteine levels observed in many patients with cardiovascular disease. However, attention is now being given to the possibility that deficiency of the various vitamins which act as co-factors for the enzymes involved in homocysteine metabolism could result in increased homocysteine concentrations. In particular, folate is required for the normal function of MTHFR, vitamin B_{12} for methionine synthase and vitamin B_6 for cystathione beta synthase.

In theory, lack of any one of these three vitamins could cause hyperhomocysteinaemia, and could therefore increase the risk of cardiovascular disease. In the Framingham Heart Study,[13] the longest observed cohort study on vascular disease, it was shown that folic acid, vitamin B_6 and vitamin B_{12} are determinants of plasma homocysteine levels, with folic acid showing the strongest association.

The question of whether increased vitamin intake can reduce cardiovascular risk was examined in the Nurse's Health Study,[14] which showed that those with the highest intake of folate had a 31% lower incidence of heart disease than those with the lowest intake. For vitamin B_6, those with the highest intake had a 33% lower risk of heart disease, while in those with the highest intake of both folate and vitamin B_6 the risk of heart disease was reduced by 45%. The risk of heart disease was reduced by 24% in those who regularly used multivitamins.

Another question is whether homocysteine levels can be lowered with folate and other B vitamins. Folic acid (250 μg daily), in addition to usual dietary intakes of folate, significantly decreased plasma homocysteine concentrations in healthy young women,[15] and breakfast cereal fortified with folic acid reduced plasma homocysteine in men and women with coronary artery disease.[16] Another study has demonstrated that the addition of vitamin B_{12} to folic acid supplements or enriched foods (400 μg folic acid daily) maximises the reduction of homocysteine.[17] Furthermore, two meta-analyses[18,19] suggest that administration of folic acid reduces plasma homocysteine concentrations and that vitamin B_{12}, but not vitamin B_6, may have an additional effect.[19]

Unfortunately, a definitive answer to the most important question – can reducing homocysteine reduce cardiovascular disease – does not yet exist due to the lack of published data. However, more data should be available during the next few years from at least six studies which are currently underway. These are designed to examine the role of folate and other B vitamins in reducing cardiovascular events.

Cancer

Marginal folate status also appears to be associated with certain cancers,[20] notably colon cancer, although it is at present unclear as to whether it is folate or some other nutritional factors that could be involved. Data, including those from two prospective studies,[21,22] and four case-control studies[23–26] indicate that an inadequate intake of folate may increase risk of colon cancer. There is also some evidence – albeit limited – that use of supplements containing folic acid could reduce the risk of colon cancer.[27,28]

Mental disorders

There is an apparent increase in mental disorders associated with reduced folate status.[29] Recent studies have found that Alzheimer's disease is associated with low blood levels of folate and vitamin B_{12} and elevated homocysteine levels.[30,31] However, whether this reduced vitamin status is a cause of the disease or occurs as a result of having the disease, is unknown.

Conclusion

There is good evidence that folic acid reduces the risk of neural tube defects, and supplementation is recommended preconceptually and during the first 12 weeks of pregnancy. There is increasing evidence that folic acid reduces elevated plasma homocysteine levels, a risk factor for cardiovascular disease. Epidemiological studies have shown an inverse relationship between serum folate levels and colon cancer. Poor folate status has also been demonstrated in some people with depression. However, controlled trials are required to determine whether supplements can reduce the risk of cancer and help to treat depression.

Precautions/contraindications

In pernicious anaemia, folic acid will correct the haematological abnormalities, but neuropathy may be precipitated. Doses of folic acid >400 μg daily are not recommended until pernicious anaemia has been ruled out.

Pregnancy and breast-feeding

No problems have been reported. Supplements are required during pregnancy and when planning a pregnancy (see Dose).

Adverse effects

Folic acid is generally considered to be safe even in high doses, but it may lead to convulsions in patients taking anticonvulsants and may also precipitate neuropathy in pernicious anaemia. Some gastrointestinal disturbance and altered sleep pattern has been reported at doses of 15 mg daily. Allergic reactions (shortness of breath, wheezing, fever, erythema, skin rash, itching) have been reported rarely.

Interactions

Drugs

Anticonvulsants: requirements for folic acid may be increased, but concurrent use of folic acid may antagonise the effects of anticonvulsants; an increase in anticonvulsant dose may be necessary in patients who receive supplementary folic acid (monitoring required).
Antibiotics: may interfere with the microbiological assay for serum and erythrocyte folic acid (falsely low results).
Colestyramine: may reduce the absorption of folic acid; patients on prolonged colestyramine therapy should take a folic acid supplement 1 h before colestyramine administration.
Methotrexate: acts as a folic acid antagonist; the risk is significant with high dose and/or prolonged use (folinic acid instead of folic acid should be used).
Oestrogens (including oral contraceptives): may reduce blood levels of folic acid.
Pyrimethamine: acts as a folic acid antagonist; the risk is significant with high dose and/or prolonged use; folic acid supplements should be given in pregnancy.
Sulfasalazine: may reduce the absorption of folic acid; requirements for folic acid may be increased.
Trimethoprim: acts as a folic acid antagonist; the risk is significant with high dose and/or prolonged use.

Nutrients

Adequate amounts of all B vitamins are required for optimal functioning; deficiency or excess of one B vitamin may lead to abnormalities in the metabolism of another.
Zinc: folic acid may reduce the absorption of zinc.

Dose

Folic acid is available in the form of tablets.

For prevention of first occurrence of NTDs in women who are planning a pregnancy, oral, 400 μg daily before conception until 12th week of pregnancy.

For prevention of recurrence of NTDs, oral, 5 mg daily before conception until 12th week of pregnancy.

For prophylaxis during pregnancy (after 12th week), oral, 200–500 μg daily.

As a dietary supplement, oral, 100–500 μg daily.

References

1 Laurence KM, James N, Miller MH, *et al.* Double-blind randomised controlled trial of folate treatment before conception to prevent recurrence of neural tube defects. *Br Med J* 1981; 282: 1509–1511.
2 Smithells RW, Seller MJ, Harris R, *et al.* Further experience of vitamin supplementation for prevention of neural tube defect recurrences. *Lancet* 1983; 1: 1027–1031.
3 Medical Research Council Vitamin Study Research Group. Prevention of neural tube defects: Results of the Medical Research Council Vitamin Study. *Lancet* 1991; 338: 131–137.
4 Czeizel AE, Dudas I. Prevention of the first occurrence of neural tube defects by periconceptual vitamin supplementation. *N Engl J Med* 1992; 327: 1832–1835.
5 Weller MM, Shapiro S, Mitchel AA, *et al.* Periconceptual folic acid exposure and risk of occurrent

neural tube defects. *JAMA* 1993; 269: 1257–1261.

6 Molloy AM, Daly S, Mills JL, *et al.* Thermolabile variant of 5,10-methylenetetrahydrofolate reductase associated with low red cell folates: Implications for folate intake recommendations. *Lancet* 1997; 349: 1591–1593.

7 Nelen WLDM, Van der Molen EF, Blom HJ, *et al.* Recurrent early pregnancy loss and genetic related disturbances in folate and homocysteine metabolism. *Br J Hosp Med* 1997; 58: 511–513.

8 Mills JL, McPartlin P, Kirke PM, *et al.* Homocysteine metabolism in pregnancies complicated by neural tube defects. *Lancet* 1995; 345: 149–151.

9 Alfthan G, Aro A, Gey KF. Plasma homocysteine and cardiovascular disease mortality. *Lancet* 1997; 349: 397.

10 Nygard O, Nordrehaug JE, Refsum H, *et al.* Plasma homocysteine levels and mortality in patients with coronary artery disease. *N Engl J Med* 1997; 337: 230–236.

11 Wald NJ, Watt HC, Law MR, *et al.* Homocysteine and ischaemic heart disease: Results of a prospective study with implications on prevention. *Arch Intern Med* 1998; 158: 862–867.

12 Weir DG, Scott JM. Homocysteine as a risk factor for cardiovascular and related disease: Nutritional implications. *Nutr Res Rev* 1998; 11: 311–338.

13 Selhub J, Jacques PF, Wilson PWF, *et al.* Vitamin status and intake as primary determinants of homocysteinaemia in an elderly population. *JAMA* 1993; 270: 2693–2698.

14 Rimm EB, Willett WC, Hu FB, *et al.* Folate and vitamin B_6 from diet and supplements in relation to risk of coronary heart disease among women. *JAMA* 1998; 279: 359–364.

15 Brouwer IA, van Dusseldorp M, Thomas CMG, *et al.* Low-dose folic acid supplementation decreases plasma homocysteine concentrations: A randomized trial. *Am J Clin Nutr* 1999; 69: 99–104.

16 Malinow MR, Duell PB, Hess DL, *et al.* Reduction of plasma homocysteine levels by breakfast cereal fortified with folic acid in patients with coronary heart disease. *N Engl J Med* 1998; 338: 1009–1015.

17 Bronstrup A, Hages M, Prinz-Langenohl R, Pietrzik K. Effects of folic acid and combinations of folic acid and vitamin B-12 on plasma homocysteine concentrations in healthy young women. *Am J Clin Nutr* 1998; 68: 1104–1110.

18 Boushey CJ, Beresford SAA, Omenn GS, Motulsky AG. A quantitative assessment of plasma homocysteine as a risk factor for vascular disease: probable benefits of increasing folic acid intake. *JAMA* 1995; 274: 1049–1057.

19 Homocysteine Lowering Trialists' Collaboration. Lowering blood homocysteine with folic acid based supplements: meta-analysis of randomised trials. *Br Med J* 1998; 316: 894–898.

20 Mason JB. Folate status: Effects on carcinogenesis. In: Bailey LB, ed. *Folates in Health and Disease*. New York: Marcel Dekker, 1995: 361–378.

21 Giovannucci E, Rimm EB, Ascherio A, *et al.* Alcohol, low methionine, low folate diets and risk of colon cancer in men. *J Natl Cancer Inst* 1995; 87: 265–273.

22 Glynn SA, Albanes D, Pietinen P, *et al.* Colorectal cancer and folate status: a nested case-control study among male smokers. *Cancer Epidemiol Biomarkers Prev* 1996; 5: 487–494.

23 Benito E, Stigglebout A, Bosch FX, *et al.* Nutritional factors in colorectal cancer risk: A case-control study in Majorca. *Int J Cancer* 1991; 49: 161–167.

24 Meyer F, White E. Alcohol and nutrients in relation to colon cancer in middle-aged adults. *Am J Epidemiol* 1993; 138: 225–236.

25 Ferraroni M, La Vecchia C, D'Avanzo B, *et al.* Selected micronutrient intake and the role of colon cancer. *Br J Cancer* 1994; 70: 1150–1155.

26 Freudenheim JL, Graham S, Marshall JR, *et al.* Folate intake and carcinogenesis of the colon and rectum. *Int J Epidemiol* 1991; 20: 368–374.

27 White E, Shannon JS, Patterson RE. Relationship between vitamin and calcium supplement use and colon cancer. *Cancer Epidemiol Biomarkers Prev* 1997; 6: 769–774.

28 Giovannucci E, Stampfer MJ, Colditz GA, *et al.* Multivitamin use, folate and colon cancer in women in the nurses' health study. *Ann Intern Med* 1998; 129: 517–524.

29 Bottiglieri ET, Crellin RF, Reynolds EH. Folates and neuropsychiatry. In: Bailey LB, ed. *Folates in Health and Disease*. New York: Marcel Dekker, 1995: 435–462.

30 Joosten E, Lesaffre E, Riezler R, *et al.* Is metabolic evidence for vitamin B_{12} and folate deficiency more frequent in elderly patients with Alzheimer's disease? *J Gerontol A Biol Sci Med* 1997; 52: M76–M79.

31 Clarke R, Smith AD, Jobst KA, *et al.* Folate, vitamin B_{12} and serum homocysteine levels in confirmed Alzheimer's disease. *Arch Neurol* 1998; 11: 1449–1455.

Gamma-oryzanol

Description

Gamma-oryzanol is one of several lipid fractions obtained from rice bran oil.

Constituents

Gamma-oryzanol is a mixture of phytosterols (plant sterols), including campesterol, cycloartanol, cycloartenol, β-sitosterol, stigmasterol, and also ferulic acid.

Action

Phytosterols appear to reduce lipid levels and ferulic acid has antioxidant properties. Gamma-oryzanol has also been suggested to have anabolic properties, but evidence is conflicting.

Possible uses

Gamma-oryzanol has been investigated for a role in lipid lowering and improving exercise performance.

Lipid lowering

Several animal studies[1–3] have shown a lipid-lowering effect with gamma-oryzanol supplementation, but one study did not.[4]

In two uncontrolled studies in humans with hyperlipidaemia, gamma-oryzanol was shown to reduce serum cholesterol levels. One study involved 80 patients with hyperlipidaemia who were given gamma-oryzanol for six months. In those with type IIa and IIb hypercholesterolaemia, serum cholesterol fell by 12% and 13%, respectively, but the reduction was significant only after three months. Plasma triglycerides reduced significantly after three months and there was a non-significant increase in high-density lipoprotein (HDL) cholesterol.[5]

In the other study, 20 patients with chronic schizophrenia with dyslipidaemia were given 300 mg gamma-oryzanol daily for 16 weeks. Both total and low-density lipoprotein (LDL) cholesterol fell significantly, but there was no significant change in HDL levels.[6]

Exercise

In a double-blind, placebo-controlled study, 22 weight-trained men were given 500 mg gamma-oryzanol daily or placebo for nine weeks. There were no differences between the groups for measures of circulating concentrations of testosterone, cortisol, oestradiol, growth hormone, insulin or beta-endorphin, blood lipids, calcium, magnesium and albumin. Resting cardiovascular variables decreased in both groups and vertical jump power and one-repetition maximum muscle strength (bench press and squat) increased in both groups. The authors concluded that gamma-oryzanol 500 mg for nine weeks did not influence either performance or physiological parameters in moderately weight-trained men.[7]

> **Conclusion**
>
> Preliminary evidence from animal studies and uncontrolled studies indicates that gamma-oryzanol may reduce serum cholesterol levels. There is no good evidence that it improves exercise performance. Further research is required.

Precautions/contraindications

None has been reported.

Pregnancy and breast-feeding

No problems have been reported, but there have not been sufficient studies to guarantee the safety of gamma-oryzanol in pregnancy and breast-feeding.

Adverse reactions

There are no long-term studies assessing the safety of gamma-oryzanol in humans. There is some evidence from a Japanese study that doses up to 600 mg daily cause dry mouth, somnolence, hot flushes, irritability and headaches.[8]

Interactions

None reported.

Dose

Gamma-oryzanol is available in the form of tablets and capsules.

The dose is not established. Dietary supplements provide 100–500 mg daily.

References

1. Seetharamaiah GS, Chandrasekhara N. Studies on hypercholesterolemic activity of rice bran oil. *Atherosclerosis* 1989; 78: 219–223.
2. Rukmini C, Raghuram TC. Nutritional and biochemical aspects of the hypolipidemic action of rice bran oil: A review. *J Am Coll Nutr* 1991; 10: 593–601.
3. Rong N, Ausman LM, Nicolosi RJ. Oryzanol decreases cholesterol absorption and fatty streaks in hamsters. *Lipids* 1997; 32: 303–309.
4. Sugano M, Tsuji E. Rice bran oil and cholesterol metabolism. *J Nutr* 1997; 127: 521S–524S.
5. Yoshino G, Kazumi T, Amano M, *et al.* Effects of gamma-oryzanol and probucol on hyperlipidemia. *Curr Ther Res* 1989; 45: 975–982.
6. Sasaki J, Takada Y, Handa K, *et al.* Effects of gamma-oryzanol on serum lipids and apolipoproteins in dyslipidemic schizophrenics receiving major tranquillisers. *Clin Ther* 1990; 12: 263–268.
7. Fry AC, Bonner E, Lewis DL, *et al.* The effects of gamma-oryzanol supplementation during resistance exercise training. *Int J Sports Nutr* 1997; 7: 318–329.
8. Takemoto T. Clinical trial of Hi-Z fine granules (gamma-oryzanol) on gastrointestinal symptoms at 375 hospitals. *Shinyaku To Rinsho* 1977; 26.

Garlic

Description

Garlic is the fresh bulb of *Allium sativum* which is related to the lily family (Liliaceae).

Constituents

The major constituents of garlic include alliin, allicin, diallyl disulphide and ajoene, but these compounds form only a small proportion of the compounds that have been isolated from crushed, cooked and dried garlic.

Alliin, present in fresh garlic, is converted by the enzyme allinase into allicin when the garlic bulb is crushed. Allicin can be converted (by heat) into diallyldisulphide which in turn is converted into various sulphide-containing substances, that cause the typical smell of garlic. Allicin and diallyldisulphide combine to form ajoene.

Possible uses

Garlic has been cultivated for thousands of years for medicinal purposes, including bites, tumours, wounds, headache, cancer and heart disease, and also as a pungent flavouring agent for cooking.

Evidence for beneficial effects of garlic is accumulating but is, as yet, incomplete. Interpretation of trials is made difficult by the fact that different forms of garlic are used and that active ingredients may be lost in processing.[1] The use of standardised, dried garlic preparations or fresh garlic appears to result in the most beneficial effects. Extracts or oils prepared by using steam distillation or organic solvents or 'odourless' garlic preparations may have little activity.[2] Any preparation which produces no odour whatsoever may be clinically ineffective, because release of the biologically active allicin has not occurred. However, allicin is rapidly destroyed even by crushing the fresh bulb, and some suggest that although allicin may be important for cholesterol lowering, it may not be important for protecting against cancer.

Cardiovascular disease

Hyperlipidaemia

Many studies have examined the potential effects of garlic on serum lipid levels. In a placebo-controlled, double-blind study of 40 patients with hypercholesterolaemia,[3] total cholesterol, triglycerides and blood pressure decreased significantly in the group receiving garlic. Daily doses of 900 mg of a garlic powder preparation (equivalent to 2700 mg fresh garlic) were administered over 16 weeks, and differences were significant after four weeks of treatment.

In a randomised, double-blind, placebo-controlled study of 42 healthy adults, 300 mg of a standardised garlic preparation three times daily showed a significantly greater reduction in total and low-density lipoprotein (LDL) cholesterol than placebo.[4] In a study of eight healthy males, ingestion of a garlic clove (approximately 3 g daily for 16 weeks) resulted in approximately a 20% reduction in serum cholesterol.[5]

In another study, serum levels of total cholesterol, LDL and triglycerides decreased significantly after administration of 400 mg garlic three times a day for a month.[5] In a study involving 56 men, administration of an aged garlic extract (7.2 g daily) resulted in a 7% reduction in total cholesterol compared with baseline and a 6% reduction compared with placebo.[6] In a multicentre, placebo-controlled, double-blind study carried out in Germany[7] using standardised dried garlic tablets, total cholesterol fell by 11%.

In 35 renal transplant patients, garlic 680 mg twice daily (equivalent to 4080 μg allicin) or placebo was administered over 12 weeks.[8] After six weeks, total and LDL cholesterol had fallen, and these changes were maintained at 12 weeks. Garlic had no effect on triglyceride or high-density lipoprotein (HDL) cholesterol levels. Yet other studies using garlic 700 mg daily for eight weeks,[9] 200 mg three times a day for 12 weeks,[10] or 1000 mg a day for 24 weeks[11] have resulted in 12–14% reductions in serum cholesterol. Other studies[12–15] demonstrated no effect of garlic on hyperlipidaemia, however.

A meta-analysis of studies[16] evaluating the effect of garlic on serum cholesterol included five of the above studies.[3,7,9–11] The garlic dose was 600–1000 mg daily for 8–24 weeks. The pooled results of the meta-analysis indicated that patients treated with garlic achieved mean total serum cholesterol concentrations of 230–290 mg/l lower than patients in placebo groups. Since the investigators used a range of dose regimens, the optimum dose for garlic could not be identified.

More recently, another meta-analysis[17] which included 13 trials, found that garlic reduced total cholesterol level from baseline significantly more than placebo. The weighted mean difference was 0.41 mmol/l (157 mg/l). However, when the trials with the highest scores for methodological quality were analysed alone, the differences in cholesterol levels between garlic and placebo were non-significant. The authors concluded that garlic is superior to placebo in reducing cholesterol levels, but the robustness of the data is questionable and any effect likely to be small. The use of garlic to treat hypercholesterolaemia was therefore debatable.

Hypertension

Several studies have evaluated the efficacy of garlic in hypertension. In a multicentre, randomised, placebo-controlled, double-blind study of 47 patients with mild hypertension, garlic powder tablets, 200 mg three times a day for 12 weeks, produced significant reductions in blood pressure as well as total cholesterol and triglycerides.[10] In an acute pilot study of nine patients with severe hypertension, single doses of 2400 mg of a garlic powder preparation (standardised to release 0.6% allicin) produced a significant reduction in diastolic blood pressure 5–14 h after administration.[18]

A meta-analysis of studies[19] evaluated the efficacy of garlic on blood pressure. Only prospective, randomised studies with two or more treatment group comparisons and a duration of at least four weeks were included, and eight studies met the defined criteria. Six of the studies were placebo-controlled, one compared garlic with a diuretic and reserpine, and another compared garlic with bezafibrate. All but one of the studies were supposedly double-blind, but with the odour of garlic being difficult to mask, it is not clear whether the studies really were blinded. All eight studies used the same dried garlic powder in doses of 600–900 mg daily (equivalent to 1.8–2.7 g of fresh garlic daily) for one to 12 months. The pooled mean reduction in systolic blood pressure was 7.7 mmHg and the pooled mean diastolic pressure 5.0 mmHg more with garlic. However, there have not been enough trials with different garlic doses for the optimum dose to be defined.

Cancer

Preliminary data from *in vitro*, animal and epidemiological studies suggest that garlic may have a protective effect in cancer development and progression. Results of epidemiological case-control studies in China[20] and Italy[21] suggest that garlic may reduce the risk of gastric cancer. Epidemiological studies cannot by themselves establish causal relationships, and prospective data on this possible effect of garlic on cancer risk are required.

Garlic consumption has been associated with a reduced risk of colon cancer in some studies,[22–24] but not others.[25] However, in another study, garlic consumption was not associated with reduced risk of stomach cancer,[25] breast cancer[26] or prostate cancer.[27] A meta-analysis of the relation between cooked garlic, raw garlic or both raw and cooked garlic on the risk of colorectal and stomach cancers showed that garlic may be associated with a protective effect against both types of cancer.[28]

Antimicrobial activity

Garlic is being investigated for antibacterial, antifungal and antiviral activity, but current evidence is too limited to recommend it for the prevention of infections.

Conclusion

There is evidence from meta-analyses that garlic supplements reduce blood cholesterol and blood pressure. However, authors of meta-analyses have criticised studies for poor methodology, small numbers of subjects, and short duration. There is preliminary evidence that garlic reduces platelet aggregation and may reduce the risk of cancer, but controlled clinical trials are needed to confirm this. Garlic has been used for centuries for antibacterial and antiviral effects. Although such effects have been demonstrated *in vitro*, controlled clinical studies are needed to confirm these findings.

Precautions/contraindications

Hypersensitivity to garlic.

Pregnancy and breast-feeding

No problems have been reported. However, there have not been sufficient studies to guarantee the safety of garlic supplements in pregnancy and breast-feeding.

Adverse effects

Unpleasant breath odour; indigestion; hypersensitivity reactions including contact dermatitis and asthma have been reported occasionally. A spinal haematoma (isolated report) has been attributed to the antiplatelet effects of garlic.

Interactions

None reported. In theory, garlic could increase bleeding with anticoagulants, aspirin and antiplatelet drugs.

Dose

Garlic supplements are available in the form of tablets and capsules.

The dose is not established, but 400–1000 mg (equivalent to 2–5 g fresh garlic or one to two cloves) daily of a standardised garlic product has been used in several studies. Dietary supplements provide 400–1000 mg dried garlic daily. Standardised products may be standardised for allicin potential. One clove of fresh garlic is equivalent to 4000 μg allicin potential.

References

1 Kleijnen J, Knipschild P, Ter Riet G. Garlic, onions and cardiovascular risk factors. A review of the evidence from human experiments with emphasis on commercially available preparations. *Br J Clin Pharmacol* 1989; 28: 533–544.
2 Mansell P, Reckless JP. Garlic. *Br Med J* 1991; 303: 379–380.
3 Vorberg G, Schneider B. Therapy with garlic: Results of a placebo-controlled, double-blind study. *Br J Clin Pract* 1990; 44 (suppl. 69): 7–11.
4 Jain AK, Vargas R, Gotzkowsky S, McMahon FG. Can garlic reduce levels of serum lipids? A controlled clinical study. *Am J Med* 1993; 94: 632–635.
5 Ali M, Thompson M. Consumption of a garlic clove a day could be beneficial in preventing thrombosis. *Prostaglandins Leukot Essent Fatty Acids* 1995; 53: 211–212.
6 Steiner M, Khan AH, Holberd D, *et al.* A double-blind crossover study in moderately hypercholesterolemic men that compared the effect of aged garlic extract and placebo administration on blood lipids. *Am J Clin Nutr* 1996; 64: 866–870.
7 Mader FH. Treatment of hyperlipidaemia with garlic-powder tablets. *Arzneimittelforschung* 1990; 40: 3–8.
8 Silagy S, Neil A. Garlic as a lipid lowering agent – a meta-analysis. *J R Coll Physicians Lond* 1994; 28: 39–45.
9 Plengvidhya C, Chinayon S, Sitprija S, *et al.* Effects of spray dried garlic preparation on primary hyperlipoproteinaemia. *J Med Ass Thai* 1988; 71: 248–252.
10 Auer W, Eiber A, Hertkorn E, *et al.* Hypertension and hyperlipidaemia: garlic helps in mild cases. *Br J Clin Pract* 1990; 44 (suppl. 69): 3–6.
11 Lau BH, Lam F, Wang-Chen R. Effect of an odor modified garlic preparation on blood lipids. *Nutr Res* 1987; 7: 139–149.
12 Luley C, Lehmann-Leo W, Moeller B, *et al.* Lack of efficacy of dried garlic in patients with

hyperlipoproteinaemia. *Arzneimittelforschung* 1986; 36: 766–768.

13 Berthold HK, Sudhop T, von Bergmann K. Effect of a garlic oil preparation on serum lipoproteins and cholesterol metabolism: a randomized controlled trial. *JAMA* 1998; 279: 1900–1902.

14 Isaacsohn JL, Moser M, Stein EA, *et al.* Garlic powder and plasma lipids and lipoproteins: A multicenter, randomized, placebo-controlled trial. *Arch Intern Med* 1998; 158: 1189–1194.

15 Simons LA, Balasubramaniam S, von Konigsmark M, *et al.* On the effect of garlic on plasma lipids and lipoproteins in mild hypercholesterolaemia. *Atherosclerosis* 1995; 113: 219–225.

16 Warshafsky S, Kamer RS, Sivak SL. Effect of garlic on total serum cholesterol: A meta-analysis. *Ann Intern Med* 1993; 119: 599–605.

17 Stevinson C, Pittler M, Ernst E. Garlic for treating hypercholesterolaemia. *Ann Intern Med* 2000; 133: 420–429.

18 McMahon GF, Vargas R. Can garlic lower blood pressure? A pilot study. *Pharmacotherapy* 1993; 13: 406–407.

19 Silagy CA, Neil HAW. A meta-analysis of the effect of garlic on blood pressure. *J Hypertens* 1994; 12: 463–468.

20 You WC, Blot WJ, Chang YS. *J Natl Cancer Inst* 1989; 81: 162–164.

21 Buiatti E, Palli D, Declari A. A case control study of gastric cancer and diet in Italy. *Int J Cancer* 1989; 44: 611–616.

22 Steinmetz KA, Kushi LH, Bostick RM, *et al.* Vegetables, fruit, and colon cancer in the Iowa Woman's Health Study. *Am J Epidemiol* 1994; 139: 1–15.

23 Witte JS, Longnecker MP, Bird CL, *et al.* Relation of vegetable, fruit, and grain consumption to colorectal adenomatous polyps. *Am J Epidemiol* 1996; 144: 1015–1025.

24 Le Marchand L, Hankin JH, Wilkens LR, *et al.* Dietary fiber and colorectal cancer risk. *Epidemiology* 1997; 8: 658–665.

25 Dorant E, van den Brandt PA, Goldbohm RA. Allium vegetable consumption, garlic supplement intake, and female breast carcinoma incidence. *Breast Cancer Res Treat* 1995; 33: 163–170.

26 Dorant E, van den Brandt PA, Goldbohm RA, *et al.* Consumption of onions and a reduced risk of stomach carcinoma. *Gastroenterology* 1996; 110: 12–20.

27 Key TJA, Silcocks PB, Davey GK, *et al.* A case-control study of diet and prostate cancer. *Br J Cancer* 1997; 76: 678–687.

28 Fleischauer AT, Poole C, Arab L. Garlic consumption and cancer prevention: Meta-analyses of colorectal and stomach cancers. *Am J Clin Nutr* 2000; 72: 1047–1052.

Ginkgo biloba

Description

Ginkgo biloba is an extract from the dried leaves of *Ginkgo biloba* (maidenhair tree). In Germany, it is one of the most frequently prescribed products for cognitive disorders.

Constituents

The leaf contains amino acids, flavonoids, and terpenoids (including bilobalide and ginkgolides A, B, C, J, M).

Action

The pharmacological properties of ginkgo biloba have been reviewed.[1,2] Ginkgo biloba extract has the following properties. It:

- antagonises platelet-activating factor (PAF), reducing platelet aggregation and decreasing the production of oxygen free radicals;[3,4]
- increases blood flow, produces arterial vasodilatation and reduces blood viscosity;[5]
- has free radical scavenging properties;[6,7] and
- may influence neurotransmitter metabolism[8].

These effects are probably due to stimulation of prostaglandin biosynthesis or by direct vasoregulatory effects on catecholamines.[6,9] In addition, ginkgo biloba acts as an antioxidant.[10]

Possible uses

Ginkgo biloba has been studied for the treatment of cerebrovascular disease and peripheral vascular insufficiency.

Memory and cognitive function

The main interest in ginkgo has focused on its use in patients with poor memory and poor cognitive function due to cerebral insufficiency, and it is licensed for this indication in Germany. A review of over 40 European clinical trials[2,11] evaluated ginkgo's efficacy in the treatment of cerebral and peripheral insufficiency. All 40 trials showed positive effects, and the authors concluded that there may have been publication bias. Of the 40 trials, eight were judged to be of good quality. The majority of studies evaluated 12 symptoms: difficulty in concentration; difficulty in memory; absent mindedness; confusion; lack of energy; tiredness; decreased physical performance; depression; anxiety; dizziness; tinnitus; and headaches. Seven of the eight trials showed statistically and clinically significant positive effects of ginkgo compared with placebo. No serious adverse effects were reported.

A meta-analysis of 11 placebo-controlled, randomised, double-blind studies (which included six of the above studies) showed that ginkgo was significantly better than placebo for all symptoms associated with cerebrovascular insufficiency of old age. Of the 11 studies, one study was inconclusive, but all the rest showed positive effects.[12]

In a double-blind, placebo-controlled study, 31 patients over the age of 50 years were randomised to receive ginkgo biloba 40 mg or placebo three times a day. Using a range of psychometric tests, ginkgo was shown to produce a significant improvement in cognitive function at both 12 and 24 weeks.[13] More recent double-blind, placebo-controlled trials have confirmed the benefits of ginkgo on memory[14] and cognitive function.[15]

Peripheral vascular disease

In the review of 40 trials,[11] 15 controlled trials evaluated the role of ginkgo in intermittent claudication and of these, two were judged to be of reasonable quality. One of these showed significant increase in walking distance tolerated before pain with ginkgo,[16] and the other trial showed a greater reduction in pain at rest.[17]

In a multicentre, randomised, double-blind, placebo-controlled study involving 74 patients with peripheral arterial occlusive disease, pain-free walking distance improved in patients given either 120 mg or 240 mg ginkgo biloba daily, with a greater improvement in the group given the higher dose.[18]

In another multicentre, double-blind, placebo-controlled trial, 111 patients with peripheral occlusive arterial disease were randomised to receive 120 mg *Ginkgo biloba* extract or placebo for 24 weeks. Pain-free walking and maximum walking distance were significantly greater in the ginkgo group, and subjective assessment by the patients showed an amelioration of complaints in both groups.[19]

Dementia

In a double-blind, placebo-controlled trial, 216 patients with Alzheimer's disease were randomised to receive either 240 mg *Ginkgo biloba* EGb 761 extract or placebo for 24 weeks. In the 156 patients who completed the study, the frequency of responders in the two groups differed significantly in favour of EGb 761. Analysis of the results on an intention-to-treat basis showed similar results, and the authors concluded that EGb 761 was beneficial in dementia of the Alzheimer type and multi-infarct dementia.[20]

A 52-week, randomised, double-blind, placebo-controlled, parallel design, multicentre study in 309 patients found that EGb 761 120 mg daily improved measures of cognitive function, daily living, and social performance and psychopathology. The authors concluded that ginkgo was safe and capable of maintaining or, in some cases improving, cognitive and social function in patients with dementia.[21] Of the 309 patients, 244 completed the study up to 26 weeks, but analysis on an intention-to-treat basis still showed significant benefits with ginkgo biloba.[22]

A review of 50 articles, of which four randomised, placebo-controlled, double-blind trials met the inclusion criteria, concluded that there is a small but significant effect of three- to six-month treatment with 120–240 mg of ginkgo biloba extract on objective measures of cognitive function in Alzheimer's disease.[23]

However, in another study of 214 elderly patients with dementia or memory impairment, who were split into three groups and given either one of two different doses of ginkgo biloba extract EGb 761 or a placebo, no differences were detected in memory function after 24 weeks.[24] The authors suggested that these results occurred because of the effort made to find a good placebo (ginkgo has a pronounced taste and smell). However, others have questioned the validity of the study, suggesting that a positive effect would have been unlikely in such a heterogeneous population where all types of memory loss were included.[25]

Ginkgo biloba has not been directly compared to conventional medicines for dementia, but improvement seems to be similar to that found with prescription drugs (e.g. donepezil, tacrine and possibly other cholinesterase inhibitors).[26,27]

Miscellaneous

Ginkgo biloba has been claimed to be of value in a number of other conditions, including asthma, tinnitus, sexual dysfunction, premenstrual syndrome and mountain sickness. However, there is only very limited evidence that it has any benefit in these conditions. A review (which included one study) of the role of ginkgo in age-related macular degeneration concluded that, although a beneficial effect was observed, only 20 people were enrolled in the trial and assessment was not masked, thus making the results equivocal.[28] Further research is needed in all these areas.

Precautions/contraindications

Ginkgo biloba extract should not be used for the treatment of disease without medical supervision. It is contraindicated in hypertension.

Conclusion
Several studies have shown that *Gingko biloba* extract may slow the progression of dementia, particularly in Alzheimer's disease. There is also some evidence that gingko improves memory and concentration in the elderly and increases pain-free walking and maximum walking distance in those with peripheral vascular disease. However, ginkgo should not be taken in any of these conditions without medical advice. There is no sound evidence that ginkgo is effective in other conditions.

Advise users to report any unusual bleeding or bruising. There is anecdotal evidence that ginkgo might be associated with seizure,[29] so until more is known, ginkgo should be avoided in epilepsy or in patients at risk of seizure. Preliminary evidence also exists that ginkgo increases insulin clearance,[30] and this should be borne in mind by monitoring blood glucose in patients with diabetes.

Pregnancy and breast-feeding

Contraindicated in pregnancy, breast-feeding and in children.

Adverse effects

There are few reports of serious toxicity. Headache, nausea, vomiting, heartburn, and diarrhoea have been reported occasionally. There have been rare reports of severe allergic reactions including skin reactions (e.g. itching, erythema and blisters) and convulsions. Ginkgo extract can decrease platelet aggregation by inhibiting platelet-activating factor, and may therefore exacerbate bleeding disorders.

Interactions

Drugs

Anticoagulants, aspirin, anti-platelet drugs: use ginkgo biloba extract with caution due to its effect on platelet-activating factor.

There is preliminary evidence that ginkgo can influence the cytochrome P450 and other drug-metabolising enzymes.[31] There are no reports of interactions, but ginkgo should be used with caution in any patients taking other medication.

Dose

Ginkgo biloba extract is available in the form of tablets, capsules and tincture. A review of 30 US ginkgo biloba products found that nearly one-quarter did have the expected chemical marker compounds for ginkgo biloba extract (e.g. flavone glycosides, terpene lactones).[32]

Most clinical trials have used a 50:1 concentrated leaf extract (EGb 761) standardised to 24% flavone glycosides and 6% terpene glycones. (A standardised 40 mg tablet should therefore contain 9.6 mg flavone glycosides and 2.4 mg terpene glycones.) Studies have used 120–240 mg daily. Dietary supplements provide 40–80 mg in a single dose.

References

1 Braquet P. The ginkgolides: platelet activating factor antagonists isolated from Ginkgo biloba: Chemistry, pharmacology and clinical applications. *Drugs of the Future* 1987; 12: 643–699.
2 Kleijnen J, Knipschild P. Ginkgo biloba for cerebral insufficiency. *Br J Clin Pharmacol* 1992; 34: 352–358.
3 Chung KF, Dent G, McCusker M, *et al*. Effect of a ginkgolide mixture (BN 52063) in antagonising skin and platelet responses to platelet activating factor in man. *Lancet* 1987; 1: 248–251.
4 Braquet P, Hosford D. Ethnopharmacology and the development of natural PAF antagonists as therapeutic agents. *J Ethnopharmacol* 1991; 32: 135–139.
5 Jung F, Morowietz C, Kiesewetter H, Wenzel E. Effect of ginkgo biloba on fluidity of blood and peripheral microcirculation in volunteers. *Arzneimittelforschung* 1990; 40: 589–593.
6 Pincemail J, Dupuis M, Nasr C. Superoxide anion scavenging effect and superoxide dismutase activity of Ginkgo biloba extract. *Experientia* 1989; 45: 708–712.
7 Robak J, Gryglewski RJ. Flavonoids are scavengers of superoxide anions. *Biochem Pharmacol* 1988; 37: 837–841.
8 Defeudis FG. Ginkgo biloba *Extract (EGb 761): Pharmacological Activities and Clinical Applications*. Paris: Editions Scientifiques, Elsevier, 1991: 78–84.

9 Nemecz G, Combest WL. Ginkgo biloba. *US Pharmacist* 1997; 22: 144–151.
10 Kobuchi H. Ginkgo biloba extract (EGB 761): Inhibitory effect of nitric oxide production in the macrophage cell line RAW 264.7. *Biochem Pharmacol* 1997; 53: 897–903.
11 Kleijnen J, Knipschild P. Ginkgo biloba. *Lancet* 1992; 340: 1136–1139.
12 Hopfenmuller W. Evidence for a therapeutic effect of Ginkgo biloba special extract: Meta-analysis of 11 clinical studies in patients with cerebrovascular insufficiency in old age. *Arzneimittelforschung* 1994; 44: 1005–1013.
13 Rai GS, Shovlin C, Wesnes KA. A double-blind, placebo-controlled study of Ginkgo biloba extract ('tanakan') in elderly outpatients with mild to moderate memory impairment. *Curr Med Res Opin* 1991; 12: 350–355.
14 Rigney U, Kimber S, Hindmarch I. The effects of acute doses of standardized Ginkgo biloba extract on memory and psychomotor performance in volunteers. *Phytother Res* 1999; 13: 408–415.
15 Mix JA, Crews WD, Jr. An examination of the efficacy of Ginkgo biloba extract Egb761 on the neuropsychologic functioning of cognitively intact older adults. *J Altern Complement Med* 2000; 6: 219–229.
16 Bauer U. 6-Month double-blind randomised clinical trial of Ginkgo biloba extract versus placebo in two parallel groups in patients suffering from peripheral arterial insufficiency. *Arzneimittelforschung* 1984; 34: 716–720.
17 Saudreau F, Serise JM, Pillet J, *et al.* Efficacité de l'extrait de Ginkgo biloba dans le traitement des artériopathies oblitérantes chroniques des membres inférieurs as stade III de la classification de fontaine. *J Mal Vasc* 1989; 14: 177–182.
18 Peters H, Kieser M, Holscher U. Demonstration of the efficacy of ginkgo biloba special extract EGb 761 on intermittent claudication – a placebo-controlled double-blind multicenter trial. *VASA* 1998; 27: 106–110.
19 Schweizer J, Hautmann C. Comparison of two dosages of ginkgo biloba extract EGb 761 in patients with peripheral arterial occlusive disease Fontaine's stage Iib: A randomised, double-blind, multicentric clinical trial. *Arzneimittelforschung* 1999; 49: 900–904.
20 Kanowski S. Proof of efficacy of the ginkgo biloba special extract EGB 761 in outpatients suffering mild to moderate primary degenerative dementia of the Alzheimer type of multi-infarct dementia. *Pharmacopsychiatry* 1996; 29: 47–56.
21 Le Bars PL. A placebo-controlled, double-blind, randomized trial of an extract of Ginkgo biloba for dementia. *JAMA* 1997; 278: 1327–1332.
22 Le Bars PL, Kieser M, Itil KZ. A 26-week analysis of a double-blind placebo-controlled trial of the ginkgo biloba extract Egb 761® in dementia. *Dement Geriatr Cogn Disord* 2000; 11: 230–237.
23 Oken BS, Storzbach DM, Kaye JA. The efficacy of Ginkgo biloba on cognitive function in Alzheimer disease. *Arch Neurol* 1998; 55: 1409–1415.
24 Van Dongen MC, van Rossum E, Kessels AG, *et al.* The efficacy of ginkgo for elderly people with dementia and age-associated memory impairment: New results of a randomized clinical trial. *J Am Geriatr Soc* 2000; 48: 1183–1194.
25 Weber W. Ginkgo not effective for memory loss in elderly. *Lancet* 2000; 356: 1389.
26 Itil TM, Eralp E, Ahmed I, *et al.* The pharmacological effects of ginkgo biloba, a plant extract, on the brain of dementia patients in comparison with tacrine. *Psychopharmacol Bull* 1998; 34: 391–397.
27 Wettstein A. Cholinesterase inhibitors and Ginkgo extracts – are they comparable in the treatment of dementia? Comparison of published placebo-controlled efficacy studies of at least six months' duration. *Phytomedicine* 2000; 6: 393–401.
28 Evans JR. Ginkgo biloba extract for age-related macular degeneration. *Cochrane Database Syst Rev* 2000; (2): CD001775.
29 US Food and Drug Administration. Special Nutritional Adverse Monitoring System. US FDA 1998. http://vm.cfscan.fda.gov/~dms/aems.html (accessed 5 December 2000).
30 Kudolo GB. The effect of 3-month ingestion of Ginkgo biloba extract on pancreatic beta-cell function in response to glucose loading in normal glucose tolerant individuals. *J Clin Pharmacol* 2000; 40: 647–654.
31 Budzinski JW, Foster BC, Vandenhoek S, *et al.* An in vitro evaluation of human cytochrome P450 3A4 inhibition by selected commercial herbal extracts and tinctures. *Phytomedicine* 2000; 7: 273–282.
32 Consumerlab. Product review. Ginkgo biloba. http://www.consumerlab.com (accessed 5 December 2000).

Ginseng

Description

Ginseng is the dried root of *Panax ginseng*. There are eight species of the genus *Panax* which are grown in the central Himalayas, China, Korea, Japan and North America. The eight species of *Panax* are: *ginseng*, *japonicus*, *notoginseng*, *pseudoginseng*, *quinquefolium*, *stipuleantus*, *trifolus* and *zingigerensis*.

Siberian, Manchurian and Brazilian ginseng are commonly referred to as 'ginseng' but do not belong to the genus *Panax*. The botanical name for Siberian ginseng is *Eleutherococcus senticocus* and for Brazilian ginseng, *Pfaffia paniculata*.

The use of precise terminology is important because the action of the different 'ginseng' varies. Some dietary supplements do not contain ginsenosides[1] because they do not contain *Panax* ginseng.

Constituents

Panax ginseng contains complex mixtures of saponins known as ginsenosides or panaxosides; at least 20 saponins have been isolated from ginseng roots. However, species vary in composition and concentration.

Eleutherococcus senticocus contains the saponins known as eleutherosides. Neither *E. senticocus* nor *Pfaffia paniculata* contain ginsenosides.

Action

Ginseng has a wide range of pharmacological effects, but their clinical significance in humans has not been fully investigated. Differences in composition of the different species lead to differences in activity.

Analgesic activity, anti-pyretic activity, anti-inflammatory activity, CNS-stimulating and CNS-depressant activity, hypotensive and hypertensive activity, histamine-like activity and antihistamine activity, hypoglycaemic activity and erythropoietic activity have been reported.[2] Opposing activities such as hypertension and hypotension are thought to be a result of different ginsenosides in one preparation.

The most consistent biochemical explanation for the effects of the ginsenosides is a facilitating influence on the hypothalamic-pituitary-adrenal axis.[3,4] Interactions with central cholinergic[5] and dopaminergic mechanisms[6] have also been demonstrated.

Possible uses

Ginseng is an ancient remedy, which has been used for thousands of years in the East. A number of extravagant claims have been made for it, including aphrodisiac and anti-ageing properties. It is not claimed to cure any specific disease, but to restore general vitality. Ginseng is claimed to be useful for:

- improving stamina;
- alleviating symptoms of tiredness and exhaustion;
- headaches;
- amnesia and mental function;
- improving libido and sexual vigour and preventing impotence;
- regulating blood pressure;
- preventing diabetes mellitus;
- preventing signs of old age and extending youth;
- improving immunity; and
- reducing the risk of cancer.

Available evidence for some of these claims has come mainly from animal studies including: increased adaptability to stress;[7] increasing stamina;[8] decreasing learning time;[9] reduction in blood pressure;[10] anti-inflammatory activity;[11] and improved sleep.[12]

Cognitive function

In an uncontrolled study in humans ginseng has been shown to increase stamina in athletes and concentration in radio operators.[13] In a double-blind, placebo-controlled trial, 60 elderly patients received a supplement containing *Panax* ginseng and vitamins and minerals or placebo daily for eight weeks. There was no difference in the ability of either the supplement or placebo to influence the rehabilitation of these patients, and the effects of the ginseng could not be separated from those of the other ingredients in the product.[14]

Diabetes

A small preliminary study[15] showed that American ginseng reduced blood sugar levels in people who had diabetes mellitus and in healthy subjects. However, because the study looked only at a single time-point, it is unclear what the results mean for real meals or prevention and treatment of diabetes. Nonetheless, the research suggests that ginseng may be useful for preventing sharp increases in blood sugar. A further study in 10 patients with type 2 diabetes showed that American ginseng reduced postprandial glycaemia, and that no more than 3 g was required to achieve reductions.[16]

A double-blind, placebo-controlled study in 36 patients with type 2 diabetes showed that ginseng therapy (100 and 200 mg) significantly reduced fasting blood glucose and elevated mood, and the 200 mg dose resulted in a statistically significant improvement in glycated haemoglobin.[17]

Cancer

Case-control[18] and cohort[19] studies in Korean subjects have shown that incidence of cancer is lower in those who consume ginseng than in those who do not.

Sexual function

A placebo-controlled (not blinded) study included 90 patients with erectile dysfunction.[20] They were randomly assigned to receive *Panax* ginseng (300 mg daily), trazodone or placebo. Patient satisfaction, libido and penile rigidity and girth were greater in the ginseng group than in the other two groups, but changes in the frequency of intercourse, premature ejaculation and morning erections were not changed in any group. None of the treatments resulted in complete remission of erectile dysfunction.

Exercise performance

Several human studies have shown an ergogenic effect in exercise, but a review concluded that such trials have been poorly controlled and not blinded, and that there is no compelling evidence that ginseng improves exercise performance in humans.[21] Double-blind, placebo-controlled trials do not support an ergogenic effect of ginseng on exercise performance.[22–24]

Conclusion

Ginseng has been used for thousands of years, but there are few controlled trials in humans. Many studies have produced conflicting results, and this may be due to lack of standardised products, variation in dosage, differences in harvest conditions of the plants, and types of ginseng used. A systematic review[25] concluded that evidence for the efficacy of ginseng for any indication is weak. The review investigated the effect of ginseng on athletic performance, psychomotor and cognitive performance, immunomodulation, diabetes mellitus and herpes. Ginseng is taken for a range of other indications, but there is little evidence that it slows the ageing process, helps mental or physical functioning in the elderly, increases exercise performance, or improves sexual function.

Precautions/contraindications

Ginseng should be avoided by children and used with caution by patients with cardiovascular disease (including hypertension), diabetes mellitus, asthma, schizophrenia and other disorders of the nervous system. Because of a possible effect on blood glucose, the effect of ginseng on glucose measurement in diabetes should be borne in mind.

Pregnancy and breast-feeding

Ginseng should be avoided.

Adverse effects

Ginseng is relatively non-toxic, but in high doses (>3 g ginseng root daily) the following symptoms may occur: insomnia, nervous excitation, euphoria; nausea and diarrhoea (especially in the morning); skin eruptions; oedema; oestrogenic effects (e.g. breast tenderness; temporary return of menstruation in post-menopausal women).[26–28]

Interactions

Drugs

Tranquillisers: ginseng may reverse the effects of sedatives and tranquillisers.
Digoxin: ginseng may increase blood levels of digoxin.[29]
Warfarin: ginseng may influence the effect of warfarin.[30,31]

Dose

Ginseng is available in the form of tablets, capsules, teas, powders and tinctures. Red ginseng is derived from steam treated ginseng roots, and white ginseng from air-dried roots. Surveys have found that the ginsenoside concentrations in different products vary enormously.[1,32] A review of 21 US products found that seven had less than the required concentration of ginsenosides, two products contained lead above acceptable levels, and eight contained unacceptable levels of quintozene and hexachlorobenzene.[33]

The dose is not established. Manufacturers tend to recommend 0.5–3 g daily of the dried root, or its equivalent.

References

1 Cui J, Garle M, Eneroth P, Bjorkhem L. What do commercial ginseng preparations contain? *Lancet* 1994; 344: 134.
2 Hikino H. Traditional remedies and modern assessment: The case for ginseng. In: Wijesekera ROB, ed. *The Medicinal Plant Industry*. Boca Raton, Florida: CRC Press, 1991.
3 Filaretov AA, Bogdanova TS, Podvigina TT, Bogdanov AL. Role of pituitary-adrenocortical system in body adaption possibilities. *Exp Clin Endocrinol* 1988; 92: 129–136.
4 Fulder S. Ginseng and the hypothalamic control of stress. *Am J Chinese Med* 1981; 9: 112–118.
5 Benishin CG, Lee R, Wang LCH, Liu HJ. Effects of ginsenoside Rb-1 on central cholinergic metabolism. *Pharmacology* 1991; 42: 223–229.
6 Watanebe H, Ohta-Himamura L, Asakura W, *et al.* Effect of *Panax* ginseng on age-related changes in the spontaneous motor activity and dopaminergic system in rat. *Jpn J Pharmacol* 1991; 55: 51–56.
7 Bittles AH, Fulder SJ, Grant EC, Nicholls W. The effect of ginseng on lifespan and stress response in mice. *Gerontology* 1979; 25: 125–131.
8 Brekhman II, Dardymov IV. New substances of plant origin which increase non-specific stress. *Ann Rev Pharmacol* 1969; 9: 419–430.
9 Saito H, Tschuiya M, Naka S, Takugi K. Effects of *Panax* ginseng root on conditioned avoidance response in rats. *Jpn J Pharmacol* 1977; 27: 509–516.
10 Lee DC, Lee MO, Kim CY, Clifford DH. Effect of ether, ethanol, and aqueous extracts of ginseng on cardiovascular function in dogs. *Can J Comp Med* 1981; 45: 182–185.
11 Yuan WX, Gui LH, Zhou JY, *et al.* Some pharmacological effects of ginseng saponins. *Zhongguo Yaoli Zuebo* 1983; 4: 124–128.
12 Lee SP, Honda K, Ho-Rhee Y, Inoue S. Chronic intake of *Panax* ginseng extract stabilises sleep and wakefulness in sleep-deprived rats. *Neurosci Lett* 1990; 111: 217–221.
13 Medvedev MA. The effect of ginseng on the working performance of radio operators. In: *Papers on the study of ginseng and other medicinal plants of the Far East, Vol. 5*. Vladivostok: Primorskoe Knizhnoe Izdatelsvo, 1963.
14 Thommessen B, Laake K. No identifiable effect of ginseng (Gericomplex) as an adjuvant in the treatment of geriatric patients. *Aging (Milano)* 1996; 8: 417–420.
15 Vuksan V, Sievenpiper JL, Koo VVY, *et al.* American ginseng (*Panax quinquefolius* L) reduces postprandial glycemia in nondiabetic subjects and subjects with type 2 diabetes mellitus. *Arch Intern Med* 2000; 160: 1009–1013.

16 Vuksan V, Stavro MP, Sievenpiper JL, *et al.* Similar postprandial glycemic reductions with escalation of dose and administration time of American ginseng in type 2 diabetes. *Diabetes Care* 2000; 23: 1221–1226.
17 Sotaniemi EA, Haapakoski E, Rautio A. Ginseng therapy in non-insulin-dependent diabetic patients. *Diabetes Care* 1995; 18: 1373–1375.
18 Yun TK, Choi SY. Preventive effect of ginseng intake against various human cancers: A case-control study on 1,987 matched pairs. *Cancer Epidemiol Biomarkers Prev* 1995; 4: 401–408.
19 Yun TK. Experimental and epidemiological evidence of the cancer preventive effects of *Panax ginseng* CA Meyer. Nutr Rev 1996; 54 (11 pt. 2): S71–S81.
20 Choi HK, Seong DH, Rha KH. Clinical efficacy of Korean red ginseng for erectile dysfunction. *Int J Impot Res* 1995; 7: 181–186.
21 Bahrke MS, Morgan WP. Evaluation of ergogenic properties of ginseng. *Sports Med* 1994; 18: 229–248.
22 Allen JD, McLung J, Nelson AG, *et al.* Ginseng supplementation does not enhance healthy adults' peak aerobic exercise performance. *J Am Coll Nutr* 1998; 17: 462–466.
23 Engels HJ, Wirth JC. No ergogenic effects of ginseng (*Panax ginseng* CA Meyer) during graded maximal aerobic exercise. *J Am Dietet Assoc* 1997; 97: 1110–1115.
24 Morris AC, Jacobs I, McLellan TM, *et al.* No ergogenic effect of ginseng ingestion. *Int J Sport Nutr* 1996; 6: 263–271.
25 Volger BK, Pittler MH, Ernst E. The efficacy of ginseng: A systematic review of randomised clinical trials. *Eur J Clin Pharmacol* 1999; 55: 567–575.
26 Siegel RK. Ginseng abuse syndrome: problems with the panacea. *JAMA* 1979; 241: 1614–1615.
27 Greenspan EM. Ginseng and vaginal bleeding. *JAMA* 1983; 249: 2018.
28 McRae S. Elevated serum digoxin levels in a patient taking digoxin and Siberian ginseng. *Can Med Assoc J* 1996; 155: 293–295.
29 Janetzky K. Probable interaction between warfarin and ginseng. *Am J Health Syst Pharm* 1997; 54: 692–693.
30 Cheng TO. Ginseng-warfarin interaction. *ACC Curr J Rev* 2000; 9: 84.
31 Palop-Larrea V, Gonzalvez-Perales JL, Catalan-Oliver C, *et al.* Metrorrhagia and ginseng. *Ann Pharmacother* 2000; 34: 1347–1348.
32 American Botanical Council. Ginseng Evaluation Program. http://www.herbalgram.org/projects/index.html (accessed 5 December 2000).
33 Consumerlab. Product review. Asian and American ginseng. http://www.consumerlab.com (accessed 5 December 2000).

Glucosamine

Description

Glucosamine is a natural substance found in mucopolysaccharides, mucoproteins and chitin. It is found in relatively high concentrations in the joints. Some foods, such as crabs, oysters and the shells of prawns are relatively rich in glucosamine, but supplements are the best source of additional glucosamine. It is available as a synthetically manufactured dietary supplement in the form of glucosamine sulphate and glucosamine hydrochloride.

Constituents

Glucosamine is a hexosamine sugar and a basic building block for the biosynthesis of glycoprotein, glycolipids, hyaluronic acid, glycosaminoglycans and proteoglycans, which are important constituents of the articular cartilage. Chondroitin sulphate (sometimes found together with glucosamine in supplements), which is synthesised by the chondrocytes, is one example of a glycosaminoglycan.

Action

Glucosamine is important for maintaining the elasticity, strength and resilience of cartilage in joints. This helps to reduce damage to the joints. In addition to supporting cartilage and other connective tissue, glucosamine enhances the production of hyaluronic acid and enhances the anti-inflammatory action of this molecule.

The mechanism of action is not known. However, the administration of glucosamine is believed to stimulate production of cartilage components and allow rebuilding of damaged cartilage. *In vitro* studies have found that glucosamine can increase mucopolysaccharide and collagen synthesis in fibroblast tissue.[1] Glucosamine also appears to activate core protein synthesis in human chondrocytes.[2]

Possible uses

Glucosamine is used to promote the maintenance of joint function and to treat pain, increase mobility, and to help repair damaged joints in individuals with osteoarthritis and other joint disorders. It is sometimes provided in supplements with chondroitin (see Chondroitin monograph), with which it may act synergistically. Both substances have anti-inflammatory activities[3,4] and both affect cartilage metabolism *in vitro*.[5,6] Animal studies have also demonstrated that glucosamine has anti-arthritic effects.[7,8]

Since 1990, about 40 studies have examined the effects of glucosamine on osteoarthritis. However, most of these have been of short duration, and many have major design flaws and critical problems with data analysis and interpretation of results. The largest randomised placebo-controlled trials to date are discussed below.

In a double-blind trial,[9] 80 in-patients with established arthritis were randomly split into two groups. The first group received two 250 mg capsules of glucosamine sulphate, and the second group an indistinguishable placebo. Each dose was given three times daily for 30 days. Articular pain, joint tenderness and restriction of movement were scored on a scale of 1 to 4 at one-week intervals. Any adverse reactions were similarly scored. Safety was monitored by haematology; results of urine analysis and occult faecal blood were recorded before and after treatment. Samples of articular cartilage from two patients of each group and from one healthy subject were submitted for scanning electron microscopy after the end of treatment. Patients treated with glucosamine sulphate experienced a reduction in overall symptoms that was almost twice as great and twice as fast as those who had placebo. The results were supported by the electron microscopy findings.

Another double-blind trial[10] used 252 out-patients who had suffered arthritis in the knee to a measurable amount for at least six months. The trial randomly allocated the patients to two groups, one receiving 250 mg tablets of glucosamine sulphate and the other placebo, three times daily. The trial was of four weeks' duration, with assessment at enrolment and weekly thereafter. A statistically significant difference between glucosamine and placebo was observed, but only after the fourth week of treatment, and the clinical significance of the difference is open to debate.

A total of 155 out-patients with osteoarthritis of the knee were involved in another double-blind trial.[11] Inclusion criteria included a requirement to have been suffering from symptoms for at least six months. The two groups, consisting of 79 and 76 patients, received 400 mg glucosamine sulphate and placebo, respectively, administered as intramuscular injection twice weekly for six weeks. Assessment was made at enrolment, at two-weekly intervals during the trial, and once after the trial had been concluded. At the end of the trial the patients were assessed by the investigator and classified as good, moderate, unchanged, or worse. Safety was monitored by a number of biochemical tests. A significant improvement in symptoms was noted compared with placebo, but this occurred only during weeks five and six of the treatment. This may have been related to the twice-weekly dosing, or to the slow onset of action. However, methodological problems of lack of randomisation and missing data, such as symptom severity at baseline, make the clinical significance of the improvement questionable, and the observed differences may be meaningless.

Other trials have compared the efficacy of glucosamine with ibuprofen[12,13] and piroxicam.[14] Oral glucosamine sulphate 500 mg three times daily was reported to be at least as effective as oral ibuprofen 400 mg three times daily in a study involving 40 patients with osteoarthritis of the knee.[12] Pain scores decreased significantly in both groups, but the onset of action was more rapid with ibuprofen, with maximum effectiveness reached after two weeks, whereas glucosamine was associated with a gradual, progressive improvement throughout the trial.

In a randomised, double-blind, parallel-group study,[13] glucosamine 500 mg three times daily was as effective as ibuprofen 400 mg three times daily for four weeks in the treatment of 200 in-patients with osteoarthritis of the knee. Again, therapeutic effect was generally obtained sooner with ibuprofen, but glucosamine was significantly better tolerated than ibuprofen. A total of six patients reported adverse effects (versus 35 with ibuprofen) and one discontinued treatment (versus seven with ibuprofen). However, the definition of treatment response as well as the short duration of the study leave the results open to debate as to their clinical significance.

Glucosamine sulphate was as effective as piroxicam alone or a combination of glucosamine and piroxicam in a randomised multicentre, double-blind, placebo-controlled trial involving 329 patients.[14] Either glucosamine sulphate 1500 mg daily, piroxicam 20 mg daily, a combination of glucosamine and piroxicam, or placebo was given for 60 days, followed by a 60-day observation period without treatment. Glucosamine appeared to have a persistent treatment effect after withdrawal compared with piroxicam, and significantly fewer adverse effects were recorded for glucosamine.

Recently, two meta-analyses[15,16] have investigated the benefits of glucosamine in the treatment of osteoarthritis. One evaluated the benefit of both glucosamine and chondroitin for osteoarthritis symptoms.[15] A meta-analysis was used combined with systematic quality assessment of clinical trials of these preparations in knee and/or hip osteoarthritis. Reviewers performed data extraction and scored each trial using a quality assessment instrument. Of the 37 trials identified, only 15 met the criteria of being double-blind (published or unpublished), randomised, placebo-controlled or of four or more weeks' duration that tested glucosamine or chondroitin for knee or hip osteoarthritis and reported extractable data on the effect of treatment on symptoms. Of the five trials analysed, only six concerned glucosamine; the remaining nine (almost all of which were manufacturer-sponsored) were judged to be of inadequate quality by the authors. Nevertheless, it was concluded that trials of glucosamine and chondroitin preparations for osteoarthritis symptoms did show moderate to large beneficial effects, but that quality issues and likely publication bias might have exaggerated these benefits.

Another meta-analysis[16] included ten trials (three of which were also included in the above meta-analysis[15]). The trials included looked at glucosamine alone – not chondroitin. The method employed was a scoring system,[17] and only five of the 10 trials achieved the arbitrary pass mark. The major problems in most of the trials in this meta-analysis were a lack of participants, a lack of detail about the randomisation process, and no monitoring of patients after the trial period had finished. Of the 10 clinical trials, six compared glucosamine sulphate with placebo. Of the remaining four trials, two compared glucosamine with ibuprofen, and the other two used glucosamine sulphate alone. The results of this meta-analysis were in broad agreement with those of the above study[15] and were positive. However, the authors concluded that the variations in study methodology made it difficult to make a firm decision as to the overall effectiveness of glucosamine for the treatment of osteoarthritis.

Precautions/contraindications

Glucosamine may alter glucose regulation/insulin sensitivity.[18,19] Consequently, patients with diabetes who wish to take glucosamine should have their glucose levels monitored.

Pregnancy and breast-feeding

No problems have been reported, but there have not been sufficient studies to guarantee the safety of glucosamine in pregnancy and breast-feeding. Glucosamine is probably best avoided.

Conclusion

Glucosamine, and also chondroitin are likely to be effective therapies for the symptoms of osteoarthritis. However, more long-term, adequately designed, rigorous, controlled studies are required before the role of glucosamine in the treatment of bone and joint disorders can be determined. In addition, trials are needed to determine whether glucosamine can modify the radiological progression of osteoarthritis. Trials so far have provided evidence on the possible efficacy of glucosamine on symptoms, but not on the underlying pathophysiology.

Adverse effects

Glucosamine is relatively non-toxic, and does not appear to be associated with serious side-effects. Side-effects reported include: constipation, diarrhoea, heartburn, nausea, drowsiness, headache and rash.

Interactions

Drugs

None is known, but in theory the effects of insulin or oral hypoglycaemic agents may be reduced.

Dose

Glucosamine is available in the form of tablets, capsules and powders as glucosamine sulphate, glucosamine hydrochloride and *N*-acetyl-D-glucosamine (NAG). A review of 10 products containing glucosamine found that all products contained the labelled amounts of glucosamine, but six out of 13 products containing glucosamine and chondroitin did not pass, all due to low chondroitin levels.[20]

The dose is not definitely established. However, a dose of glucosamine sulphate 500 mg three times a day (1500 mg daily) has been used in most studies, and this is the dose that is recommended by many manufacturers.

References

1 McCarty MF. The neglect of glucosamine as treatment for osteoathritis. *Med Hypotheses* 1994; 42: 323–327.
2 Bassleer C, Henroitin Y, Franchimont P. In vitro evaluation of drugs proposed as chondroprotective agents. *Int J Tissue React* 1992; 14: 231–241.
3 Sentnikar I, Cereda R, Pacini MA, Revel L. Antireactive properties of glucosamine sulphate. *Arzneimittelforschung* 1991; 41: 157–161.
4 Ronca F, Palmieri L, Panicucci P, Ronca G. Anti-inflammatory activity of chondroitin sulphate. *Osteoarth Cart* 1998; 6 (suppl. A): 14–21.
5 Bassleer CT, Combal JP, Bougaret S, Malaise M. Effects of chondroitin sulphate and interleukin-1 beta on human articular chondrocytes cultivated in clusters. *Osteoarth Cart* 1998; 6: 196–204.
6 Bassleer CT, Rovati L, Franchimont P. Stimulation of proteoglycan production by glucosamine sulphate in chondrocytes isolated from human osteoarthritic articular cartilage in vitro. *Osteoarth Cart* 1998; 6: 427–434.
7 Setnikar I, Pacini MA, Revel L. Antiarthritic effects of glucosamine sulfate studied in animal models. *Arzneimittelforschung* 1991; 41: 542–545.
8 Uebelhart D, Thonar EJ, Zhang J, Williams JM. Protective effect of exogenous chondroitin 4,6-sulfate in the acute degradation of articular cartilage in the rabbit. *Osteoarth Cart* 1998; 6 (suppl. A): 6–13.
9 Drovanti A, Bignamini AA, Rovati AL. Therapeutic activity of oral glucosamine sulphate in osteoarthritis: A placebo controlled double blind investigation. *Clin Ther* 1980; 3: 260–272.
10 Noack W, Fischer M, Forster K, *et al.* Glucosamine in osteoarthritis of the knee. *Osteoarth Cart* 1994; 2: 51–59.
11 Reichelt A, Forster KK, Fischer M, *et al.* Efficacy and safety of intramuscular glucosamine sulphate in osteoarthritis of the knee. *Arzneimittelforschung* 1994; 44: 75–80.
12 Vaz AL. Double-blind clinical evaluation of the relative efficacy of ibuprofen and glucosamine sulphate in the management of osteoarthritis of the knee in outpatients. *Curr Med Res Opin* 1983; 3: 145–149.
13 Muller-Fassbender H, Bach G, Haase W, *et al.* Glucosamine sulphate compared with ibuprofen in osteoarthritis of the knee. *Osteoarth Cart* 1994; 2: 61–69.
14 Rovati LC, Giacovelli G, Annefeld M, *et al.* A large, randomized, placebo-controlled, double-blind study of glucosamine sulfate vs piroxicam and vs their association on the kinetics of the symptomatic effect in knee osteoarthritis (abstract). *Osteoarth Cart* 1994; 2 (suppl. 1): 56.
15 McAlindon TE, LeValley MP, Gulin JP, Felson DT. Glucosamine and chondroitin for treatment of osteoarthritis: A systematic quality assessment and meta-analysis. *JAMA* 2000; 283: 169–175.
16 Kayne SB, Wadeson K, MacAdam A. Glucosamine – an effective treatment for osteoarthritis? A meta-analysis. *Pharm J* 2000; 265: 759–763.
17 Kleijnen J, Knipschild P, ter Riet G. Clinical trials of homoeopathy. *Br Med J* 1991; 302: 316–323.
18 Balkan B, Dunning BE. Glucosamine inhibits glucokinase in vitro and produces a glucose-specific impairment of in vivo insulin secretion in rats. *Diabetes* 1994; 43: 1173–1179.
19 Shankar R.R, Zhu JS, Baron AD. Glucosamine infusion in mice mimics the beta-cell dysfunction of non-insulin dependent diabetes mellitus. *Metab Clin Exp* 1998; 47: 573–577.
20 Consumerlab. Product review. Glucosamine and chondroitin. http://www.consumerlab.com (accessed 5 December 2000).

Grape seed extract

Description

Grape seed extract is an extract from the tiny seeds of red grapes.

Constituents

Grape seed extract is a source of oligomeric proanthocyanidin complexes (OPCs), sometimes known as proanthocyanidins, which are one of the categories of flavonoids (see p. 88). Proanthocyanidins are polyphenol oligomers derived from flavan-3-ols and flavan-3,4-diols. Grape seed extract contains OPCs made up of dimers or trimers of catechin and epicatechin. Additional active ingredients in grape seed extract include essential fatty acids and tocopherols.

Proanthocyanidins used to be known as pycnogenols. Pycnogenol, itself, is a trademark for a specific proanthocyanidin derived from maritime pine bark. It can be used instead of grape seed extract, but tends to be more expensive.

Action

Grape seed is a potent antioxidant. Proanthocyanidins are thought to:[1]

- neutralise free radicals, including hydroxyl groups and lipid peroxides, blocking lipid peroxidation and stabilising cell membranes;
- inhibit the destruction of collagen by stabilising the activity of 1-antitrypsin, which inhibits the activity of destructive enzymes such as elastin and hyaluronic acid (this is thought to prevent fluid exudation by allowing red blood cells to cross the capillaries);
- inhibit the release of inflammatory mediators, such as histamine and prostaglandins; and
- inhibit platelet aggregation.

In addition, they are thought to have antibacterial, antiviral and anticarcinogenic actions.

Possible uses

Grapeseed extract is promoted as an antioxidant to prevent coronary heart disease and stroke, and to strengthen fragile capillaries and improve circulation to the extremities. It is promoted for the treatment of conditions associated with poor vascular function such as diabetes mellitus, varicose veins, impotence and tingling in the arms and legs. Anecdotally it has been reported to be useful for treating inflammatory conditions, varicose veins and cancer. It has also been suggested to be useful for helping to prevent macular degeneration and cataracts.

Cardiovascular disease

Oral administration of proanthocyanidins from grape seed extract reduced serum cholesterol in a high-cholesterol animal feed model.[2] Specifically, it prevented the increase of total and low-density lipoprotein (LDL) cholesterol.

In a double-blind study, 71 patients with peripheral venous insufficiency received 300 mg daily OPCs from grape seed. A reduction in functional symptoms was observed in 75% of the treated patients compared to 41% of the patients given a placebo.[3]

In a double-blind clinical trial, a group of elderly patients with either spontaneous or drug-induced poor capillary resistance were treated with 100–150 mg OPCs from grape extract daily, or placebo. There was a significant improvement in capillary resistance in the treated group after approximately two weeks.[4]

> **Conclusion**
> Preliminary evidence suggests that grape seed extract might lower lipid levels and improve symptoms of venous insufficiency and capillary resistance. However, there are no well-controlled studies, and evidence for efficacy is promising but not yet robust.

Precautions/contraindications

No known contraindications, but based on the potential pharmacological activity of OPCs (i.e. that they may inhibit platelet aggregation), grape seed extract should be used with caution in patients with a history of bleeding or haemostatic disorders. It is probably wise to discontinue use 14 days before any surgery, including dental surgery.

Pregnancy and breast-feeding

No problems have been reported, but there have not been sufficient studies to guarantee the safety of grape seed extract in pregnancy and breast-feeding.

Adverse effects

None reported. However, there are no long-term studies assessing the safety of grape seed extract.

Interactions

Drugs

None reported, but in theory, bleeding tendency may be increased with anticoagulants, aspirin and anti-platelet drugs.

Dose

Grape seed extract is available in the form of tablets and capsules. Supplements should be standardised (and labelled) to contain 92–95% proanthocyanidins or OPCs.

The dose is not established, but doses of 100–300 mg daily have been used in studies.

References

1 Murray M, Pizzorono J. Procyanidolic oligomers. In: Murray M, Pizzorono J, eds. *The Textbook of Natural Medicine*, 2nd edn. London: Churchill Livingstone, 1999: 899–902.

2 Tebib K, Bessanicon P, Roaunet J. Dietary grape seed tannins affect lipoproteins, lipoprotein lipases and tissue lipids in rats fed hypercholesterolemic diets. *J Nutr* 1994; 124: 2451–2457.

3 Thebaut JF, Thebaut P, Vin F. Study of Endotolon in functional manifestations of peripheral venous insufficiency. *Gaz Med France* 1985; 92: 96–100.

4 Dartenuc JY, Marache P, Choussat H. Capillary resistance in geriatry. A study of a microangioprotector – Endotolon. *Bord Med* 1980; 13: 903–907.

Green-lipped mussel

Description

Green-lipped mussel is an extract of the green-lipped mussel (*Perna canaliculata*), which is a salt-water shellfish indigenous to New Zealand.

Constituents

Green-lipped mussel extract contains a weak prostaglandin inhibitor that exerts an anti-inflammatory effect, as well as amino acids, fats, carbohydrates and minerals.

Possible uses

Green-lipped mussel extract is claimed to be effective in the treatment of rheumatoid arthritis. The small number of human studies published have generally shown that green-lipped mussel is not effective in arthritis,[1–3] but two studies have shown positive effects.[4,5] Evidence to show that green-lipped mussel works is equivocal.

Adverse effects

Green-lipped mussel extract is relatively non-toxic, but allergic reactions (e.g. gastrointestinal discomfort, nausea and flatulence) have been reported occasionally.

Dose

Green-lipped mussel extract is available in the form of capsules.

The dose is not established; dietary supplements provide approximately 1 g per daily dose.

References

1 Caughey DE, Grigor RR, Caughey EB. *Perna canaliculus* in the treatment of rheumatoid arthritis. *Eur J Rheumatol Inflamm* 1983; 6: 197–200.
2 Huskisson EC, Scott J, Bryans R. Seatone is ineffective in arthritis. *Br Med J* 1981; 282: 1358–1359.
3 Larkin JG, Capell HA, Sturrock RD. Seatone in rheumatoid arthritis: A six-month placebo-controlled study. *Ann Rheum Dis* 1985; 44: 199–201.
4 Gibson RG, Gibson SL. Seatone in arthritis. *Br Med J* 1981; 282: 1795.
5 Gibson RG, Gibson SL, Conway V, Chapell D. *Perna canaliculus* in the treatment of arthritis. *Practitioner* 1980; 224: 955–960.

Green tea extract

Description

Green tea is prepared from the steamed and dried leaves of *Camellia sinensis*. Green tea is different from black tea in that black tea is produced from leaves that have been withered, rolled, fermented and dried. The lack of fermentation gives green tea its unique flavour and also preserves the naturally present flavonoids, which are antioxidants.

Constituents

Green tea contains flavonoids, a large group of polyphenolic compounds with antioxidant properties. Of the flavonoids found in green tea, catechins make up 30–50% of the dry tea leaf weight. These include epigallocatechin gallate, epicatechin and epicatechin gallate. Green tea also contains flavonols, tannins, minerals, free amino acids, and methylxanthines (caffeine, theophylline and theobromine).

Action

Green tea appears to have the following effects:

- An antioxidant effect; green tea may protect against oxidative damage to cells and tissues.
- A chemoprotective effect that is attributed to the catechins. These compounds are thought to inhibit cell proliferation. *In vitro* studies have shown that green tea polyphenols induce programmed cell death (apoptosis) in human cancer cells[1,2] and block tumour growth by inhibition of tumour necrosis factor-α as well as a variety of other potential anti-cancer effects.[3–7] Animal studies have also shown the inhibitory effect of green tea against carcinogens.[8–10]
- Antibacterial and antiviral activity. *In vitro* studies have shown that green tea polyphenols block the growth of bacteria that cause diarrhoea[11] and viruses that cause influenza.[12]
- Reduction of serum cholesterol.
- Reduction in low-density lipoprotein (LDL) cholesterol oxidation. Two *in vitro* studies[13,14] showed that green tea can inhibit oxidation of LDL.
- Inhibition of platelet aggregation.

Possible uses

Green tea has been investigated mainly for supposed protective effects in cancer and cardiovascular disease.

Cancer

A review of 31 epidemiological studies[6] of green tea consumption and cancer risk showed no overall consistent effect. Of the total studies reviewed, 17 showed reduced cancer risk, seven increased risk, three no association and five an increased risk. Of the 10 studies on stomach cancer, six suggested a reduced risk and three an increased risk. Of the nine studies on colorectal cancer, four suggested a reduced risk and three an increased risk. Both studies on bladder cancer showed a reduced risk, and two out of the three studies on pancreatic cancer showed reduced risk. Studies examining oesophageal cancer showed mixed results, but very hot or scalding tea was associated with increased risk.

In a study of 472 Japanese women with stage I, II and III breast cancer,[15] the level of green tea consumption before clinical diagnosis of cancer was evaluated. Increased consumption of green tea was significantly associated with decreased numbers of axillary lymph node metastases among premenopausal patients with stage I and II breast cancer and increased expression of progesterone receptor and oestrogen receptor in postmenopausal patients. In a follow-up study, increased consumption of green tea was correlated with reduced recurrence of stage I and II breast cancer; the recurrence rate was 16.7% among those consuming five or more cups daily, or 24.3% in those consuming four or less cups daily. However, no improvement was seen in women with stage III breast cancer.

Green tea may block the frequency of sister chromatid exchange (SCE), a biomarker of mutagenesis. A study in 52 Korean smokers[16] showed that SCE rates were significantly higher in smokers than non-smokers. However, the frequency of SCE in smokers who consumed green tea was comparable with that of non-smokers.

Cardiovascular disease

A cross-sectional study of the effects of drinking green tea on cardiovascular and liver disease[17] in 1371 Japanese men (aged >40 years) showed that increased green tea consumption was associated with reduced serum concentrations of total cholesterol and triglyceride and an increased proportion of high-density lipoprotein (HDL) cholesterol with a decreased proportion of LDL and very-low-density lipoprotein (VLDL) cholesterol. In addition, increased consumption of green tea was associated with reduced concentrations of hepatic markers in serum (aspartate aminotransferase, alanine transferase and ferritin).

However, another cross-sectional study in 371 individuals from five districts of Japan[18] showed that green tea was not associated with serum concentrations of total cholesterol, triglycerides and HDL cholesterol.

Another study examined the relation between green tea consumption and arteriographically determined coronary atherosclerosis.[19] The subjects were 512 patients (302 men, 210 women) aged 30 years or more who had undergone coronary arteriography for the first time between September 1996 and August 1997. Green tea consumption tended to be inversely associated with coronary atherosclerosis in men but not in women.

Conclusion
Green tea has been investigated for protective effects in cancer and cardiovascular disease. However, results from studies so far have been conflicting.

Precautions/contraindications

There are no known contraindications, but based on the potential pharmacological activity of polyphenols (i.e. that they may inhibit platelet aggregation), green tea extract should be used with caution in patients with a history of bleeding or haemostatic disorders. It is probably wise to discontinue use 14 days before any surgery, including dental surgery.

Pregnancy and breast-feeding

No problems have been reported, but there have been insufficient studies to guarantee the safety of green tea supplements in pregnancy and breast-feeding.

Adverse effects

None has been reported. However, some people are allergic to green tea. There is a lack of tolerance and safety data on supplements of this substance, although green tea has been consumed safely in China for more than 4000 years.

Interactions

Drugs

None is known, but in theory, bleeding tendency may be increased with anticoagulants, aspirin and anti-platelet drugs.

Dose

Green tea is available in the form of capsules as well as tea for drinking.

The dose is not established, but doses of 250–300 mg daily have been used. Supplements should be standardised (and labelled) to contain 50–97% polyphenols, containing per dose at least 50% (-)epigallocatechin-3-gallate. Four to six cups of freshly brewed green tea should provide similar levels of polyphenols.

References

1 Ahmad N, Feyes DK, Niemenen AL, *et al*. Green tea constituent epigallocatechin-3-gallate and induction of apoptosis and cell cycle arrest in human carcinoma cells. *J Natl Cancer Inst* 1997; 89: 1881–1886.
2 Hibasami H, Komiya T, Achiwa Y, *et al*. Induction of apoptosis in human stomach cancer cells by green tea catechins. *Oncol Rep* 1998; 5: 527–529.
3 Kuroda Y, Hara Y. Antimutagenic and anticarcinogenic activity of tea polyphenols. *Mutat Res* 1999; 436: 69–97.
4 Leanderson P, Faresjo AO, Tagesson C. Green tea polyphenols inhibit oxidant-induced DNA strand breakage in cultured lung cells. *Free Radical Biol Med* 1997; 310: 235–242.
5 Fujiki H, Suganuma M, Okabe S, *et al*. Mechanistic findings of green tea as cancer preventive for humans. *Proc Soc Exp Biol Med* 1999; 220: 225–228.
6 Bushman JL. Green tea and cancer in humans: a review of the literature. *Nutr Cancer* 1998; 31: 151–159.
7 Nihal A, Hasan M. Green tea polyphenols and cancer: biological mechanisms and practical implications. *Nutr Rev* 1999; 57: 78–83.
8 Yang CS, Yang GY, Landau JM, *et al*. Tea and tea polyphenols inhibit cell proliferation, lung tumorigenesis and tumour progression. *Exp Lung Res* 1998; 24: 629–639.
9 Wang ZY, Huang MT, Ferraro T, *et al*. Inhibitory effect of green tea in the drinking water on tumorigenesis by ultraviolet light and 12-O-tetradecanoylphorbol-13-acetate in the skin of SKH-1 mice. *Cancer Res* 1992; 52: 1162–1170.
10 Paschka GA, Butler R, Young CY. Induction of apoptosis in prostate cancer lines by the green tea component (-)epigallocatechin-3-gallate. *Cancer Lett* 1998; 130: 1–7.
11 Shetty M, Subbannaya K, Shivananda PG. Antibacterial activity of tea (*Camellia sinensis*) and coffee (*Coffee arabica*) with special reference to *Salmonella typhimurium*. *J Commun Dis* 1994; 26: 147–150.
12 Nakayama M, Suzuki K, Toda M, *et al*. Inhibition of the infectivity of influenza virus by tea polyphenols. *Antiviral Res* 1993; 21: 289–299.
13 van het Kof KH, de Boer HS, Wiseman SA, *et al*. Consumption of green or black tea does not increase resistance of low-density lipoprotein to oxidation in humans. *Am J Clin Nutr* 1997; 66: 1125–1132.
14 Yokozawa T, Dong E. Influence of green tea and its three major components upon low density lipoprotein oxidation. *Exp Toxicol Pathol* 1997; 49: 329–335.
15 Nakachi K, Suemasu K, Suga K, *et al*. Influence of drinking green tea on breast cancer malignancy among Japanese patients. *Jpn J Cancer Res* 1998; 89: 254–261.
16 Lee IP, Kim JH, Kang MH, *et al*. Chemoprotective effect of green tea (*Camellia sinensis*) against cigarette smoke-induced mutations (SCE) in humans. *J Cell Biochem Suppl* 1997; 27: 68–75.
17 Imai K, Nakachi K. Cross-sectional study of effects of drinking green tea on cardiovascular and liver disease. *Br Med J* 1995; 310: 693–696.
18 Tsubono Y, Tsugane S. Green tea intake in relation to serum lipid levels in middle-aged Japanese men and women. *Ann Epidemiol* 1997; 7: 280–284.
19 Sasazuki S, Kodama H, Yoshimasu K, *et al*. Relation between green tea consumption and the severity of coronary atherosclerosis among Japanese men and women. *Ann Epidemiol* 2000; 10: 401–408.

Guarana

Description

Guarana is produced from the seeds of a South American shrub, *Paullinia cupana*, which are dried and powdered.

Constituents

Guarana contains a substance named guaranine (a synonym for caffeine). It also contains theobromine, theophylline and tannins.

Action

Guarana acts as a CNS stimulant, increases heart rate and contractility, increases blood pressure, inhibits platelet aggregation, stimulates gastric acid secretion, causes diuresis, relaxes bronchial smooth muscle and stimulates the release of catecholamines.

Possible uses

Guarana is claimed to:

- improve mental alertness, endurance, vitality, immunity, stamina in athletes and sexual drive;
- retard ageing;
- alleviate migraine, diarrhoea, constipation and tension; and
- act as an appetite suppressant to aid slimming.

Because of its caffeine content, guarana is likely to be effective when taken as a CNS stimulant, but it has not been subjected to controlled trials. There is no good evidence that guarana improves stamina and performance in athletes. There is insufficient reliable information about the effectiveness of guarana for other indications.

Precautions/contraindications

Guarana should be avoided by people with heart conditions, peptic ulcer, anxiety disorders, renal impairment. It should also not be taken within 2 h of bedtime.

Pregnancy and breast-feeding

Guarana should be avoided during pregnancy and breast-feeding.

Adverse effects

High doses of guarana may cause insomnia, nervousness, irritability, palpitations, gastric irritation, flushing and elevated blood pressure.

Interactions

None has been reported.

Dose

Guarana is available in the form of tablets and capsules either in isolation or with vitamins and minerals in other dietary supplements.

The dose is not established. Guarana should not be recommended. Dietary supplements provide 50–200 mg.

Iodine

Description

Iodine is an essential trace element.

Human requirements

See Table 1 for Dietary Reference Values for iodine.

Intakes

In the UK, the average adult daily diet provides: for men, 251 μg; for women, 184 μg.

Action

Iodine is an essential part of the thyroid hormones, thyroxine (T_4) and triiodothyronine (T_3).

Dietary sources

See Table 2 for dietary sources of iodine.

Table 1 Dietary Reference Values for iodine (μg/day)
EU RDA (for labelling purposes) = 150 μg

Age	UK		USA		WHO	Europe
	LNRI	RNI	RDA	UL	RNI	PRI
0–3 months	40	50	110[1]	–	50	–
4–6 months	40	60	110[1]	–	50	–
7–12 months	40	60	130	–	50	50
1–3 years	40	70	90	200	90	70
4–6 years	50	100	–	–	90	90
4–8 years	–	–	90	300	–	–
7–10 years	55	110	–	–	120	100
9–13 years	–	–	120	600	–	–
14–18 years	–	–	150	900	–	–
Males and females						
11–14 years	65	130	–	–	150	120
15–18 years	70	140	–	–	150	130
19–50+	70	140	150	1100	150	130
Pregnancy	*	*	220	1100[2]	200	*
Lactation	*	*	290	1100[2]	200	*

*No increment.
[1]Adequate Intakes (AIs).
[2]aged <18 years, 90 μg daily.
UL = Tolerable Upper Intake Level.

Table 2 Dietary sources of iodine

Food portion	Iodine content (μg)
Milk and dairy products	
½ pint (280 ml) milk, whole, semi–skimmed or skimmed	*45*
1 pot yoghurt (150 g)	*90*
Cheese (50 g)	*25*
Fish	
Cod, cooked (150 g)	**150**
Haddock, cooked (150 g)	**300**
Mackerel, cooked (150 g)	**200**
Plaice, cooked (150 g)	*50*

Excellent sources (**bold**); good sources (*italics*).
Note: Iodised salt contains 150 μg/5 g.

Metabolism

Absorption

Inorganic iodine is rapidly and efficiently absorbed. Organically bound iodine is less well absorbed.

Distribution

Iodine is transported to the thyroid gland (for the synthesis of thyroid hormones), and to a lesser extent to the salivary and gastric glands.

Elimination

Excretion of inorganic iodine is mainly via the urine. Some organic iodine is eliminated in the faeces. Iodine is excreted in the breast milk.

Deficiency

Iodine deficiency leads to goitre and hypothyroidism.

Possible uses

Supplements containing iodine may be required by vegans (strict vegetarians who consume no dairy products). In a study in Greater London which included 38 vegans,[1] intakes of iodine in the vegan individuals were below the Dietary Reference Values. The authors of the study concluded that the impact of these low iodine intakes should be studied further, and that vegans should use appropriate dietary supplements. A further study[2] confirmed a markedly reduced iodine intake with a lactovegetarian diet compared with an ordinary diet.

Precautions/contraindications

None has been reported.

Pregnancy and breast-feeding

Doses exceeding the RDA should not be used (they may result in abnormal thyroid function in the infant).

Adverse effects

High iodine intake may induce hyperthyroidism (particularly in those over the age of 40 years) and toxic modular goitre or hypothyroidism in autoimmune thyroid disease. There is a risk of hyperkalaemia with prolonged use of high doses. Toxicity is rare with intakes below 5000 μg daily and extremely rare at intakes below 1000 μg daily.

Hypersensitivity reactions including, headache, rashes, symptoms of head cold, swelling of lips, throat and tongue, arthralgia (joint pain) have been reported.

Interactions

Drugs

Antithyroid drugs: iodine may interfere with thyroid control.

Dose

Iodine is available mostly as an ingredient in multivitamin and mineral products.

Dietary supplements will usually provide 50–100% of the RDA.

References

1 Draper A, Lewis J, Malhotra N, Wheeler E. The energy and nutrient intakes of different types of vegetarian: A case for supplements? *Br J Nutr* 1993; 69: 3–19.
2 Remer T, Neubert A, Manz F. Increased risk of iodine deficiency with vegetarian nutrition. *Br J Nutr* 1999; 81: 45–49.

Iron

Description

Iron is an essential trace mineral.

Human requirements

See Table 1 for Dietary Reference Values of iron.

Table 1 Dietary Reference Values for iron (mg/day)

EU RDA (for labelling purposes) = 14 mg

Age	UK			USA		WHO	Europe
	LNRI	EAR	RNI	RDA	UL	RNI	PRI
0–3 months	0.9	1.3	1.7	0.27[2]	40	–	–
4–6 months	2.3	3.3	4.3	0.27[2]	40	8.5	–
7–12 months	4.2	6.0	7.8	11	40	8.5	6
1–3 years	3.7	5.3	6.9	7	40	5.0	4
4–6 years	3.3	4.7	6.1	–	–	5.5	4
4–8 years	–	–	–	10	40	–	–
7–10 years	4.7	6.7	8.7	10	–	9.5	6
9–13 years	–	–	–	8	40	–	–
Males							
11–14 years	6.1	8.7	11.3	–	–	15.0	10
15–18 years	6.1	8.7	11.3	–	–	9.0	13
14–18 years	–	–	–	11	45	–	–
19–50+ years	4.7	6.7	8.7	8	45	9.0	9
Females							
11–14 years	8.0	11.4	14.8[1]	–	–	16.0	18–22
14–18 years	–	–	–	15	45	–	–
15–50+ years	8.0	11.4	14.8[1]	–	–	12.5	17–21
19–50+ years	–	–	–	18	45	–	–
50+ years	4.7	6.7	8.7	8	45	9.5	8
Pregnancy	*	*	*	27	45	*	*
Lactation	*	*	*	9[3]	45	10.5	10
Postmenopause				8			
Premenopause				18			

*No increment.
[1]Insufficient level for women who have high menstrual losses who may need iron supplements.
[2]Adequate Intakes (AIs).
[3]aged <18 years, 10 mg daily.
UL = Tolerable Upper Intake Level.

Intakes

In the UK, the average adult daily diet provides: for men 14.5 mg; for women, 12.9 mg. Dietary iron consists of haem and non-haem iron; in animal foods, about 40% of the iron is haem iron and 60% is non-haem iron; all the iron in vegetable products is non-haem iron.

Action

Iron is a component of haemoglobin, myoglobin and many enzymes which are involved in a variety of metabolic functions, including transport and storage of oxygen, the electron transport chain, DNA synthesis and catecholamine metabolism.

Dietary sources

See Table 2 for dietary sources of iron.

Metabolism

Absorption

Absorption of iron occurs principally in the duodenum and proximal jejunum. Absorption of food iron varies between 5 and 15%. Haem iron is more efficiently absorbed than non-haem iron. Body iron content is regulated mainly through changes in absorption.

Distribution

Iron is transported in the blood bound to the protein transferrin, and is stored in the liver, spleen and bone marrow as ferritin and haemosiderin.

Elimination

The body has a limited capacity to eliminate iron, and iron can accumulate in the body to toxic amounts. Small amounts are excreted in the faeces, urine, skin, sweat, hair, nails and menstrual blood.

Bioavailability

The absorption of non-haem iron is enhanced by concurrent ingestion of meat, poultry and fish, and by various organic acids, especially ascorbic acid; it is inhibited by phytates (found in bran and high-fibre cereals), tannins (found in tea and coffee), egg yolk and by some drugs and nutrients (see Interactions). Ferrous salts are more efficiently absorbed than ferric salts.

Deficiency

Iron deficiency leads to microcytic, hypochromic anaemia. Symptoms include fatigue, weakness, pallor, dyspnoea on exertion and palpitations. Non-haematological effects include impairment in work capacity, intellectual performance, neurological function and immune function, and, in children, behavioural disturbances. Gastrointestinal symptoms are also fairly common and the fingernails may become lustreless, brittle, flattened and spoon-shaped.

Possible uses

Requirements may be increased and/or supplements needed in:

- infants and children from the age of 6 months to 4 years;
- early adolescence;
- the female reproductive period;
- pregnancy; and
- vegetarians.

Precautions/contraindications

Iron supplements should be avoided in: conditions associated with iron overload (e.g. haemochromatosis, haemosiderosis, thalassaemia); gastrointestinal disease, particularly inflammatory bowel disease, intestinal stricture, diverticulitis and peptic ulcer.

Pregnancy and breast-feeding

The Reference Nutrient Intake for iron during pregnancy is no greater than for other adult women. Requirements during pregnancy are partly offset by lack of menstruation and partly by increased efficiency of absorption. Routine iron supplementation is not required in pregnancy, but iron status should be monitored.

Table 2 Dietary sources of iron

Food portion	Iron content (mg)	Food portion	Iron content (mg)
Breakfast cereals		**Liver, lamb's, cooked (90 g)**	**9**
1 bowl All-Bran (45 g)	**5**	**Kidney, lamb's, cooked (75 g)**	**9**
1 bowl Bran Flakes (45 g)	**9**		
1 bowl Corn Flakes (30 g)	*2*	**Fish**	
1 bowl Muesli (95 g)	**5**	**Cockles (80 g)**	**21**
2 pieces Shredded Wheat	*2*	**Mussels (80 g)**	**6**
1 bowl Special K (35 g)	*4*	*Pilchards, canned (105 g)*	*2.8*
1 bowl Start (30 g)	**5**	*Sardines, canned (70 g)*	*3*
1 bowl Sultana Bran (35 g)	**5**		
2 Weetabix	*3*	**Vegetables**	
		Green vegetables, average, boiled (100g)	*1.5*
Cereal products		Potatoes, boiled (150 g)	0.5
Bread, brown, 2 slices	*1.5*	*1 small can baked beans (200 g)*	*3*
white[1], 2 slices	1	*Lentils, kidney beans or other pulses (105 g)*	*2*
wholemeal, 2 slices	*2*	**Dahl, chickpea (155 g)**	**5**
1 chapati	*1.5*	*Soya beans, cooked (100 g)*	*3*
1 naan	*3.5*		
Pasta, brown, boiled (150 g)	*2.0*	**Fruit**	
white, boiled (150 g)	1.0	*8 dried apricots*	*2*
Rice, brown, boiled (165 g)	0.7	*4 figs*	*2.5*
white, boiled (165 g)	0.3	*½ an avocado pear*	*1.5*
		Blackberries (100 g)	1
Dairy products		Blackcurrants (100 g)	1
1 egg, size 2 (60 g)	1		
		Nuts	
Meat		20 almonds	1
Red meat, roast (85 g)	*2.5*	10 Brazil nuts	1
1 beef steak (155 g)	**5.4**	1 small bag peanuts (25 g)	0.5
Minced beef, lean, stewed (100 g)	**3**		
1 chicken leg (190 g)	*1*	*Milk chocolate (100 g)*	*1.6*
		Plain chocolate (100 g)	*2.4*

[1]White bread is supplemented with additional iron in the UK.
Excellent sources (**bold**); good sources (*italics*).

Adverse effects

Iron supplements may cause gastrointestinal irritation, nausea and constipation, which may lead to faecal impaction, particularly in the elderly. Patients with inflammatory bowel disease may suffer exacerbation of diarrhoea. Any reduced incidence of side-effects associated with modified-release preparations may be due to the fact that only small amounts of iron are released in the intestine. Liquid iron preparations may stain the teeth.

Interactions

Drugs

Antacids: reduced absorption of iron; give 2 h apart.
Bisphosphonates: reduced absorption of bisphosphonates; give 2 h apart.
Co-careldopa: reduced plasma levels of carbidopa and levodopa.
Levodopa: absorption of levodopa may be reduced.

Methyldopa: reduced absorption of methyldopa.
Penicillamine: reduced absorption of penicillamine.
4-Quinolones: absorption of ciprofloxacin, norfloxacin and ofloxacin reduced by oral iron; give 2 h apart.
Tetracyclines: reduced absorption of iron and vice-versa; give 2 h apart.
Trientine: reduced absorption of iron; give 2 h apart.

Nutrients

Calcium: calcium carbonate or calcium phosphate may reduce absorption of iron; give 2 h apart (absorption of iron in multiple formulations containing iron and calcium is not significantly altered).
Copper: large doses of iron may reduce copper status and vice-versa.
Manganese: reduced absorption of manganese.
Vitamin E: large doses of iron may increase requirement for vitamin E; vitamin E may impair haematological response to iron in patients with iron-deficiency anaemia.
Zinc: reduced absorption of iron and vice-versa.

Dose

Iron is best taken on an empty stomach, but food reduces the possibility of stomach upsets; oral liquid preparations should be well diluted with water or fruit juice and drunk through a straw.

As a dietary supplement, 10–20 mg daily.

Note: doses are given in terms of elemental iron; patients should be advised that iron supplements are not identical and provide different amounts of elemental iron; iron content of various iron salts commonly used in supplements is shown in Table 3.

Table 3 Iron content of commonly used iron supplements

Iron salt	Iron (mg/g)	Iron (%)
Ferrous fumarate	330	33
Ferrous gluconate	120	12
Ferrous glycine sulphate	180	18
Ferrous orotate	150	15
Ferrous succinate	350	35
Ferrous sulphate	200	20
Ferrous sulphate, dried	300	30
Iron amino acid chelate	100	10

Isoflavones

Description

Isoflavones belong to the class of compounds known as flavonoids, and are found principally in soya beans and products made from them, including soya flour, soya milk, tempeh and tofu. They are present in varying amounts depending on the type of soya product and how it is processed. Isoflavones are also found in dietary supplements.

Constituents

The principal isoflavones in the soya bean are genistein, daidzein and glycetin, which are present mainly as glycosides. After ingestion, the glycosides are hydrolysed in the large intestine by the action of bacteria to release genistein, daidzein and glycetin. Daidzein can be metabolised by the bacteria in the large intestine to form either equol, which is oestrogenic or O-desmethylangolensin, which is non-oestrogenic, while genistein is metabolised to the non-oestrogenic P-ethyl phenol. Variation in the ability to metabolise daidzein could therefore have an influence on the health effects of isoflavones.

Action

Isoflavones are naturally occurring weak oestrogens, also known as phyto-oestrogens, which are capable of binding to oestrogen receptors where, depending on the hormonal status of the individual, they seem to exert either oestrogenic or anti-oestrogenic effects. Premenopausally, isoflavones may therefore be anti-oestrogenic, while postmenopausally they could act oestrogenically, although further research is required to confirm this concept.

There are two types of oestrogen receptors – alpha and beta – and different tissues appear to have different ratios of each type. Thus, alpha receptors appear to predominate in breast, uterus and ovary, while beta receptors appear to predominate in prostate, bone and vascular tissue. Phyto-oestrogens, although less potent than endogenous or synthetic oestrogens, have been shown to bind to beta oestrogen receptors, raising the possibility that phyto-oestrogens could produce beneficial effects on, for example, bone and vascular tissue, without causing adverse effects on the breast and ovary.

In addition to these hormonal effects, animal and *in-vitro* evidence indicates that isoflavones arrest growth of cancer cells through inhibition of DNA replication, interference of signal transduction pathways, and reduction in the activity of various enzymes. Isoflavones also exhibit antioxidant effects, suppress angiogenesis and inhibit the actions of various growth factors and cytokines.[1]

Possible uses

Isoflavones have been investigated for a potential role in cardiovascular disease, cancer, osteoporosis and menopausal symptoms.

Cardiovascular disease

Products containing soya protein have been shown to reduce both total and low-density lipoprotein (LDL) cholesterol in some – but not all – studies in animals and humans with raised cholesterol levels. The mechanisms by which soya foods could reduce cholesterol are being investigated, but may include enhancement of bile acid secretion and reduced cholesterol metabolism. Other mechanisms, independent of cholesterol lowering, by which soya could be cardioprotective, include reduction of platelet aggregation and clot formation, and inhibition of atherosclerosis by an antioxidant effect and by inhibiting cell adhesion and proliferation in the arteries.[2] However, further studies are required to confirm these possibilities.

In addition, the question of which constituents of soya are actually responsible for lipid lowering is under discussion, and it is not certain that isoflavones are the components responsible for any beneficial effect. Animal studies specifically comparing the effects of isoflavone-rich soya with isoflavone-free soya on a range of blood lipids have produced conflicting results.

A meta-analysis of 38 controlled clinical trials looking at the effects of soya protein on serum lipid levels in humans showed that there was a statistically significant association between soya protein intake and improvement in serum lipid levels.[3] Of the 38 trials, 34 reported a reduction in serum cholesterol, and overall there was a 9.3% decrease in total cholesterol, a 12.9% decrease in LDL cholesterol and a 10.5% decrease in triacylglycerols. High-density lipoprotein (HDL) cholesterol was increased, but this change was not significant.

A double-blind, randomised trial of six months' duration involving 66 postmenopausal women with hypercholesterolaemia found that compared to control, soya protein providing either 56 mg or 90 mg isoflavones significantly reduced non-HDL cholesterol and raised HDL cholesterol, with no change in total cholesterol.[4]

The effects of consuming a soya protein beverage powder compared with a casein supplement was evaluated in 20 male subjects who were randomly allocated into the two groups.[5] There were no significant differences in total and HDL cholesterol or in platelet aggregation between the groups, possibly because the men were normocholesterolaemic at entry into the study.

Soya protein was found to enhance the effect of a low-fat, low-cholesterol diet by reducing serum LDL cholesterol and increasing the ratio of LDL cholesterol to HDL cholesterol in men with both normal and high serum lipid levels.[6]

In a double-blind, placebo-controlled trial involving 156 healthy men and women, soya protein providing 62 mg isoflavones was associated with a significant reduction in total and LDL cholesterol compared with isoflavone-free soya protein (the placebo).[7] Moreover, soya protein providing 37 mg isoflavones was also associated with a decrease in total and LDL cholesterol, but the reduction was significant only in those subjects with a baseline LDL exceeding 4.24 mmol/l. There was no effect on HDL levels or triacylglycerols. Soya protein providing a lower dose of isoflavones (27 mg daily) had no effect on any of the measured indices. In subjects with baseline LDL levels between 3.62 and 4.24 mmol/l there was no significant effect of any dose of isoflavones.

A further study, involving 81 men with moderate hypercholesterolaemia (total serum cholesterol 5.7–7.7 mmol/l), found that soya protein (20 g daily, providing 37.5 mg isoflavones) reduced non-HDL cholesterol by 2.6% and total cholesterol by 1.8% after six weeks.[8]

A study in 13 premenopausal women with normal serum cholesterol levels found that total cholesterol, HDL cholesterol and LDL cholesterol levels changed significantly across menstrual cycle phases. During specific phases of the cycle, soya protein providing 128.7 mg isoflavones significantly lowered LDL cholesterol by 7.6–10.0%, the ratio of total to HDL cholesterol by 10.2%, and the ratio of LDL to HDL cholesterol by 13.8%. Despite the high intake of isoflavones, the changes in lipid concentrations were small, but the authors concluded that over a lifetime the small effects observed could slow the development of atherosclerosis and reduce the risk of coronary heart disease (CHD) in women with normal cholesterol levels.[9]

A preliminary study in six subjects investigated the effect of soya (providing genistein 12 mg and daidzein 7 mg) daily for two weeks on the resistance of LDL to oxidation, since it appears that LDL has to be oxidised before it can damage the arteries. The results from this small study indicated that isoflavones could offer protection against LDL oxidation.[10]

A randomised, cross-over study in 24 subjects compared a soya-free diet with a diet enriched with soya (providing a daily amount of 1.9 mg or 66 mg of isoflavones). The aim was to investigate the effects of the diets on biomarkers of lipid peroxidation and resistance of LDL to oxidation, since oxidative damage to lipids may be involved in the aetiology of atherosclerosis and cardiovascular disease. The diet high in isoflavones reduced lipid peroxidation and increased the resistance of LDL to oxidation.[11]

Studies giving isoflavones in tablet form have yielded less positive results than those using soya protein. Forty six men and 13 postmenopausal women not taking hormone replacement therapy, all with average serum cholesterol levels, participated in a randomised, double-blind, placebo-controlled trial of two-way parallel design and eight weeks' duration. One tablet containing 55 mg isoflavones (predominantly in the form of genistein) or placebo was taken daily. Post intervention, there were no significant differences in total, LDL and HDL cholesterol and lipoprotein(a).[12]

Another trial, this time in 14 premenopausal women, found that a supplement providing isoflavones 86 mg daily for two months produced no change compared with placebo in plasma concentrations of total cholesterol and triacylglycerol, nor in the oxidisability of LDL.[13] A further study in 20 healthy postmenopausal women (age 50–70 years) with evidence of endothelial dysfunction, found that a soyabean tablet providing 80 mg of isoflavones daily for eight weeks produced no significant effects on plasma lipids compared with placebo.[14]

The effects of dietary isoflavone supplementation using a purified red clover supplement (containing approximately: biochanin A 26 mg, formononetin 16 mg, daidzein 0.5 mg and genistein 1 mg per tablet) at doses of one to two tablets daily were compared with placebo in a three-period, randomised, double-blind, ascending-dose study in 66 postmenopausal women with moderately elevated plasma cholesterol levels (5.0–9.0 mmol/l).[15] Each of the three treatment periods lasted for four weeks. The dietary supplement did not significantly alter plasma total cholesterol, LDL or HDL cholesterol or plasma triglycerides.

Cancer

Epidemiological studies have shown that populations with high intakes of soya foods – such as in China, Japan and other Asian countries – usually have a lower risk of cancers of the breast, uterus, prostate and colon.[16,17] Experimental evidence from *in vitro* and animal studies on the effects of isoflavones on cancerous cells[18–20] has led to the suggestion that isoflavones might reduce the risk of cancer in humans.

Substantial reduction in risk of breast cancer has been reported among women with high intakes of phyto-oestrogens (as evidenced from urinary excretion).[21] Lower urinary daidzein and genistein concentrations were found in postmenopausal women with recently diagnosed breast cancer compared with controls.[22] Isoflavones appear to protect against cancer by influences on growth factor, malignant cell proliferation and cell differentiation. However, most clinical studies have not specifically examined the relationship between isoflavone intake and cancer risk, so definitive data are not available. Clinical trials in prostate cancer are in progress, and studies in breast cancer are being considered.

Osteoporosis

There is some evidence from animal studies that soya isoflavones preserve bone mineral density.[23,24] A preliminary study in 66 hypercholesterolaemic, postmenopausal women supplemented with soya protein (providing either 1.39 mg isoflavones/g protein or 2.2 mg/g protein) or placebo for six months showed that the higher dose of isoflavones was associated with a significant increase in bone mineral density at the lumbar spine site.[25] The lower dose was not associated with any change in bone mineral density. HDL cholesterol (the beneficial type) increased significantly with both soya treatments.

More recently, a study examined the effects of 24-week consumption of soya protein isolate with isoflavones (80.4 mg daily) on bone loss in perimenopausal women.[26] The randomised, double-blind study showed that soya isoflavones attenuated the reduction in lumbar spine bone mineral density and bone mineral content, both of which occurred in the control group.

Some studies conducted with ipriflavone, a synthetic isoflavone, available as a dietary supplement, found that ipriflavone reduced bone loss in postmenopausal women.[27–29] Currently, a number of further studies are underway looking at the effect of soya protein or isoflavone supplements on bone health.

Menopausal symptoms

Reduction of oestrogen production in middle-aged women is associated with symptoms of the menopause, such as hot flushes, vaginal dryness and atrophic vaginitis, and is also thought to contribute to the increased risk of CHD and osteoporosis. The main symptoms of the menopause were once thought to occur universally, but women in some countries (such as Japan) appear to experience symptoms such as hot flushes less frequently than women in western countries[30] and far fewer Japanese women use hormone replacement therapy post-menopausally.[31]

Several preliminary studies on the effects of administration of soya isoflavones on menopausal symptoms indicate possible benefit, but the overall evidence is inconclusive. One study involved 58 postmenopausal women with at least 14 hot flushes a week.[32] They received either 45 g soya flour or wheat flour each day as a supplement to their regular diet over 12 weeks in a randomised, double-blind design. Hot flushes decreased in both groups (45% in the soya group and 25% in the controls), with a rapid response in the soya group at six weeks. Menopausal symptoms also decreased significantly in both groups. The authors concluded that the lack of difference between the two groups could be due either to a strong placebo effect, or to a decline with time in symptoms.

Another study provides more persuasive information. A total of 145 postmenopausal women were randomised to receive either three servings of soya foods daily or control for 12 weeks.[33] Menopausal symptom scores, hot flushes and vaginal dryness decreased by 50, 54 and 60%, respectively, in women on the soya diet. These three parameters also fell in the control group, but only the reduction in menopausal symptom score was significant.

More recently, a double-blind, placebo-controlled study involved 104 postmenopausal women who were randomised to receive 60 g soya protein isolate, containing 76 mg isoflavones, or a control.[34] In comparison with placebo, subjects on the soya supplement reported statistically fewer mean number of flushes per 24 h after four, eight and 12 weeks. By week three, the treated group experienced a 26% reduction in the mean number of hot flushes, a 33% reduction by week 4, and by week 12 a 45% reduction compared with 30% in the control group.

Conclusion

Many studies have evaluated the effects of isoflavones on cardiovascular disease, cancer, osteoporosis and menopausal symptoms. However, data are inconclusive on whether potential beneficial effects are attributable to isoflavones alone or to other components in the foods that contain them. The most convincing data to date relate to those of soya foods containing isoflavones – rather than dietary supplements – on plasma lipid levels. Moreover, effects seem to be greater in individuals with high cholesterol levels than in those with levels in the normal range.

Data on the ability of isoflavones to protect against various cancers (including breast cancer) and osteoporosis are, as yet, inconclusive. Results of some research support the value of isoflavones in reducing menopausal symptoms such as hot flushes, but several studies have found no differences between those treated with isoflavones and controls. Contrary to claims being made for supplements containing these compounds, there is insufficient evidence to say that they can be used as a substitute for hormone replacement therapy during the menopause.

Precautions/contraindications

Use with caution in individuals at risk of hormone-dependent cancers.

Pregnancy and breast-feeding

No problems have been reported, but there have not been sufficient studies to guarantee the safety of isoflavones in pregnancy and breast-feeding. Because of their hormonal effects, isoflavones are probably best avoided.

Adverse effects

Soya foods have been consumed in Asian cultures for centuries. However, studies to assess the long-term safety of supplemental soya protein isolates or isoflavone supplements are necessary. In addition, isoflavones are oestrogenic – albeit weakly so – and there is some evidence that they may stimulate cancer cell proliferation in women with breast cancer.[35] Until more is known about these compounds, women with breast cancer should consult their doctors before taking isoflavones.

Interactions

None is known. Women using hormonal medication should seek medical advice before taking these supplements.

Dose

Isoflavones are available in the form of tablets and capsules.

The dose is not established. Dietary supplements containing mixed isoflavones provide 50–100 mg in a dose.

References

1 Potter JD, Steinmetz K. Vegetables, fruit and phytoestrogens as preventive agents. In: Stewart BW, McGregor D, Kleihues P, eds. *Principles of Chemoprevention*. Lyons, France: International Agency for Research on Cancer, 1996: 61–90.

2 Setchell KDR. Phytoestrogens: The biochemistry, physiology, and implications for human health of soy isoflavones. *Am J Clin Nutr* 1998; 68: 1333S–1346S.

3 Anderson JW, Johnstone BW, Cook-Newell ME. Meta-analysis of the effects of soy protein intake on serum lipids. *N Engl J Med* 1995; 333: 276–282.

4 Baum JA, Teng H, Erdman JW, Jr, *et al*. Long-term intake of soy protein improves blood lipid profiles and increases mononuclear cell low-density-lipoprotein receptor messenger RNA in hypercholesterolemic, postmenopausal women. *Am J Clin Nutr* 1998; 68: 545–551.

5 Gooderham MH, Adlercreutz H, Ojala ST, *et al*. A soy protein isolate rich in genistein and daidzein and its effects on plasma isoflavone concentration, platelet aggregation, blood lipids and fatty acid composition of plasma phospholipid in normal men. *J Nutr* 1996; 126: 2000–2006.

6 Wong W, O'Brian Smith E, Stuff JE, *et al*. Cholesterol-lowering effect of soy protein in normocholesterolemic and hypercholesterolemic men. *Am J Clin Nutr* 1998; 68: 1385S–1389S.

7 Crouse JR, III, Morgan T, Terry JG, *et al*. Soy protein containing isoflavones reduces plasma concentrations of lipids. *Arch Intern Med* 1999; 159: 2070–2076.

8 Teixera SR, Potter SM, Weigel R, *et al*. Effects of feeding 4 levels of soy protein for 3 and 6 weeks on blood lipids and apolipoproteins in moderately hypercholesterolemic men. *Am J Clin Nutr* 2000; 71: 1077–1084.

9 Merz-Demlow BE, Duncan AM, Wangen KE, *et al*. Soy isoflavones improve plasma lipids in normocholesterolemic, premenopausal women. *Am J Clin Nutr* 2000; 71: 1462–1469.

10 Tikkanen MJ, Wahala K, Ojala S, *et al*. Effect of soybean phytoestrogen intake on low density lipoprotein oxidation resistance. *Proc Natl Acad Sci USA* 1998; 95: 3106–3110.

11 Wiseman H, O'Reilly JD, Adlercreutz H, *et al*. Isoflavone phytoestrogens consumed in soy decrease F_2-isoprostane concentrations and increase resistance of low-density lipoprotein to oxidation in humans. *Am J Clin Nutr* 2000; 72: 395–400.

12 Hodgson JM, Puddey IB, Beilin LJ, *et al*. Supplementation with isoflavonoid phytoestrogens does not alter serum lipid concentrations: A randomized controlled trial in humans. *J Nutr* 1998; 128: 728–732.

13 Samman S, Lyons Wall PM, Chan GS, *et al*. The effect of supplementation with isoflavones on plasma lipids and oxidisability of low density lipoprotein in premenopausal women. *Atherosclerosis* 1999; 147: 277–283.

14 Simons LA, von Koningsmark M, Simons J, Celermajer DS. Phytoestrogens do not influence lipoprotein levels or endothelial function in healthy, postmenopausal women. *Am J Cardiol* 2000; 85: 1297–1301.

15 Howes JB, Sullivan D, Lai N, *et al*. The effects of dietary supplementation with isoflavones from red

clover on the lipoprotein profiles of postmenopausal women with mild to moderate hypercholesterolaemia. *Atherosclerosis* 2000; 152: 143–147.

16 Messina MJ, Persky V, Setchell KD, *et al.* Soy intake and cancer risk: a review of the in vitro and in vivo data. *Nutr Cancer* 1994; 21: 113–131.

17 Goodman MT, Wilkens LR, Hankin JH, *et al.* Association of soy and fiber consumption with the risk of endometrial cancer. *Am J Epidemiol* 1997; 146: 294–306.

18 Barnes S. Effect of genistein on in vitro and in vivo models of cancer. *J Nutr* 1995; 125: 777S–783S.

19 Hawrylewicz EJ, Zapata JJ, Blair WH. Soy and experimental cancer. *J Nutr* 1995; 125: 698S–708S.

20 Kennedy AR. The evidence for soybean products as cancer preventive agents. *J Nutr* 1995; 125: 733S–743S.

21 Ingram D, Sanders K, Kolybaba M, Lopez D. Case-control study of phyto-estrogens and breast cancer. *Lancet* 1997; 350: 990–994.

22 Murkies A, Dalais FS, Briganti EM, *et al.* Phyto-estrogens and breast cancer in postmenopausal women: A case control study. *Menopause* 2000; 7: 289–296.

23 Arjmandi BH, Alekel L, Hollis BW, *et al.* Dietary soybean protein prevents bone loss in an ovariectomized rat model of osteoporosis. *J Nutr* 1996; 126: 161–167.

24 Anderson JJ, Ambrose WW, Garner SC. Biphasic effects of genistein on bone tissue in the ovariectomized, lactating rat model. *Proc Soc Exp Biol Med* 1998; 217: 345–350.

25 Potter SM, Baum JA, Teng H, *et al.* Soy protein and isoflavones: their effects on blood lipids and bone mineral density in postmenopausal women. *Am J Clin Nutr* 1998; 68: 1375S–1379S.

26 Alekel DL, St Germain A, Peterson CT, *et al.* Isoflavone-rich soy protein isolate attenuates bone loss in the lumbar spine of perimenopausal women. *Am J Clin Nutr* 2000; 72: 844–852.

27 Agnusdei D, Crepaldi G, Isaia G, *et al.* A double-blind, placebo-controlled diet of ipriflavone for prevention of postmenopausal spinal bone loss. *Calcif Tissue Int* 1997; 61: 142–147.

28 Gambacciani M, Ciaponi M, Cappagli B, *et al.* Effects of combined low dose of the isoflavone derivative ipriflavone and estrogen replacement on bone mineral density and metabolism in postmenopausal women. *Maturitas* 1997; 28: 75–81.

29 Ohta H, Komukai S, Makita K, *et al.* Effects of 1-year ipriflavone treatment on bone mineral density and bone metabolic markers in postmenopausal women with low bone mass. *Horm Res* 1999; 51: 178–183.

30 Lock M. Contested meanings of the menopause. *Lancet* 1991; 337: 1270–1272.

31 Kurzer MS, Xu X. Dietary phytoestrogens. *Annu Rev Nutr* 1997; 17: 353–381.

32 Murkies AL, Lombard C, Strauss BJG, *et al.* Dietary flour supplementation decreases post-menopausal hot flushes: Effect of soy and wheat. *Maturitas* 1995; 21: 189–195.

33 Brzezinski A, Aldercreutz H, Shaoul R, *et al.* Short-term effects of phytoestrogen-rich diet on postmenopausal women. *J North Am Menopause Soc* 1997; 4: 89–94.

34 Albertazzi P, Pansini F, Bonaccorsi G, *et al.* The effect of dietary soy supplementation on hot flushes. *Obstet Gynecol* 1998; 91: 6–11.

35 McMichael-Phillips DF, Harding C, Morton M, *et al.* Effects of soy-protein supplementation on epithelial proliferation in the histologically normal human breast. *Am J Clin Nutr* 1998; 68: 1431S–1436S.

Kelp

Description

Kelp is a long-stemmed seaweed, derived from various species (e.g. *Fucus, Laminaria)* of brown algae, known as preparation of dried seaweed of various species.

Constituents

Kelp is a source of several minerals and trace elements, especially iodine.

Possible uses

Kelp is claimed to be a slimming aid (some herbal products containing kelp are licensed in the UK for this purpose). Its main use is as a source of iodine.

Precautions/contraindications

Kelp should be avoided in patients with thyroid disease, unless recommended by a doctor. It may be contaminated with toxic trace elements (e.g. antimony, arsenic, lead, strontium).

Pregnancy and breast-feeding

Avoid (contaminants – see Precautions).

Adverse effects

Kelp may impair the control of hypothyroidism and hyperthyroidism. Nausea and diarrhoea have been reported occasionally.

Interactions

See Iodine monograph.

Dose

Kelp is available in the form of capsules, tablets, powder and liquid.

The dose is not established. Dietary supplements contain 200–500 mg kelp. The iodine content is variable and not always quoted on the label.

Lecithin

Description and nomenclature

Lecithin is a phospholipid and is known as phosphatidylcholine.

Constituents

Lecithin is composed of phosphatidyl esters, mainly phosphatidylcholine, phosphatidyl-ethanolamine, phosphatidylserine and phosphatidylinositol. It also contains varying amounts of other substances such as fatty acids, triglycerides and carbohydrates. One teaspoon (3.5 g) lecithin granules provides on average: energy 117 kJ (28 kcal), phosphatidylcholine 750 mg, phosphatidylinositol 500 mg, choline 100 mg, inositol 100 mg, phosphorus 110 mg.

Human requirements

Lecithin is not an essential component of the diet. It is synthesised from choline.

Action

Lecithin is a source of choline (see Choline monograph) and inositol. It is an essential component of cell membranes and a precursor to acetylcholine.

Dietary sources

Soya beans, peanuts, liver, meat, eggs.

Metabolism

About 50% of ingested lecithin enters the thoracic duct intact. The rest is degraded to glycerophosphorylcholine in the intestine, and then to choline in the liver. Plasma choline levels reflect lecithin intake.

Deficiency

Not established.

Possible uses

Lecithin is claimed to be beneficial in the treatment of disease related to impaired cholinergic function (see Choline monograph). It has also been claimed to be of benefit in lowering serum cholesterol levels and improving memory. It is sometimes taken for dementia and Alzheimer's disease.

Cholesterol

An open clinical trial in the 1970s showed that oral lecithin in large doses (20–30 g daily) led to a significant reduction in cholesterol concentration in one out of the three healthy subjects studied and three out of the seven people with hypercholesterolaemia.[1]

However, in a double-blind study, 20 hyperlipidaemic men were randomised to receive frozen yoghurt, frozen yoghurt with 20 g soya bean lecithin or frozen yoghurt with 17 g sunflower oil. Sunflower oil was used to control for the increased intake in energy and linoleic acid from the lecithin. Lecithin treatment had no independent effect on serum lipoprotein or plasma fibrinogen levels in this group of men.[2]

Alzheimer's disease

A double-blind, placebo-controlled, cross-over study in 11 out-patients with Alzheimer's disease found that lecithin 10 g three times a day for three months was associated with an improvement in tests of learning ability, but there was no improvement in any of the psychological tests used.[3]

Two further double-blind studies (one in patients with Alzheimer's disease,[4] one in normal adults[5]) showed no effect of lecithin on memory.

Another double-blind, randomised controlled trial in 53 subjects with probable Alzheimer's disease involved the use of lecithin and tacrine or lecithin and placebo for 36 weeks. No clinically relevant improvement was found in any of the groups over 36 weeks.[6]

Conclusion
Controlled clinical trials have provided no evidence that lecithin lowers cholesterol or helps to improve memory in patients with Alzheimer's disease. Claims for the value of lecithin in lowering blood pressure and also in hepatitis, gallstones, psoriasis and eczema are unsubstantiated. Further trials are needed to assess the role of lecithin.

Precautions/contraindications

None is known.

Pregnancy and breast-feeding

No problems have been reported, but there have not been sufficient studies to guarantee the safety of lecithin (in amounts greater than those found in foods) in pregnancy and breast-feeding.

Adverse effects

None reported.

Interactions

None reported.

Dose

Lecithin is available in the form of tablets, capsules and powder. Lecithin supplements provide between 20 and 90% phosphatidylcholine (depends on the product).

The dose is not established. On current evidence, lecithin is unlikely to be useful. Product manufacturers recommend 1200–2400 mg daily.

References

1 Simons LA, Hickie JB, Ruys J. Treatment of hypercholesterolaemia with oral lecithin. *Aust NZ J Med* 1977; 7: 262–266.
2 Oosthuizen W, Vorster HH, Vermaak WJ, *et al.* Lecithin has no effect on serum lipoprotein, plasma fibrinogen and macromolecular protein complex levels in hyperlipidaemic men in a double-blind controlled study. *Eur J Clin Nutr* 1998; 52: 419–424.
3 Etienne P, Dastoor D, Gauthier S, *et al.* Alzheimer disease: Lack of effect of lecithin treatment for 3 months. *Neurology* 1981; 31: 1552–1554.
4 Brinkman SD, Smith RC, Meyer JS, *et al.* Lecithin and memory training in suspected Alzheimer's disease. *J Gerontol* 1982; 37: 4–9.
5 Harris CM, Dysken MW, Fovall P, Davis JM. Effect of lecithin on memory in normal adults. *Am J Psychiatry* 1983; 140: 1010–1012.
6 Maltby N, Broe GA, Creasey H, *et al.* Efficacy of tacrine and lecithin in mild to moderate Alzheimer's disease: Double-blind trial. *Br Med J* 1994; 308: 879–883.

Magnesium

Description

Magnesium is an essential mineral. It is the second most abundant intracellular cation in the body.

Human requirements

See Table 1 for Dietary Reference Values for magnesium.

Intakes

In the UK, the average daily diet provides: for males, 336 mg; females, 250 mg.

Action

Magnesium is an essential co-factor for enzymes requiring adenosine 5′-triphosphate (ATP) (these are involved in glycolysis, fatty acid oxidation and amino acid metabolism). It is also required for: the synthesis of RNA and replication of DNA; neuromuscular transmission; and calcium metabolism.

Dietary sources

See Table 2 for dietary sources of magnesium.

Metabolism

Absorption

Absorption of magnesium occurs principally in the jejunum and ileum by active carrier-mediated processes (partly dependent on vitamin D and parathyroid hormone) and by diffusion.

Distribution

Magnesium is widely distributed in the soft tissues and skeleton.

Elimination

Excretion is largely via the urine (magnesium homeostasis is controlled mainly by the kidneys), with unabsorbed and endogenously secreted magnesium in the faeces. Small amounts are excreted in saliva and breast milk.

Bioavailability

Bioavailability appears to be enhanced by vitamin D, but is decreased by phytates and non-starch polysaccharides (dietary fibre).

Deficiency

Signs and symptoms include: hypocalcaemia and hypokalaemia; muscle spasm, tremor and tetany; personality changes, lethargy and apathy; convulsions, delirium and coma; anorexia, nausea, vomiting, abdominal pain and paralytic ileus; cardiac arrhythmias, tachycardia and sudden cardiac death.

Possible uses

Magnesium has been investigated for a role in cardiovascular disease (including hypertension), diabetes mellitus, migraine, osteoporosis and premenstrual syndrome (PMS).

Cardiovascular disease

Magnesium deficiency has been associated with cardiovascular disease, and some epidemiological data have suggested a reduced mortality from coronary artery disease in populations

Table 1 Dietary Reference Values for magnesium (mg/day)

EU RDA (for labelling purposes) = 14 mg

Age	UK			USA	WHO	European
	LNRI	EAR	RNI	RDA	RNI	acceptable range
0–3 months	30	40	55	30	–	–
4–6 months	40	50	60	30	–	–
7–9 months	45	60	75	75	–	–
10–12 months	45	60	80	75	–	–
1–3 years	50	65	85	80	–	–
4–6 years	70	90	120	–	–	–
4–8 years	–	–	–	130	–	–
7–10 years	115	150	200	–	–	–
9–13 years	–	–	–	240	–	–
Males						
11–14 years	180	230	280	–	–	–
14–18 years	–	–	–	410	–	–
15–18 years	190	250	280	–	–	–
19–50+years	190	250	300	–	200–300	150–500
19–30 years	–	–	–	400	–	–
31–70+ years	–	–	–	420	–	–
Females						
11–14 years	180	230	280	–	–	–
14–18 years	–	–	–	360	–	–
15–18 years	190	250	300	360	–	–
19–50 years	190	250	300	–	200–300	150–500
50+ years	150	200	270	–	–	–
19–30 years	–	–	–	310	–	–
31–70+ years	–	–	–	320	–	–
Pregnancy	*	*	*	360–400	–	–
Lactation	–	–	+50	320–360	–	–

*No increment.

US Tolerable Intake Level = 350 mg daily.

living in hard-water areas compared with those living in soft-water areas. Other data, however, have indicated no such association, and a large cohort study[1] in which 2512 older men have been followed for 10 years also provided no evidence of a protective role for magnesium in coronary heart disease (CHD).

There is, as yet, insufficient evidence to argue that the UK population has a significant amount of 'subclinical' magnesium deficiency, which is a contributing factor to the high prevalence of CHD.

Marginal magnesium status has been implicated in myocardial infarction, but reduced serum magnesium levels found in some myocardial infarct patients may be a result of the infarction rather than the cause of it. However, one double-blind, placebo-controlled study in patients with acute myocardial infarction showed reduced serum triglyceride concentrations and tendencies toward increased high-density lipoprotein concentrations after oral magnesium supplementation.[2]

Some controlled studies have suggested that intravenous magnesium given early after

Table 2 Dietary sources of magnesium

Food portion	Magnesium content (mg)
Breakfast cereals	
1 bowl All-Bran (45 g)	*90*
1 bowl Bran Flakes (45 g)	*50*
1 bowl Corn Flakes (30 g)	5
1 bowl Muesli (95 g)	*90*
2 pieces Shredded Wheat	*50*
2 Weetabix	*50*
Cereal products	
Bread, brown, 2 slices	40
white, 2 slices	15
wholemeal, 2 slices	*60*
1 chapati	30
Pasta, brown, boiled (150 g)	*60*
white, boiled (150 g)	25
Rice, brown, boiled (165 g)	*60*
white, boiled (165 g)	15
Milk and dairy products	
½ pint (280 ml) milk, whole, semi-skimmed or skimmed	35
1 pot yoghurt (150 g)	30
Cheese (50 g)	12
1 egg, size 2 (60 g)	10
Meat and fish	
Meat, cooked (100 g)	25
Liver, lamb's, cooked (90 g)	20
Kidney, lamb's, cooked (75 g)	20
White fish, cooked (150 g)	30
Pilchards, canned (105 g)	40
Sardines, canned (70 g)	35
Shrimps (80 g)	*49*
Tuna, canned (95 g)	30
Vegetables	
Green vegetables, average, boiled (100g)	20
Potatoes, boiled (150 g)	20
1 small can baked beans (200 g)	*60*
Lentils, kidney beans or other pulses (105 g)	*50*
Fruit	
1 banana	35
1 orange	20
Nuts	
20 almonds	*50*
10 Brazil nuts	*80*
30 hazelnuts	*50*
30 peanuts	*70*

Excellent sources (**bold**); good sources (*italics*).
Note: Hard drinking water may contribute significantly to intake.

suspected myocardial infarction could reduce the frequency of serious arrhythmias and mortality. However, magnesium has been given as a prescription medicine in these cases, and not as a dietary supplement.

Blood pressure

There is some evidence that magnesium reduces blood pressure.[3] A 20 mmol increase in daily magnesium intake resulted in a diastolic blood pressure fall of 3.4 mmHg in a trial on Dutch women.[4] A reduction in blood pressure occurred with a low-sodium, high-potassium, high-magnesium salt in older patients with mild to moderate hypertension and suggested that the increased magnesium intake could have contributed to the fall in blood pressure.[5]

However, another study[6] showed that magnesium supplementation did not have an additive hypotensive effect in mild hypertensive subjects on a reduced sodium intake. Another group,[7] using a double-blind, randomised crossover design, detected no fall in blood pressure with magnesium supplementation, despite a significant increase in plasma magnesium concentration.

More recent double-blind, placebo-controlled trials[8,9] have shown no effect of magnesium supplementation (300–360 mg) on blood pressure in healthy subjects and those with mild to moderate hypertension.[10]

Diabetes mellitus

Magnesium modulates glucose transport across cell membranes, and is a co-factor in various pathways involving enzymatic oxidation. Individuals with diabetes, especially those with glycosuria and ketoacidosis, may have excessive urinary losses of magnesium.[11,12] Hypomagnesaemia is common in these patients and can potentially cause insulin resistance.[13] One study has shown that insulin secretory capacity improved with dietary magnesium supplementation for four weeks.[14] The effect of diabetes on tissue content of magnesium is variable, and cannot always be predicted from serum magnesium measurements. Epidemiologically, magnesium deficiency has been associated with diabetic neuropathy,[15] and although there is no evidence to indicate that magnesium supplementation can alter this complication, the magnesium status of patients at risk of magnesium depletion (e.g. those on thiazides) should be assessed. However, monitoring is difficult and a dose for patients with diabetes mellitus has not been established.

In an open trial, 11 patients with type 1 diabetes and persistently low erythrocyte magnesium levels were given 450 mg magnesium following an intravenous loading dose of magnesium. During intravenous loading, plasma magnesium decreased and erythrocyte magnesium increased. Supplementation did not normalise magnesium status, and there were no significant changes in glycated haemoglobin or serum lipid levels. The authors concluded that chronic magnesium depletion may occur in type 1 diabetes and that it is difficult to replete and maintain body stores.[16]

In a double-blind, placebo-controlled trial, 128 Brazilian patients with type 2 diabetes were randomised to receive 497 mg magnesium, 994 mg magnesium or placebo. At the start of the study 47.7% of the patients had low plasma magnesium and 31.1% had low magnesium levels in the mononucleocytes. Intracellular magnesium was significantly lower than in the normal population and was lower in those with peripheral neuropathy than in those without. However, there was no correlation between plasma and intracellular magnesium and glycaemic control. In the groups on placebo and lower-dose magnesium, neither a change in plasma nor intracellular magnesium occurred and there was no change in glycaemic control. The higher dose magnesium was associated with an increase in plasma and intracellular magnesium and a significant fall in fructosamine plasma levels.[17]

In a placebo-controlled (not blinded) study, involving 50 patients with type 2 diabetes, supplementation with 360 mg magnesium daily over three months increased plasma magnesium and urinary magnesium excretion, but had no effect on glycaemic control or lipid concentration.[18]

Premenstrual syndrome

Reduced magnesium levels have been reported in women affected by premenstrual syndrome. An Italian double-blind, randomised study[19] in 32 women showed that a supplement of 360 mg magnesium daily improved premenstrual symptoms related to mood changes. More recently, a randomised, double-blind, placebo-controlled study[20] in 38 women showed no effect of magnesium supplementation (200 mg daily) in the first month, but symptoms including weight gain, swelling of extremities, breast tenderness and abdominal bloating, improved during the second month. A further study[21] of one month's duration in 44 women showed that magnesium 200 mg daily plus vitamin B_6 50 mg daily produced a modest effect on anxiety-related premenstrual symptoms.

Migraine

There is some evidence that magnesium supplementation is effective in migraine, but results from studies are equivocal. Thus, oral magnesium was effective in reducing the frequency of migraine in a 12-week placebo-controlled, double-blind study.[22] There was also a reduction in the average duration of pain and need for acute medication, although these changes were not significant. However, in another similar study, magnesium had no effect.[23]

Osteoporosis

Magnesium is a constituent of bone, and supplementation has been shown to increase bone density in individuals with osteoporosis. Increased magnesium intake is associated with a lower decline in bone mineral density after the menopause.[24] Supplements have been shown to decrease markers of bone turnover in young men[25] but not young women.[26] Bone density increased in patients with gluten-sensitive enteropathy and associated osteoporosis,[27] and also in menopausal women[28] who were given oral magnesium.

Athletes

Magnesium supplementation has been suggested to improve athletic performance. In one double-blind, placebo-controlled study,[29] magnesium (507 mg daily versus 246 mg daily) improved muscular strength, and in another similar study[30] swimming, running and cycling performance was improved. However, in a two-week study,[31] athletes taking magnesium 500 mg daily did not demonstrate improved performance or reduced muscle tiredness.

Conclusion

Epidemiological studies show an association between marginal magnesium status and cardiovascular disease and hypertension. However, the effect of supplementation is equivocal and any effect appears to be small. Patients with diabetes often have poor magnesium status, but supplementation does not appear to have an effect on glucose control, possibly because it is difficult to replete and maintain adequate magnesium levels. Preliminary evidence suggests that magnesium could reduce the frequency and pain of migraine and may help the symptoms of premenstrual syndrome. There is no good evidence that magnesium improves performance in athletes.

Precautions/contraindications

Doses exceeding the RDA are best avoided in renal impairment.

Pregnancy and breast-feeding

No problems reported with normal intakes.

Adverse effects

Toxicity from oral ingestion is unlikely in individuals with normal renal function. Doses of 3–5 g have a cathartic effect.

Interactions

Drugs

Alcohol: excessive alcohol intake increases renal excretion of magnesium.
Loop diuretics: increased excretion of magnesium.
4-Quinolones: may reduce absorption of 4-quinolones; give 2 h apart.
Tetracyclines: may reduce absorption of tetracyclines; give 2 h apart.
Thiazide diuretics: increased excretion of magnesium.

Dose

Magnesium is available in the form of tablets and capsules. It is available in isolation, in combination with calcium (and sometimes with vitamin D) and in multivitamin and mineral preparations.

The dose is not established. Dietary supplements provide 100–500 mg per dose.

References

1 The Caerphilly and Speedwell Collaborative Group. Caerphilly and Speedwell collaborative heart disease studies. *J Epidemiol Community Health* 1994; 38: 235–238.
2 Rasmussen HS, Aurup P, Goldstein K, *et al*. Influence of magnesium substitution therapy on blood lipid composition in patients with ischaemic heart disease: A double-blind, placebo controlled study. *Arch Intern Med* 1989; 149: 1050–1053.
3 Widman L, Webster PO, Stegmayr BK, Wirell M. The dose-dependent reduction in blood pressure through administration of magnesium. *Am J Hypertension* 1993; 6: 41–45.
4 Witteman JCM, Grobbee DE, Derkx FHM, *et al*. Reduction of blood pressure with oral magnesium

supplementation in women with mild to moderate hypertension. *Am J Clin Nutr* 1994; 60: 129–135.

5 Geleijnse JM, Witteman JCM, Bak AAA, *et al.* Reduction in blood pressure with a low sodium, high potassium, high magnesium salt in older subjects with mild to moderate hypertension. *Br Med J* 1994; 309: 436–440.

6 Nowson CA, Morgan TO. Magnesium supplementation in mild hypertensive patients on a moderately low sodium diet. *Clin Exp Pharmacol Physiol* 1989; 16: 299–302.

7 Cappuccio FP, Markandu ND, Beynon GW, *et al.* Lack of effect of oral magnesium on high blood pressure: A double-blind study. *Br Med J* 1985; 291: 235–238.

8 Sacks FM, Willet WC, Smith A, *et al.* Effect on blood pressure of potassium, calcium and magnesium in women with low habitual intake. *Hypertension* 1998; 31: 131–138.

9 Yamamoto ME, Applegate WB, Klag MJ, *et al.* Lack of blood pressure effect with calcium and magnesium supplementation in adults with high-normal blood pressure: Reports from phase I of the Trials of Hypertension Prevention (TOHP). Trials of Hypertension Prevention (TOHP) Collaborative Research Group. *Ann Epidemiol* 1995; 5: 96–107.

10 Ferrara LA, Iannuzzi R, Castaldo A, *et al.* Long-term magnesium supplementation in essential hypertension. *Cardiology* 1992; 81: 25–33.

11 Fujii S, Takemura T, Wada M, *et al.* Magnesium levels in plasma, erythrocyte and urine in patients with diabetes mellitus. *Horm Metab Res* 1982; 14: 161–162.

12 McNair P, Christensen MS, Christiansen C, *et al.* Renal hypomagnesaemia in human diabetes mellitus: Its relation to glucose homeostasis. *Eur J Clin Invest* 1982; 12: 81–85.

13 Jain AP, Gupta NN, Kumar A. Some metabolic effects of magnesium in diabetes mellitus. *J Assoc Physicians India* 1976; 24: 827–831.

14 Paolisso G, Passariello N, Pizza G, *et al.* Dietary magnesium supplements improve β-cell response to glucose and arginine in elderly non-insulin dependent diabetic subjects. *Acta Endocrinol* 1989; 121: 16–20.

15 McNair P, Christiansen C, Madsbad S, *et al.* Hypomagnesaemia, a risk factor in diabetic nephropathy. *Diabetes* 1978; 27: 1075–1077.

16 De Leeuw I, Engelen W, Vertommen J, *et al.* Effect of intensive IV + oral magnesium supplementation on circulating ion levels, lipid parameters, and metabolic control in Mg-depleted insulin-dependent diabetic patients (IDDM). *Magnes Res* 1997; 10: 135–141.

17 Lima M de L, Cruz T, Pousada JC, *et al.* The effect of magnesium supplementation in increasing doses on the control of type 2 diabetes. *Diabetes Care* 1998; 21: 682–686.

18 de Valk HW, Verkaaik R, van Rijn HJ, *et al.* Oral magnesium supplementation in insulin-requiring Type 2 diabetic patients. *Diabetic Med* 1998; 15: 503–507.

19 Facchinetti F, Borella P, Sances G, *et al.* Oral magnesium successfully relieves premenstrual mood changes. *Obstet Gynecol* 1991; 78: 177–181.

20 Walker AF, De Souza MC, Vickers MF, *et al.* Magnesium supplementation alleviates premenstrual symptoms of fluid retention. *J Womens Health* 1998; 7: 1157–1165.

21 De Souza MC, Walker AF, Robinson PA, Bolland K. A synergistic effect of a daily supplement for 1 month of 200 mg magnesium plus 50 mg vitamin B6 for the relief of anxiety related premenstrual symptoms: A randomized, double-blind, crossover study. *J Womens Health Gend Based Med* 2000; 9: 131–139.

22 Peikert A, Wilimzig C, Kohne-Volland R. Prophylaxis of migraine with oral magnesium: results from a progressive multi-center, placebo-controlled and double blind randomized study. *Cephalagia* 1996; 16: 257–263.

23 Pfaffenrath V, Wessely P, Meyer C. Magnesium in the prophylaxis of migraine – a double blind, placebo-controlled study. *Cephalagia* 1996; 16: 436–440.

24 Tucker AK, Hannan MT, Chen H. Potassium, magnesium, and fruit and vegetable intakes are associated with greater bone mineral density in elderly men and women. *Am J Clin Nutr* 1999; 69: 727–736.

25 Dimai HP, Porta S, Wirnsberger G. Daily oral magnesium supplementation suppresses bone turnover in young adult males. *J Clin Endocrinol Metab* 1998; 83: 2742–2748.

26 Doyle L, Flynn A, Cashman K. The effect of magnesium supplementation on biochemical markers of bone metabolism or blood pressure in healthy young adult females. *Eur J Clin Nutr* 1999; 53: 255–261.

27 Rude RK, Olerich M. Magnesium deficiency: possible role in osteoporosis associated with gluten-sensitive enteropathy. *Osteoporosis Int* 1996; 6: 453–461.

28 Stendig-Limberg G, Tepper R, Leichter R. Trabecular bone density in a two year controlled trial of peroral magnesium in osteoporosis. *Magnes Res* 1993; 6: 155–163.

29 Brilla LR, Haley TF. Effect of magnesium supplementation on strength training in humans. *J Am Coll Nutr* 1992; 11: 326–329.

30 Golf SW, Bender S, Gruttner J. On the significance of magnesium in extreme physical stress. *Cardiovasc Drugs Ther* 1998; 12 (suppl. 2): 197–202.

31 Weller E, Backert P, Meinck HM. Lack of effect of oral Mg-supplementation on magnesium in serum, blood cells, and calf muscle. *Med Sci Sport Exerc* 1998; 30: 1584–1591.

Manganese

Description

Manganese is an essential trace mineral.

Human requirements

No Reference Nutrient Intake or Estimated Average Requirement has been set for manganese in the UK, but a safe and adequate intake is, for adults, 1.4 mg daily; infants, 16 μg daily. There is no EU or US RDA.

In the USA, the daily Adequate Intakes (AIs) are: adults aged 19–70+ years, males 2.3 mg, females 1.8 mg, pregnancy 2 mg, lactation 2.6 mg; 14–18 years, males 2.2 mg, females 1.6 mg; children aged 9–13 years, males 1.9 mg, females 1.6 mg; 4–8 years, 1.5 mg; 1–3 years, 1.2 mg; infants aged 7–12 months, 0.6 mg; 0–6 months, 0.003 mg. Daily Upper Tolerable Intake Levels (ULs) are: adults aged 19–70+ years (including pregnancy and lactation), 11 mg; 14–18 years (including pregnancy and lactation), 9 mg; children aged 9–13 years, 6 mg; 4–8 years, 3 mg; 1–3 years, 2 mg.

Intakes

In the UK, the average adult diet provides 4.6–5.4 mg daily.

Action

Manganese activates several enzymes, including hydroxylases, kinases, decarboxylases and transferases. It is also a constituent of several metalloenzymes, such as arginase, pyruvate carboxylase, and also superoxide dismutase which protects cells from free radical attack. It may also have a role in the regulation of glucose homeostasis and in calcium mobilisation.

Dietary sources

See Table 1 for dietary sources of manganese.

Metabolism

Absorption

Absorption of manganese occurs throughout the length of the small intestine, probably via a saturable carrier mechanism, but absorptive efficiency is believed to be poor.

Distribution

Manganese is transported in the blood bound to plasma proteins. Organs with the highest concentrations include the liver, kidney and pancreas, but 25% of the body pool is found within the skeleton. Homeostasis is maintained by hepatobiliary and intestinal secretion.

Elimination

Manganese is eliminated primarily in the faeces.

Bioavailability

Bioavailability of manganese appears to be enhanced by vitamin C and meat-containing diets, but is decreased by iron and non-starch polysaccharides (dietary fibre). Although large amounts of manganese are contained in tea, it is essentially unavailable to humans.

Deficiency

Manganese deficiency in individuals consuming mixed diets is very rare. Symptoms thought to be associated with deficiency (which have occurred only on semi-purified diets) include weight loss, dermatitis, hypocholesterolaemia,

Table 1 Dietary sources of maganese

Food portion	Manganese content (mg)
Cereal products	
Bread, brown, 2 slices	**1.0**
white, 2 slices	0.3
wholemeal, 2 slices	**1.5**
Milk and dairy products	
Milk and cheese	Traces
Meat and fish	
Meat and fish	Traces
Lamb's liver, cooked (90 g)	0.4
Vegetables	
1 small can baked beans (200 g)	0.6
Lentils, kidney beans or other pulses (105 g)	**1–1.5**
Green vegetables, average, boiled (100g)	0.2
Fruit	
1 banana	0.5
Blackberries, stewed (100 g)	**1.5**
Pineapple, canned (150 g)	**1.5**
Nuts	
20 almonds	0.3
10 Brazil nuts	0.4
30 hazelnuts	**1.0**
30 peanuts	0.7
Tea, 1 cup	0.3

Note: Some other foods (e.g. breakfast cereals) contain significant quantities, but there is no reliable information on the amount. Excellent sources (>1 mg/portion) (**bold**).

depressed growth of hair and nails and reddening of black hair.

Possible uses

Diabetes

Manganese has been claimed to be useful in diabetes mellitus. A relationship between dietary manganese and carbohydrate metabolism in humans has been suggested.[1] This report described the case of a diabetic patient resistant to insulin therapy who responded to oral manganese with a consistent drop in blood glucose levels. However, there is insufficient evidence to warrant recommendation of manganese supplements to patients with diabetes.

Miscellaneous

Manganese supplements have also been used to treat inflammatory conditions such as rheumatoid arthritis on the basis that manganese supplementation has been shown to raise levels of superoxide dismutase, which may protect against oxidative damage.[2]

Precautions/contraindications

No problems reported.

Pregnancy and breast-feeding

No problems reported at normal doses.

Adverse effects

Manganese is essentially non-toxic when administered orally. Toxic reactions in humans occur only as the result of the chronic inhalation of large amounts of manganese found in mines and some industrial plants. Signs include severe psychiatric abnormalities and neurological disorders similar to Parkinson's disease.

Interactions

None reported.

Dose

Manganese is available in the form of tablets and capsules.

The dose is not established. Dietary supplements provide 5–50 mg per dose.

References

1 Rubenstein AH, Levin NW, Elliot GA. Manganese-induced hypoglycaemia. *Lancet* 1962; 2: 1348–1351.
2 Pasquier C. Manganese containing superoxide dismutase deficiency in polymorphonuclear lymphocytes in rheumatoid arthritis. *Inflammation* 1984; 8: 27–32.

Melatonin

Description

Melatonin is a hormone synthesised by the pineal gland. It is synthesised from tryptophan, which is converted to serotonin, and this in turn is converted to melatonin. Melatonin is secreted in a 24-h circadian rhythm, regulating the normal sleep–wake periods. Secretion starts as soon as darkness falls, normally peaking between 02:00 and 04:00, and synthesis is inhibited by exposure to light. Daily output is greatest in young adults; production declines after the age of 20 years.

Action

Melatonin has a role in the regulation of sleep, and as a supplement it can reset the sleep–wake cycle and help to promote sleep. In addition, it regulates the secretion of growth hormone and gonadotrophic hormones, and it has antioxidant activity. It may also have anticancer properties.

Possible uses

Melatonin has been investigated for jet lag, sleeping difficulties and cancer prevention.

Jet lag

A small double-blind, placebo-controlled trial involved 17 volunteers who flew from London to San Francisco, where they stayed for two weeks before returning. For three days before returning to London, subjects were given 5 mg melatonin or placebo at 18:00 local time. Following their return to Britain, the dose was continued for four more days between 14:00 and 16:00. On day seven, the volunteers were asked to rate their jet lag, and those taking melatonin reported significantly less severe jet lag than those taking placebo.[1]

In another similar study, 20 subjects flew eastwards from Auckland, New Zealand, to London and returned after three weeks. Subjects took either melatonin 5 mg or placebo for the first journey and vice-versa for the return journey. Less jet lag was experienced in the volunteers taking melatonin.[2]

In a further double-blind placebo-controlled trial, 52 flight crew were randomly assigned to three groups: early melatonin (5 mg melatonin for three days before arrival, continuing for five days after returning home), late melatonin (placebo for three days, followed by melatonin 5 mg for five days) and placebo. The flight was from Los Angeles to New Zealand, and all subjects began taking capsules at 07:00 to 08:00 Los Angeles time (corresponding to 02:00 to 03:00 New Zealand time) two days before departure and continued for five days after arrival in New Zealand. Subjects in the late melatonin group reported less jet lag and sleep disturbance than placebo, while those in the early melatonin group reported a worse recovery than the placebo group. The authors concluded that the timing of melatonin appeared to influence the subjective symptoms of jet lag.[3]

In another double-blind, placebo-controlled study 257 subjects on a flight from New York to Oslo were randomised to receive either 5 mg melatonin or placebo at bedtime, 0.5 mg melatonin at bedtime or 0.5 mg melatonin taken on a shifting schedule. In this study melatonin showed no difference over placebo. However, the authors acknowledged that the study had various limitations, including the fact that the subjects stayed only four days at their destination before flying back, and may not have had enough time to adapt to the new time. In addition, time of sleep onset at night, awakening in the morning and daytime sleepiness were assessed rather than night-time sleep disturbance, and it is night-time disturbance which is most associated with jet lag. Moreover, subjects knew that they had three out of four chances of receiving melatonin, and the placebo effect may have been quite large, diluting the influence of melatonin.[4]

In a study in baboons (which have similar sleep patterns to those of humans), various doses of melatonin were given at various times of day to see if melatonin shifted circadian rhythms. Activity patterns of the baboons was constantly monitored in a darkened room. Melatonin did not shift circadian rhythms, but it did induce sleep when given at night. However, the same dose given during the day did not cause sleep.[5] The authors concluded that melatonin does not shift circadian phase in baboons using doses similar to those prescribed for treating human circadian system disorders, suggesting that melatonin may not help to overcome the effects of jet lag.

Sleep disorders

In a study of six healthy young men, doses of 0.3 mg and 1 mg melatonin given at night produced acute hypnotic effects. There were no residual hypnotic effects the next morning, as shown from the results on mood and performance tests carried out by the volunteers.[6]

In a double-blind, placebo-controlled, crossover study, 12 elderly patients were randomised to receive 2 mg controlled-release melatonin daily for three weeks. There were no differences in sleep time, but a reduction in time to onset of sleep, and an increase in sleep quality as measured by wrist actigraphy.[7]

In a further double-blind, placebo-controlled, cross-over study, 14 patients with insomnia (aged 55–80 years) received 0.5 mg melatonin either as an immediate-release dose 30 min before bedtime, a controlled-release dose 30 min before bedtime, an immediate-release dose 4 h after bedtime, or placebo. Each trial lasted for two weeks with two-week washout periods. All melatonin trials resulted in significant reductions in time to sleep onset, but no improvement in sleep quality and no increase in sleep time.[8]

Cancer

A group of 80 patients with advanced solid tumours, all of whom refused chemotherapy or who had not responded to previous chemotherapy, were randomised to receive either interleukin 2 (IL-2) or IL-2 and melatonin (40 mg) starting one week before IL-2. Melatonin increased the anti-tumour activity of IL-2, resulting in accelerated tumour regression rate, increased progression-free survival and longer overall survival in these patients.[9]

In a small preliminary study involving 14 women with metastatic breast cancer, melatonin was shown to increase the effects of tamoxifen.[10]

In a controlled study, 50 patients with brain metastases caused by solid neoplasms were randomised to receive supportive care alone (steroids and anticonvulsants) or supportive care plus melatonin 20 mg daily. Survival at one year, free from tumour progression, and mean survival time were significantly higher in the melatonin group.[11]

In another study, 80 patients with metastatic tumours were randomised to receive chemotherapy or chemotherapy plus melatonin (20 mg daily). Melatonin was associated with a significant reduction in the frequency of thrombocytopenia, malaise and asthenia, and a non-significant trend towards less stomatitis and neuropathy compared with controls. However, melatonin had no effect on alopecia and vomiting.[12]

Precautions/contraindications

Caution in taking melatonin (as any other sleep therapy) for prolonged periods without medical assessment of the patient. People should not drive or operate machinery after taking melatonin. Melatonin should be avoided in women wishing to conceive (large doses may inhibit ovulation); in children and in patients with mental illness, including depression.

Conclusion
Melatonin has been promoted widely for the prevention and treatment of jet lag and sleep disorders. For jet lag, melatonin appears promising, but results from studies on supplements and sleep have been conflicting. Reduced secretion has also been associated with cancer, and preliminary research suggests that melatonin may reduce adverse effects associated with chemotherapy and increase survival time. Reduced secretion has also been linked with cardiovascular disease, epilepsy and depression, but its role as a potential supplement in these conditions is unclear.

Pregnancy and breast-feeding

Melatonin should be avoided in pregnancy.

Adverse effects

No known toxicity or serious side-effects, but the effects of long-term supplementation are unknown. However, there have been reports of headaches, abdominal cramp, inhibition of fertility and libido, gynaecomastia, exacerbation of symptoms of fibromyalgia, and also sleep disturbance. In addition, there have been reports of increased seizures in children suffering from neurological disorders. Inhibition of ovulation has been observed with high doses, but melatonin should not be used as a contraceptive.

Interactions

No data are available, but in theory melatonin may be additive with medication that causes CNS depression. In addition, beta-blockers inhibit melatonin release, and this may be the mechanism by which beta-blockers cause sleep disturbance. Other drugs, including fluoxetine, ibuprofen and indometacin may also reduce nocturnal melatonin secretion.

References

1 Arendt J, Aldhous M, Marks V. Alleviation of jet lag by melatonin: Preliminary results of controlled double blind trial. *Br Med J* 1986; 292: 1170.
2 Petrie K, Conaglen JV, Thompson L, Chamberlain K. Effect of melatonin on jet lag after long haul flights. *Br Med J* 1989; 298: 705–707.
3 Petrie K, Dawson AG, Thompson L, *et al.* A double-blind trial of melatonin as a treatment for jet lag in international cabin crew. *Biol Psychiatry* 1993; 33: 526–530.
4 Spitzer RL, Terman M, Williams JBW, *et al.* Jet lag: Clinical features, validation of a new syndrome-specific scale, and lack of response to melatonin in a randomised, double-blind trial. *Am J Psychiatry* 1999; 156: 1392–1396.
5 Hao H, Rivkees S. Melatonin does not shift circadian phase in baboons. *J Clin Endocrinol Metab* 2000; 85: 3618–3622
6 Zhdanova IV, Wurtman RJ, Lynch HJ, *et al.* Sleep inducing effects of low doses of melatonin ingested in the evening. *Clin Pharmacol Ther* 1995; 57: 552–558.
7 Garfinkel D, Laudon M, Nof D, *et al.* Improvement of sleep quality in elderly people by controlled release melatonin. *Lancet* 1995; 346: 541–544.
8 Hughes RJ, Sack RJ, Lewy AJ. The role of melatonin and circadian phase in age-related sleep maintenance insomnia: Assessment in a clinical trial of melatonin replacement. *Sleep* 1998; 21: 52–58.
9 Lissoni P, Barni S, Tancini G, *et al.* A randomised study with subcutaneous low-dose interleukin 2 alone vs. interleukin 2 plus the pineal neurohormone melatonin in advanced solid neoplasms other than renal cancer and melanoma. *Br J Cancer* 1994; 69: 196–199.
10 Lissoni P, Barni S, Meregalli S, *et al.* Modulation of cancer endocrine therapy by melatonin: A phase II study of tamoxifen plus melatonin in metastatic breast cancer patients progressing under tamoxifen alone. *Br J Cancer* 1995; 71: 854–856.
11 Lissoni P, Barni S, Ardizzoia A, *et al.* A randomised study with the pineal hormone melatonin versus supportive care alone in patients with brain metastases due to solid neoplasms. *Cancer* 1994; 73: 699–701.
12 Lissoni P, Tancini G, Barni S, *et al.* Treatment of cancer chemotherapy-induced toxicity with the pineal hormone melatonin. *Support Cancer Care* 1997; 5: 126–129.

Molybdenum

Description

Molybdenum is an essential ultratrace mineral.

Human requirements

No Reference Nutrient Intake or Estimated Average Requirement has been set for molybdenum in the UK but a safe and adequate daily intake is, for adults, 50–400 µg; infants, children and adolescents, 0.5–1.5 µg/kg.

In the USA, the Recommended Daily Allowances (RDAs) are: adults aged 19–70+ years, 45 µg; pregnancy and lactation, 50 µg daily; 14–18 years, 43 µg; children aged 9–13 years, 34 µg; 4–8 years, 22 µg; 1–3 years, 17 µg. Adequate Intakes (AIs) are, daily: infants aged 7–12 months, 3 µg; 0–6 months, 2 µg. Tolerable Upper Intake Levels (ULs) are, daily: adults aged 19–70+ years (including pregnancy and lactation), 2000 µg; 14–18 years (including pregnancy and lactation), 1700 µg; children aged 9–13 years, 1100 µg; 4–8 years, 600 µg; 1–3 years, 300 µg.

Intakes

Average adult intakes of molybdenum are 120–140 µg daily (USA figures).

Action

Molybdenum functions as an essential co-factor for several enzymes, including: aldehyde oxidase (oxidises and detoxifies various pyrimidines, purines and related compounds which are involved in DNA metabolism); xanthine oxidase/dehydrogenase (catalyses the formation of uric acid); sulphite oxidase (involved in sulphite metabolism).

Dietary sources

The richest sources of molybdenum include milk and milk products, dried beans and peas, wholegrain cereals and liver and kidney.

Metabolism

Absorption

Molybdenum is readily absorbed, but the mechanism of absorption is uncertain.

Distribution

Molybdenum is transported in the blood loosely attached to erythrocytes and binds specifically a_2-macroglobulin. The highest concentrations are found in the liver and kidney.

Elimination

Excretion of molybdenum is mainly via the kidneys, but significant amounts are eliminated in the bile.

Deficiency

A precise description of molybdenum deficiency in humans has not been clearly documented. Evidence so far has been limited to a single patient on long-term total parenteral nutrition, who developed hypermethioninaemia, decreased urinary excretion of sulphate and uric acid, and increased urinary excretion of sulphite and xanthine. In addition, the patient suffered irritability and mental disturbances that progressed into coma. Supplementation with molybdenum improved the clinical condition and normalised uric acid production.

Possible uses

None established.

Adverse effects

Molybdenum is a relatively non-toxic element. High dietary intakes (10–15 mg daily) have been associated with elevated uric acid concentrations in blood and an increased incidence of gout, and may also result in impaired bioavailability of copper and altered metabolism of nucleotides.

Dose

Molybdenum is available mainly in multivitamin and mineral supplements.

There is no established dose.

N-Acetyl cysteine

Description

N-Acetyl cysteine (NAC) is a derivative of the dietary amino acid, L-cysteine. It is a source of sulphydryl groups and, as such, can stimulate the synthesis of reduced glutathione (GSH), an endogenous antioxidant. It has been in clinical use for more than 30 years as a mucolytic agent for a variety of respiratory conditions, but is now available as a dietary supplement.

Action

By stimulating the production of GSH, NAC acts as an antioxidant. It also helps to protect the liver from various toxicants and is used in high dosage for the treatment of paracetamol-induced toxicity. NAC also chelates heavy metals such as cadmium, lead and mercury, and may be useful for the treatment of heavy metal toxicity.

Possible uses

NAC is promoted for influenza, bronchitis and the management of symptoms related to HIV and cancer.

Respiratory conditions

Oral NAC has been used since the 1960s for the treatment of bronchitis and it has also been advocated as a prophylactic in patients with chronic bronchitis. Various trials have also reported that supplementation many reduce the duration of bronchitic exacerbations.

In a study in nine patients for four weeks,[1] regular use of NAC 200 mg three times a day resulted in no significant differences in lung function, mucociliary clearance curves or sputum viscosity compared with placebo. In another study involving 181 patients randomised to receive either NAC 200 mg three times a day or placebo for five months in a double-blind manner, the number of exacerbations of bronchitis and the total number of days taking an antibiotic was reduced in the NAC group compared with placebo, but the differences were not significant.[2]

A further study in 526 patients suffering from chronic bronchitis found no significant differences between NAC and placebo in the number of exacerbations, but there was a significant reduction with NAC in the number of days patients were incapacitated.[3] Yet another double-blind, randomised, placebo controlled trial found that NAC tablets 300 mg three times a day were associated with a significant reduction in the number of sick leave days after four months of treatment during the winter. After six months the number of sick leave days and exacerbations of bronchitis remained lower in the NAC group, but the differences were not significant.[4]

An open, randomised study involving 169 patients with chronic obstructive pulmonary disease (COPD) found that NAC 600 mg daily plus standard treatment compared with placebo plus standard treatment was associated with a reduction in the number of sick leave days and exacerbations.[5]

A meta-analysis of nine double-blind, placebo-controlled trials of oral NAC in chronic bronchopulmonary disease concluded that a prolonged course of NAC prevents acute exacerbations of chronic bronchitis, thus possibly reducing morbidity and health-care costs.[6]

Influenza

In a randomised, double-blind study, 262 subjects, 62% of whom had chronic, but non-respiratory, degenerative disease (e.g. cardiovascular disease, diabetes, arthritis) received either NAC 1200 mg daily or placebo for six months. In the NAC group, there was a significant reduction in influenza-like episodes, severity of illness and length of time confined to bed as compared with the placebo group.[7] However, NAC did not prevent subclinical influenza infection (as assessed by antibody response to A/H_1N_1 virus), but the authors concluded that it reduced the incidence of clinically apparent disease.

HIV

In general, HIV-positive individuals have low levels of cysteine and GSH, and it has been suggested that NAC may benefit these patients by raising GSH levels,[8] but evidence for the value of NAC supplementation is equivocal.

In a double-blind, placebo-controlled trial, 45 HIV-positive patients on retroviral therapy were randomised to receive 800 mg NAC or placebo for four months. In the NAC group, cysteine levels increased from their low pre-treatment levels, and TNF-α levels fell. In addition the decline in CD4+ lymphocyte count found at the start of the study was less severe in the NAC group compared with placebo.[9]

NAC has also been investigated in combination with trimethoprim-sulphamethoxazole in the prophylaxis of *Pneumocystis carinii* in HIV-positive patients.[10,11] It has been suggested that adverse reactions to the antibiotics are due to low GSH levels in these patients, which may be improved by NAC supplementation. However, NAC did not reduce the risk of adverse reactions to trimethoprim-sulphamethoxazole in either study.

Cancer

Preliminary *in vitro* studies have indicated that NAC could have a role in the prevention and management of some forms of cancer. In a large randomised trial, 2592 patients (60% with head and neck cancer and 40% with lung cancer), most of whom were previous or current smokers, received either vitamin A (300 000 units daily for one year, followed by 150 000 units daily during the second year), NAC (600 mg daily for two years), both compounds, or placebo.[12] However, there was no benefit in terms of survival, event-free survival or second primary tumours with either vitamin A or NAC.

> **Conclusion**
> NAC may be useful as prophylaxis in patients with chronic bronchitis. There is preliminary evidence from one study that it may also reduce symptoms of influenza in older people. Preliminary studies in HIV-positive patients suggest that NAC may improve the clinical picture in such patients, although further research is required. *In vitro* studies have indicated that NAC might reduce the risk of cancer, although one large study has shown no significant benefits in this respect.

Precautions/contraindications

None reported.

Pregnancy and breast-feeding

No problems have been reported, but there have not been sufficient studies to guarantee the safety of NAC in pregnancy and breast-feeding.

Adverse effects

None reported, but there are no long-term studies assessing the safety of NAC. It has been used since the 1970s with few side-effects (e.g. mild gastrointestinal side-effects and skin rash). Such adverse effects that have been noted have occurred mainly with large oral doses of NAC given for paracetamol poisoning.

Interactions

None reported.

Dose

NAC is available in the form of tablets.

The dose is not established (for use as a supplement). Clinical trials have used 600–1200 mg daily.

References

1 Millar AB, Pavia D, Agnew JE, *et al.* Effect of oral *N*-acetylcysteine on mucus clearance. *Br J Dis Chest* 1985; 79: 262–266.
2 British Thoracic Society Research Committee. Oral *N*-acetylcysteine and exacerbation rates in patients with chronic bronchitis and severe airways obstruction. *Thorax* 1985; 40: 832–835.
3 Parr GD, Huitson A. Oral Fabrol (oral *N*-acetyl cysteine) in chronic bronchitis. *Br J Dis Chest* 1987; 81: 341–348.
4 Rasmussen JB, Glennow C. Reduction in days of illness after long-term treatment with *N*-acetylcysteine controlled-release tablets in patients with chronic bronchitis. *Eur Respir J* 1988; 1: 341–345.
5 Pela R, Calcagni AM, Subiaco S, *et al.* *N*-Acetylcysteine reduces the exacerbation rate in patients with moderate to severe COPD. *Respiration* 1999; 66: 495–500.
6 Granjean EM, Berthet P, Ruffmann R, Leuenberger P. Efficacy of oral long-term *N*-acetylcysteine in chronic bronchopulmonary disease: A meta-analysis of published double-blind, placebo-controlled clinical trials. *Clin Ther* 2000; 22: 209–221.
7 De Flora S, Grassi C, Carati L. Attenuation of influenza-like symptomatology and improvement of cell-mediated immunity with long-term *N*-acetyl cysteine treatment. *Eur Resp J* 1997; 10: 1535–1541.
8 Herzenbeg LA, De Rosa SC, Dubs JG, *et al.* Glutathione deficiency is associated with impaired survival in HIV disease. *Proc Natl Acad Sci USA* 1997; 94: 1967–1972.
9 Akerlund B, Jarstrand C, Lindeke B, *et al.* Effect of *N*-acetylcysteine (NAC) treatment on HIV-1 infection: a double-blind placebo-controlled trial. *Eur J Clin Pharmacol* 1996; 50: 457–461.
10 Akerlund B, Tynell E, Bratt G, *et al.* *N*-Acetylcysteine treatment and the risk of toxic reactions to trimethoprim-sulphamethoxazole in primary *Pneumocystis carinii* prophylaxis in HIV-infected patients. *J Infect* 1997; 35: 143–147.
11 Walmsley SL, Khorasheh S, Singer J, *et al.* A randomised trial of *N*-acetylcysteine for prevention of trimethoprim-sulphamethoxazole hypersensitivity reactions in *Pneumocystis carinii* pneumonia prophylaxis (CTN 057). Canadian HIV Trials Network 057 Study Group. *J Acquir Immune Defic Syndr Hum Retrovir* 1998; 19: 498–505.
12 Van Zandwiijk N, Dalesio O, Pastorino U, *et al.* EUROSCAN, a randomized trial of vitamin A and *N*-acetylcysteine in patients with head and neck cancer or lung cancer. For the European Organization for Research and Treatment of Cancer Head and Neck and Lung Cancer Cooperative Groups. *J Natl Cancer Inst* 2000; 92: 977–986.

Niacin

Description

Niacin is a water-soluble vitamin of the vitamin B complex.

Nomenclature

Niacin is a generic term used to describe the compounds that exhibit the biological properties of nicotinamide. It occurs in food as nicotinamide and nicotinic acid. It is sometimes known as niacinamide.

Units

Requirements and food values for niacin are the sum of the amounts of nicotinic acid and nicotinamide. Niacin is also obtained in the body from the amino acid tryptophan. On average, 60 mg tryptophan is equivalent to 1 mg niacin.

> Niacin (mg equivalents) = nicotinic acid (mg) + nicotinamide (mg) + tryptophan (mg)/60

Human requirements

Niacin requirements depend on energy intake; values are therefore given as mg/1000 kcal and also as total values based on estimated average energy requirements for the majority of people in the UK (Table 1).

Intakes

In the UK, the average adult daily diet provides (niacin equivalents): for men, 42 mg; for women, 30.9 mg.

Action

Nutritional

As a vitamin, niacin functions as a component of two co-enzymes, nicotinamide adenine dinucleotide (NAD) and nicotinamide adenine dinucleotide diphosphate (NADP). These co-enzymes participate in many metabolic processes including glycolysis, tissue respiration, lipid, amino acid and purine metabolism.

Pharmacological

In doses in excess of nutritional requirements, nicotinic acid (but not nicotinamide) reduces serum cholesterol and triglycerides by inhibiting the synthesis of very-low-density proteins (VLDL), which are the precursors of low-density lipoproteins (LDL). Nicotinic acid also causes direct peripheral vasodilatation.

Dietary sources

See Table 2 for dietary sources of niacin.

Metabolism

Absorption

Both nicotinamide and nicotinic acid are absorbed in the duodenum by facilitated diffusion (at low concentrations) and by passive diffusion (at high concentrations).

Distribution

Conversion of niacin to its co-enzymes occurs in most tissues.

Table 1 Dietary Reference Values for niacin (nicotinic acid equivalent)

EU RDA = 18 mg

Age	UK				USA	WHO	Europe
	LNRI[1]	EAR[1]	RNI[1]	RNI[2]	RDA[2]	RNI[2]	PRI[2]
0–6 months	4.4	5.5	6.6	3	2	5.4	–
7–12 months	4.4	5.5	6.6	5	3	5.4	5
1–3 years	4.4	5.5	6.6	8	6	9.0	9
4–6 years	4.4	5.5	6.6	11	–	12.1	11
4–8 years	–	–	–	–	8	–	–
7–10 years	4.4	5.5	6.6	12	–	14.5	13
9–13 years	–	–	–	–	12	–	–
Males							
11–14 years	4.4	5.5	6.6	15	–	19.1	15
15–18 years	4.4	5.5	6.6	18	–	20.3	18
19–50 years	4.4	5.5	6.6	17	–	18.8	18
50+ years	4.4	5.5	6.6	16	–	19.8	18
14–70+ years	–	–	–	–	16	–	–
Females							
11–14 years	4.4	5.5	6.6	12	–	16.4	14
15–18 years	4.4	5.5	6.6	14	–	15.2	14
19–50 years	4.4	5.5	6.6	13	–	14.5	14
50+ years	4.4	5.5	6.6	12	–	14.5	14
14–70+ years	–	–	–	–	14	–	–
Pregnancy	*	*	*	–	18	+2.3	*
Lactation	*	*	+2.3	+2	17	+3.7	+2

*No increment.
[1] mg/1000 kcal.
[2] mg/day.
US Tolerable Upper Intake Level (UL) = 35 mg daily for adults aged >18 years.

Elimination

Elimination occurs mainly via the urine. Niacin appears in breast milk.

Bioavailability

Niacin is remarkably stable and can withstand reasonable periods of heating, cooking and storage with little loss. Bioavailability of niacin from cereals may be low, but much of the niacin in breakfast cereals comes from fully available synthetic niacin added to fortify such products.

Deficiency

Niacin deficiency (rare in the UK) may lead to pellagra. Early signs of deficiency are vague and non-specific, and may include reduced appetite, weight loss, gastrointestinal discomfort, weakness, irritability and inability to concentrate. Signs of more advanced deficiency include sore mouth, glossitis and stomatitis. The severe deficiency state of pellagra is characterised by dermatitis (predominantly in the areas of skin exposed to sunlight), dementia (associated with confusion, disorientation, seizures and hallucinations) and diarrhoea.

Table 2 Dietary sources of niacin

Food portion	Niacin content[1] (mg)	Food portion	Niacin content[1] (mg)
Breakfast cereals		1 pot yoghurt (150 g)	1.5
1 bowl All-Bran (45 g)	*6.5*	Cheese (50 g)	1.5
1 bowl Bran Flakes (45 g)	*7.5*	*1 egg, size 2 (60 g)*	*2.5*
1 bowl Corn Flakes (30 g)	*5.0*		
1 bowl Muesli (95 g)	**8.0**	**Meat and fish**	
1 bowl Start (40 g)	**10.0**	**Beef, roast (85 g)**	**10.0**
2 pieces Shredded Wheat	*3.0*	**Lamb, roast (85 g)**	**10.0**
2 Weetabix	*6.0*	**Pork, roast (85 g)**	**10.0**
		1 chicken leg portion	**16.0**
Cereal products		**Liver, lamb's, cooked (90 g)**	**18.0**
Bread, brown, 2 slices	*3.0*	**Kidney, lamb's, cooked (75 g)**	**11.5**
white, 2 slices	*2.5*	**Fish, cooked (150 g)**	**10–15**
wholemeal, 2 slices	*4.0*		
1 chapati	*2.5*	**Vegetables**	
1 naan	*5.0*	*Peas, boiled (100 g)*	*2.5*
1 white pitta bread	*2.5*	Potatoes, boiled (150 g)	1.5
Pasta, brown, boiled (150 g)	*3.5*	*1 small can baked beans (200 g)*	*2.6*
white, boiled (150 g)	2.0	Chickpeas, cooked (105 g)	2.0
Rice, brown, boiled (160 g)	*3.0*	Red kidney beans (105 g)	2.0
white, boiled (160 g)	2.0	Dahl, lentil (150 g)	1.5
2 heaped tablespoons wheatgerm	1.5		
		Nuts	
Milk and dairy products		*30 peanuts*	*6.5*
½ pint (280 ml) milk, whole, semi-skimmed or skimmed	*2.5*		
½ pint (280 ml) soya milk	1.5	**Yeast**	
		Brewer's yeast (10 g)	1.5
		Marmite, spread on 1 slice bread	*3.5*

[1]Niacin equivalents (includes both preformed niacin and niacin obtained from tryptophan).
Excellent sources (**bold**); good sources (*italics*).

Possible uses

Despite claims made for niacin, it is of unproven value in arthritis, alcohol dependence, schizophrenia and other mental disorders unrelated to niacin deficiency. Nicotinic acid is prescribable on the NHS for hyperlipidaemia, but should not be sold as a supplement for this purpose.

Precautions/contraindications

Large doses of niacin are best avoided in: gout (may increase uric acid levels); peptic ulcer (large doses may activate an ulcer); liver disease (large doses cause deterioration). Large doses should also be used with caution in diabetes mellitus. However, one study[1] suggests that lipid modifying doses can safely be used in patients with diabetes. Supplements containing nicotinic acid should not be used as a cholesterol-lowering agent without medical advice.

Pregnancy and breast-feeding

No problems reported.

Adverse effects

Both nicotinamide and nicotinic acid can be toxic in excessive amounts, but the effects are somewhat different.

Nicotinamide

In normal doses, nicotinamide is not toxic, but chronic administration at doses of 3 g daily for periods greater than three months may cause nausea, headaches, heartburn, fatigue, sore throat, dry hair, dry skin and blurred vision.

Nicotinic acid

Acute flushing (at doses of 100–200 mg, but reduced risk with sustained-release preparation), pounding headache, dizziness, nausea, vomiting, pruritus; occasionally decreased glucose tolerance and increased uric acid levels; rarely hepatic impairment (risk may be increased with sustained-release preparations) and hypertension.

Interactions

Drugs

Lipid-lowering drugs: increased risk of rhabdomyolysis and myopathy (combined therapy should include careful monitoring).

Nutrients

Adequate amounts of all B vitamins are required for optimal functioning; deficiency or excess of one B vitamin may lead to abnormalities in the metabolism of another.

Dose

Nicotinamide is available in the form of tablets, but is found mainly in multivitamin and mineral products.

Dietary supplements generally provide 30–50 mg daily.

Reference

1 Elam MB, Hunninghake DB, Davis KB, *et al.* Effect of niacin on lipid and lipoprotein levels and glycemic control in patients with diabetes and peripheral arterial disease. *JAMA* 2000; 284: 1263–1270.

Octacosanol

Description

Octacosanol is the main component of policosanol, which is isolated from sugar cane wax. Octacosanol has also been isolated from *Eupolyphaga sinensis,* some *Euphorbia* species, *Acacia modeseta, Serenoa repens* and other plants, including whole grains, fruit and vegetables. It is a 28-carbon long-chain alcohol.

Action

Octacosanol appears to have a lipid-lowering effect, and there is some evidence (albeit limited) that octacosanol may improve muscle endurance.

Possible uses

Octacosanol has been claimed to be protective against cardiovascular disease, for improving endurance in athletes, and to be beneficial in patients with Parkinson's disease.

Cardiovascular disease

Animal studies have shown that policosanol reduces serum lipids,[1–3] platelet aggregation[4] and atherosclerosis,[5,6] and that it may help to protect against cerebral ischaemia.[7]

Platelet aggregation

In a double-blind, placebo-controlled study, 37 healthy volunteers were randomised to receive either placebo or policosanol 10 mg daily for seven days, 20 mg daily for the next seven days, then 40 mg daily for the next seven days. Platelet aggregation (induced by adenosine 5′-diphosphate (ADP) and adrenaline (epinephrine)) reduced as the dose of policosanol increased, with significant effects observed after the second and third but not the first dose level. Coagulation time remained unchanged during the trial.[8]

In a further randomised, placebo-controlled, double-blind study involving healthy volunteers, policosanol (5, 10, 25 and 50 mg) administered orally, inhibited platelet aggregation (induced by ADP and epinephrine (adrenaline)), and at a dose of 20 mg daily for seven days the inhibition was significant. A modest effect on collagen-induced platelet aggregation was observed only at the highest dose (50 mg daily), while the lowest dose (5 mg daily) was ineffective. Policosanol did not affect coagulation time.[9] Further studies in healthy volunteers[10] and those with type II hypercholesterolaemia[11] have shown similar effects on platelet aggregation.

A randomised, double-blind, placebo-controlled study was carried out in 43 healthy volunteers to compare the effects of policosanol (20 mg daily), aspirin (100 mg daily) and combination therapy (policosanol 20 mg daily plus aspirin 100 mg daily) on platelet aggregation. With policosanol platelet aggregation induced by ADP, epinephrine (adrenaline) and collagen was significantly reduced. Aspirin reduced platelet aggregation induced by collagen and epinephrine (adrenaline), but not by ADP. Combined therapy significantly inhibited platelet aggregation by all agonists. Coagulation time did not change during the trial. The authors concluded that policosanol (20 mg daily) was as effective as aspirin (100 mg daily), and that combination therapy showed some advantages over the respective monotherapies.[12]

Lipid lowering

A pilot single-blind, randomised, placebo-controlled trial was conducted in 23 middle-aged out-patients with well-documented chronic coronary heart disease (CHD) and primary or marginal hyperlipidaemia. Twelve patients received 1 mg policosanol twice a day, and 11 patients received placebo. The treated group showed a significant reduction in total (14.8%) and LDL (15.6%) cholesterol. The authors stated there was also a clinical tendency in five out of 12 of the treated patients towards improvement of CHD.[13]

In a two-year, double-blind, randomised, placebo-controlled trial involving 69 patients with total and LDL cholesterol poorly controlled by diet, octacosanol 5 mg twice a day was associated with a 25% reduction in LDL cholesterol and an 18% reduction in total cholesterol. Ratios of LDL to HDL cholesterol were also reduced. All changes were significant and were maintained throughout the two years of the study.[14]

Another double-blind, placebo-controlled trial in 29 patients with non-insulin-dependent diabetes mellitus (NIDDM) and hypercholesterolaemia found that 10 mg policosanol daily significantly reduced total cholesterol by 17.5% and LDL cholesterol by 21.8%, non-significantly reduced triglycerides by 6.6%, and non-significantly raised HDL cholesterol by 11.3%. Glycaemic control was unaffected, and no adverse effects were attributable to policosanol. The authors concluded that policosanol is safe and effective in patients with NIDDM and hypercholesterolaemia.[15]

A further double-blind, randomised study comparing the effect of policosanol (10 mg daily; 55 patients) with the two HMG-CoA reductase inhibitors, lovastatin (20 mg daily; 26 patients) or simvastatin (10 mg daily; 25 patients), showed that LDL cholesterol was reduced by 24% with policosanol, by 22% with lovastatin and by 15% with simvastatin. HDL cholesterol was increased in the policosanol group, but not in the two groups using HMG-CoA reductase inhibitors.[16]

A similar study comparing policosanol (10 mg daily) with acipimox (750 mg daily), involving 63 patients, showed that policosanol reduced total cholesterol and LDL cholesterol by 15.8% and 21%, respectively, and raised the ratio of LDL to HDL cholesterol by 15.8%. Acipimox reduced both total cholesterol and LDL cholesterol by 7.5%.[17]

A further study comparing policosanol (10 mg daily) and pravastatin (10 mg daily) showed reductions in total and LDL cholesterol with policosanol of 13.9% and 19.3%, respectively, and raised the LDL:HDL cholesterol ratio by 28.3%. Pravastatin lowered total cholesterol by 11.8% and LDL cholesterol by 15.6%. Policosanol reduced platelet aggregation to a greater extent than pravastatin. The authors concluded that policosanol (10 mg daily) produces more favourable effects on serum lipids and platelet aggregation than pravastatin (10 mg daily).[18] A further study comparing policosanol (10 mg daily) with lovastatin (20 mg daily) in 53 patients showed similar effects on serum lipid levels.[19]

Further studies have shown that policosanol reduced serum total and LDL cholesterol and raised HDL cholesterol in a study involving 437 individuals with type II hypercholesterolaemia and additional coronary risk factors,[20] and in a study involving 69 healthy subjects, policosanol decreased the susceptibility of LDL cholesterol to oxidation *in vitro*.[21] Similar influences on cholesterol with policosanol have been shown in a trial involving 244 postmenopausal women with hypercholesterolaemia.[22]

Parkinson's disease

Octacosanol has been evaluated in patients with mild to moderate Parkinson's disease. In a double-blind cross-over trial, 10 patients received either 5 mg octacosanol or placebo (both three times a day) for six weeks. Only three patients had improved significantly at the study's end. Some responded slightly or had no disease progression during the study. Activities of daily living and mood improved, but physical endurance and parkinsonian symptoms did not. One patient experienced dizziness and another experienced exacerbation of dyskinesias. The authors concluded that octacosanol might be beneficial for patients with mild Parkinson's disease, but that the benefit is likely to be small and less than that exerted by existing treatments.[23]

Amyotrophic lateral sclerosis

Anecdotally, octacosanol has been claimed to improve symptoms of amyotrophic lateral sclerosis (ALS), but a placebo-controlled, double-blind, cross-over trial in which patients received either 40 mg octacosanol or placebo for three months and then the groups were crossed over showed no difference between octacosanol and placebo.[24]

Athletes

Octacosanol is now being widely advertised for enhancing performance in athletes, particularly in the USA and Australia. However, there are almost no supporting data.

One study in 33 male student athletes (20 controls, 13 supplemented) showed that a pre-packed supplementation containing 29 supplements including 2000 μg octacosanol was associated with a decrease in body fat and increase in muscle girth measurement, indicating the formation of lean body mass. However, the study was not blinded, the diet not controlled, and the pre-pack contained a variety of ingredients in addition to octacosanol.[25]

Another study in 16 subjects (students and lecturers in physical education) measured grip strength, chest strength, and reaction time to both auditory and visual stimuli. Following supplementation with 1000 μg octacosanol for eight weeks, only grip strength and reaction time to visual stimuli were improved.[26]

> **Conclusion**
> A number of human studies have now been conducted with policosanol, and have shown benefits in lipid lowering and platelet aggregation compared with placebo. They have also shown similar effects to various lipid-lowering drugs. However, most of the studies have been conducted by one research group in Havana, Cuba. There is very little evidence that octacosanol is useful for athletes.

Precautions/contraindications

None documented.

Pregnancy and breast-feeding

No problems have been reported, but there have not been sufficient studies to guarantee the safety of octacosanol in pregnancy and breast-feeding. The effects are unknown, and octacosanol is best avoided.

Adverse effects

None reported, but there are no long-term studies assessing the safety of octacosanol. In a trial investigating the effects of placebo and policosanol, 5 mg, 10 mg and 20 mg daily, policosanol was said by the authors to be well tolerated with no disturbances of blood or clinical biochemistry. Adverse effects were found to be mild and transient with no differences between the groups.[27]

Interactions

None documented. A study in rats showed that adding policosanol to warfarin therapy did not enhance the prolongation of bleeding time induced by warfarin alone.[28]

Dose

Octacosanol is available in the form of tablets and capsules.

The dose is not established. Doses used in studies have varied from 1 to 20 mg policosanol daily.

References

1 Arruzazabala ML, Carbajal D, Mas R, *et al.* Cholesterol-lowering effect of policosanol in rabbits. *Biol Res* 1994; 27: 205–208.
2 Menendez R, Amor AM, Gonzalez RM, *et al.* Effect of policosanol on the hepatic cholesterol biosynthesis of normocholesterolemic rats. *Biol Res* 1996; 29: 253–257.
3 Menendez R, Arruzazabala ML, Mas R, *et al.* Cholesterol-lowering effect of policosanol on rabbits with hypercholesterolaemia induced by a wheat starch-casein diet. *Br J Nutr* 1997; 77: 923–932.
4 Arruzazabala ML, Carbajal D, Mas R, *et al.* Effects of policosanol on platelet aggregation in rats. *Thromb Res* 1993; 69: 321–327.
5 Noa M, Mas R, de la Rosa MC, *et al.* Effect of policosanol on lipofundin-induced atherosclerotic lesions in rats. *J Pharm Pharmacol* 1995; 47: 289–291.
6 Arruzazabala ML, Noa M, Menendez R, *et al.*

Protective effect of policosanol on atherosclerotic lesions in rabbits with exogenous hypercholesterolaemia. *Braz J Med Biol Res* 2000; 33: 835–840.

7 Molina V, Arruzazabala ML, Carbajal D, *et al.* Effect of policosanol on cerebral ischemia in Mongolian gerbils. *Braz J Med Biol Res* 1999; 32: 1269–1276.

8 Arruzazabala ML, Valdes S, Mas R, *et al.* Effect of policosanol successive dose increases on platelet aggregation in healthy volunteers. *Pharmacol Res* 1996; 34: 181–185.

9 Valdes S, Arruzazabala ML, Fernandez L, *et al.* Effect of policosanol on platelet aggregation in healthy volunteers. *Int J Clin Pharmacol Res* 1996; 16: 67–72.

10 Carbajal D, Arruzazabala ML, Valdes S, *et al.* Effect of policosanol on platelet aggregation and serum levels of arachidonic acid metabolites in healthy volunteers. *Prostaglandins Leukot Essent Fatty Acids* 1998; 58: 61–64.

11 Arruzazabala ML, Mas R, Molina V, *et al.* Effect of policosanol on platelet aggregation in type II hypercholesterolemic patients. *Int J Tissue React* 1998; 20: 119–124.

12 Arruzazabala ML, Valdes S, Mas R, *et al.* Comparative study of policosanol, aspirin and the combination therapy policosanol-aspirin on platelet aggregation in healthy volunteers. *Pharmacol Res* 1997; 36: 293–297.

13 Batista J, Stusser R, Saez F, *et al.* Effect of policosanol on hyperlipidemia and coronary heart disease in middle-aged patients. A 14-month pilot study. *Int J Clin Pharmacol Ther* 1996; 34: 134–137.

14 Canetti M, Moreira M, Mas R, *et al.* A two-year study on the efficacy and tolerability of policosanol in patients with type II hyperlipoproteinaemia. *Int J Clin Pharmacol Ther* 1995; 15: 159–165.

15 Torres O, Agramonte AJ, Illnait J, *et al.* Treatment of hypercholesterolemia in NIDDM with policosanol. *Diabetes Care* 1995; 18: 393–397.

16 Prat H, Roman O, Pino E. Comparative effects of policosanol and two HMG-CoA reductase inhibitors on type II hypercholesterolemia. *Rec Med Chil* 1999; 127: 286–294.

17 Alcocer L, Fernandez L, Campos E, *et al.* A comparative study of policosanol versus acipimox in patients with type II hypercholesterolemia. *Int J Tissue React* 1999; 21: 85–92.

18 Castano G, Mas R, Arruzazabala ML, *et al.* Effect of policosanol and pravastatin on lipid profile, platelet aggregation and endothelemia in older hypercholesterolemic patients. *Int J Clin Pharmacol Res* 1999; 19: 105–116.

19 Crespo N, Illnait J, Mas R, *et al.* Comparative study of the efficacy and tolerability of policosanol and lovastatin in patients with hypercholesterolemia and noninsulin dependent diabetes mellitus. *Int J Clin Pharmacol Res* 1999; 19: 117–127.

20 Mas R, Castano G, Illnait J, *et al.* Effects of policosanol in patients with type II hypercholesterolemia and additional risk factors. *Clin Pharmacol Ther* 1999; 65: 439–447.

21 Menendez R, Mas R, Amor AM, *et al.* Effects of policosanol treatment on the susceptibility of low density lipoprotein (LDL) isolated from healthy volunteers to oxidative modification in vitro. *Br J Clin Pharmacol* 2000; 50: 255–262.

22 Castano G, Mas R, Fernandez L, *et al.* Effects of policosanol on postmenopausal women with type II hypercholesterolemia. *Gynecol Endocrinol* 2000; 14: 187–195.

23 Snider SR. Octacosanol in Parkinsonism. *Ann Neurol* 1984; 16: 273 (letter).

24 Norris FH, Denys EH, Fallat RJ. Trial of octacosanol on amyotrophic lateral sclerosis. *Neurology*, 1986; 36: 1263–1264.

25 Cockerill DL, Bucci LR. Increases in muscle girth and decreases in body fat associated with a nutritional supplement program. *Chiro Sports Med* 1987; 1: 73–76.

26 Saint-John M, McNaughton L. Octacosanol ingestion and its effects on metabolic responses to submaximal cycle ergometry, reaction time, and chest and grip strength. *Int Clin Nutr Rev* 1986; 6: 81–87.

27 Pons P, Rodriguez M, Robaina C, *et al.* Effects of successive dose increases of policosanol on the lipid profile of patients with type II hypercholesterolaemia and tolerability to treatment. *Int J Clin Pharmacol Res* 1994; 14: 27–33.

28 Carbajal D, Arruzazabala ML, Valdes, S *et al.* Interaction of policosanol-warfarin on bleeding time and thrombosis in rats. *Pharmacol Res* 1998; 38: 89–91.

Pangamic acid

Description and nomenclature

An alternative name for pangamic acid is vitamin B_{15}, but it is not an officially recognised vitamin. Pangamic acid is the name given to a product originally claimed to contain D-gluconodimethyl aminoacetic acid, which was obtained from apricot kernels and later from rice bran.

Constituents

The composition of supplements is undefined, but they may contain one or more of the following substances: calcium gluconate, glycine, *N*,*N*-dimethylglycine and *N*,*N*-diisopropylamine dichloroacetate; (*N*,*N*-diisopropylamine dichloroacetate has pharmacological activity).

Dietary sources

Apricot kernels, brewer's yeast, liver, wheatgerm, bran and wholegrains.

Possible uses

Research by Soviet sports scientists focused attention on pangamic acid, but very little research has been done in other countries. Pangamic acid is claimed to enhance athletic performance and to be beneficial in cardiovascular disease, asthma and diabetes mellitus. Scientific studies show no evidence of therapeutic efficacy for pangamic acid.

Precautions/contraindications

Pangamic acid should not be taken at all by anyone.

Adverse effects

Pangamic acid may be mutagenic and thus potentially able to cause cancer. It may cause occasional transient flushing of the skin.

Dose

Pangamic acid should be avoided. Dietary supplements are rarely available in UK high-street outlets, but may be available on the Internet.

Pantothenic acid

Description

Pantothenic acid is a water-soluble B complex vitamin.

Human requirements

See Table 1 for Dietary Reference Values for pantothenic acid.

Intakes

In the UK, the average adult diet provides 5.1 mg daily.

Action

Pantothenic acid functions mainly as a component of co-enzyme A and acyl carrier protein. Co-enzyme A has a central role as a co-factor for enzymes involved in the metabolism of lipids, carbohydrates and proteins; it is also required for the synthesis of cholesterol, steroid hormones, acetylcholine and porphyrins. As a component of acyl carrier protein, pantothenic acid is involved in various transfer reactions and in the assembly of acetate units into longer-chain fatty acids.

Dietary sources

See Table 2 for dietary sources of pantothenic acid.

Metabolism

Absorption

Absorption occurs in the small intestine.

Distribution

Pantothenic acid is widely distributed in body tissues (particularly in the liver, adrenal glands, heart and kidneys) mainly as co-enzyme A.

Table 1 Dietary Reference Values for pantothenic acid (mg/day)

EU RDA = 6 mg

Age	UK safe intake	USA AI	European acceptable range
0–6 months	1.7	1.7	–
7–12 months	1.7	1.8	–
1–3 years	1.7	2.0	–
4–10 years	3–7	–	–
4–8 years	–	3.0	–
9–13 years	–	4.0	–
Males and females			
11–50+ years	3–7	–	3–12
14–70+ years	–	5.0	–

Table 2 Dietary sources of pantothenic acid

Food portion	Pantothenic acid content (mg)
Breakfast cereals	
1 bowl All-Bran (45 g)	0.7
1 bowl Bran Flakes (45 g)	0.7
1 bowl Corn Flakes (30 g)	0.1
1 bowl Muesli (95 g)	**1.1**
2 pieces Shredded Wheat	0.4
2 Weetabix	0.3
Cereal products	
Bread, brown, 2 slices	0.2
white, 2 slices	0.2
wholemeal, 2 slices	0.4
1 chapati	0.1
Milk and dairy products	
½ pint (280 ml) milk, whole, semi-skimmed or skimmed	0.8
1 pot yoghurt (150 g)	0.6
Cheese (50 g)	0.2
1 egg, size 2 (60 g)	**1.0**
Meat and fish	
Beef, roast (85 g)	0.5
Lamb, roast (85 g)	0.5
Pork, roast (85 g)	0.8
1 chicken leg portion	**1.5**
Liver, lamb's, cooked (90 g)	**7.0**
Kidney, lamb's, cooked (75 g)	**4.0**
Fish, cooked (150 g)	0.5
Vegetables	
1 small can baked beans (200 g)	0.4
Chickpeas, cooked (105 g)	0.3
Red kidney beans (105 g)	0.2
Peas, boiled (100 g)	0.1
Potatoes, boiled (150 g)	0.6
Green vegetables, average, boiled (100g)	0.2
Fruit	
1 banana	0.5
1 orange	0.6
Nuts	
30 peanuts	0.7
Yeast	
Brewer's yeast (10 g)	**1.0**

Excellent sources (>1 mg/portion) (**bold**).

Elimination

About 70% is excreted unchanged in the urine and 30% in the faeces.

Bioavailability

Bioavailability may be reduced by some drugs (see Interactions) and high fat intake, but increased by a diet high in protein.

Deficiency

Deficiency has not been clearly identified in humans consuming a mixed diet.

Possible uses

Pantothenic acid has been used for a wide range for disorders such as acne, alopecia, allergies, burning feet, asthma, grey hair, dandruff, cholesterol lowering, improving exercise performance, depression, osteorathritis, rheumatoid arthritis, multiple sclerosis, stress, shingles, ageing and Parkinson's disease. It has been investigated in clinical trials for arthritis, cholesterol lowering and exercise performance.

Arthritis

In an uncontrolled trial, patients treated with pantothenate 12.5 mg twice a day showed a limited, variable improvement within one to two weeks of therapy, which ended upon discontinuation of therapy.[1] In a double-blind, placebo-controlled trial,[2] 94 patients with arthritis (of whom 27 had rheumatoid arthritis) were randomised to receive large doses of calcium pantothenate (titrated up from 500 mg daily to 2000 mg daily) or a placebo for eight weeks. There was no significant reduction in either group in the duration of morning stiffness or disability, but both groups experienced significant relief from pain. When the subjects with rheumatoid arthritis were analysed separately, the group receiving pantothenate showed statistically significant reduction in morning stiffness, disability and pain compared with placebo.

Cholesterol lowering

A double-blind, placebo-controlled, cross-over study in 29 patients with various types of dyslipidaemia found that 900 mg pantothenic acid daily reduced total and LDL cholesterol in type IIb hyperlipidaemia with varying effects in type IV patients.[3]

Exercise performance

Two double-blind, placebo-controlled studies with pantothenic acid in runners[4] and cyclists[5] showed that pantothenic acid had no effect on exercise performance.

> **Conclusion**
> Research is too limited to be able to make recommendations for pantothenic acid.

Precautions/contraindications

None reported.

Pregnancy and breast-feeding

No problems reported.

Adverse effects

No adverse effects except for occasional diarrhoea have been reported in humans.

Interactions

Drugs

Alcohol: excessive alcohol intake may increase requirement for pantothenic acid.

Oral contraceptives: may increase requirement for pantothenic acid.

Nutrients

Adequate amounts of all B vitamins are required for optimal functioning; deficiency or excess of one B vitamin may lead to abnormalities in the metabolism of another.

Dose

Pantothenic acid and calcium pantothenate are available in the form of tablets and capsules, but they are found mainly in multivitamin and mineral preparations.

The dose is not established. Dietary supplements contain up to 100 mg daily.

References

1 Annand J. Pantothenic acid and OA. *Lancet* 1963; 2: 1168.
2 General Practitioner Research Group. Calcium pantothenate in arthritic conditions: A report from the General Practitioner Research Group. *Practitioner* 1980; 224: 208–211.
3 Gaddi A, Descovich GC, Noseda G, *et al.* Controlled evaluation of pantethine, a natural hypolipemic compound, in patients with hyperlipidaemia. *Atherosclerosis* 1984; 50: 73–83.
4 Nice C, Reeves AG, Brinck-Johnsen T, *et al.* The effects of pantothenic acid on human exercise capacity. *J Sports Med Phys Fitness* 1984; 24: 26–29.
5 Webster MJ. Physiological and performance responses to supplementation with thiamin and pantothenic acid derivatives. *Eur J Appl Physiol* 1998; 77: 486–491.

Para-amino benzoic acid

Description and nomenclature

Para-amino benzoic acid (PABA) is a member of the vitamin B complex, but is not an officially recognised vitamin.

Dietary sources

Brewer's yeast, liver, wheatgerm, bran and wholegrains.

Possible uses

PABA is claimed to prevent greying hair and to be useful as an anti-ageing supplement. It has been used in digestive disorders, arthritis, insomnia and depression. There is no convincing scientific evidence available.

A derivative of PABA is used topically as a sunscreen agent; this is effective in the prevention of sunburn.

Adverse effects

Toxicity is low, but high doses (>30 mg) may cause anorexia, nausea, vomiting, liver toxicity, fever, itching and skin rash.

Interactions

Drugs

Sulphonamides: kill bacteria by mimicking PABA; supplements containing PABA should be avoided while taking these drugs.

Dose

PABA is available in the form of tablets and capsules.

There is no established dose. Supplements are not justified. Dietary supplements provide 100–500 mg per dose.

Phosphatidylserine

Description

Phosphatidylserine belongs to a class of fat-soluble compounds called phospholipids. Phospholipids are essential components of cell membranes, with high concentrations found in brain. Phosphatidylserine is the most abundant phosphoplipid in the brain.

Action

Phosphatidylserine helps to ensure fluidity, flexibility and permeability in cell membranes. It stimulates the release of various transmitters, such as acetylcholine and dopamine, and enhances ion transport and increases the number of neurotransmitter receptor sites in the brain.

Possible uses

Phosphatidylserine is claimed to be useful in enhancing memory, treating depression and the prevention of age-related neurotransmitter defects.

Age-related cognitive decline

A double-blind, randomised, controlled study was conducted in 42 hospitalised demented patients, in which half the patients received 300 mg phosphatidylserine and the other half placebo. The trial lasted for six weeks. Two distinct rating scales were used: the Crighton Scale and the Peri Scale. Results showed a trend towards improvement in the treated patients and analysis of covariance showed a significant treatment effect on the Peri Scale. The results at the end of treatment were compared with results obtained three weeks later and there was still a significant difference on the Peri Scale, indicating – according to the authors – a drug-related effect.[1]

The effects of phosphatidylserine on cognitive, affective and behavioural symptoms were studied in a group of elderly women with depressive disorders. The treatment was not blinded or randomised. Patients were treated with placebo for 15 days followed by phosphatidylserine (300 mg daily) for 30 days. Changes in depression, memory and general behaviour were measured according to four different scales before and after placebo, and after treatment. Depressive symptoms were marked before placebo, did not change after placebo, and were significantly reduced by phosphatidylserine treatment. There was also improvement in memory (recall, long-term retrieval), but there were no changes in plasma levels of various neurochemicals.[2]

In a double-blind, placebo-controlled study, 149 patients with age-associated memory impairment were treated with phosphatidylserine 300 mg or placebo for 12 weeks. The supplemented subjects improved relative to placebo on performance tests related to learning and memory tasks of daily life. Analysis of subgroups showed that subjects who performed at a relatively low level prior to treatment were most likely to respond to phosphatidylserine. The authors concluded that phosphatidylserine may be a promising candidate for treating memory loss in later life.[3]

In a double-blind, placebo-controlled study, 51 patients with probable Alzheimer's disease were treated with phosphatidylserine (300 mg daily) or placebo for 12 weeks. Two rating scales were used to assess the patients, and after 12 weeks, the treated group improved on three of the 12 variables on one scale and five of the 25 variables on the other scale. Family members rated significant improvements with phosphatidylserine after six and nine weeks but not at 12 weeks. The authors stressed that phosphatidylserine might be helpful in patients with early-stage disease, but might have no effect in middle and later stages.[4]

In a double-blind, placebo-controlled crossover study, 33 patients with mild primary degenerative dementia received either phosphatidylserine 300 mg daily or placebo for eight weeks. Clinical global rating scales showed significantly more patients improving with phosphatidylserine than placebo. However, there were no significant improvements in dementia rating scale or psychometric tests.[5]

A double-blind, placebo-controlled study involving 494 elderly patients (aged 65–93 years) with moderate to severe cognitive decline were randomised to receive either phosphatidylserine 300 mg daily or placebo for six months. Sixty-nine patients dropped out of the trial. Patients were examined before the study, and at three and six months after. Statistically significant improvements in the treated group compared with placebo were observed in terms of both behavioural and cognitive parameters.[6]

Physical stress

In a double-blind trial, eight healthy men underwent three experiments with a bicycle ergometer. Before the exercise, each subject received intravenously 50 or 75 mg of phosphatidylserine or placebo. Blood samples were collected before and after the exercise and analysed for adrenaline (epinephrine), noradrenaline (norepinephrine), dopamine, adrenocorticotrophin, cortisol, growth hormone, prolactin and glucose. Physical stress induced a clear-cut increase in plasma adrenaline, noradrenaline, adrenocorticotrophic hormone (ACTH), cortisol, growth hormone and prolactin, whereas no significant change was found in plasma dopamine and glucose. Pretreatment with both 50 mg and 75 mg phosphatidylserine significantly blunted the ACTH and cortisol responses to physical stress.[7]

In a study using the same exercise protocol in the same research centre, nine healthy men were treated for three 10-day periods with placebo, 400 mg and 800 mg phosphatidylserine daily. Oral phosphatidylserine rather than the intravenous formulation was used. Phosphatidylserine 800 mg significantly blunted the ACTH and cortisol responses to physical exercise. The authors concluded that chronic oral administration of phosphatidylserine might counteract stress-induced activation of the hypothalamic-pituitary-adrenal axis in men.[8]

Conclusion

There is evidence from controlled trials that phosphatidylserine improves memory and other symptoms of cognitive decline in elderly patients. There is also some limited evidence that phosphatidylserine attenuates the cortisol response to exercise. However, this response is a natural phenomenon, and interfering with it might delay recovery in athletes. Further research is required to ascertain whether or not phosphatidylserine is beneficial in athletes.

Precautions/contraindications

None documented.

Pregnancy and breast-feeding

No problems have been reported, but there have not been sufficient studies to guarantee the safety of phosphatidylserine in pregnancy and breast-feeding.

Adverse effects

No known toxicity or side-effects, but there are no long-term studies assessing the safety of phosphatidylserine. Concerns have been expressed about phosphatidylserine supplements derived from bovine brain tissue with regard to diseases such as bovine spongiform encephalopathy (BSE). Hence, supplements based on soya protein have been developed. The two supplements are slightly different and there has been discussion about whether they have the same level of efficacy. Most research to date has been conducted with bovine-based supplements. Preliminary research in animals suggests that the effects are similar, but further work needs to be done in this area.

Dose

Phosphatidylserine is available in the form of tablets, capsules and powder.

The dose is not established. Doses used in studies have been 300 mg daily in investigations on cognitive function, and up to 800 mg daily in studies on physical stress. Supplements provide 100–800 mg daily.

References

1 Delwaide PJ, Gyselynck-Mambourg AM, Hurlet A, *et al.* Double-blind randomized controlled study of phosphatidylserine in senile demented patients. *Acta Neurol Scand* 1986; 73: 136–140.

2 Maggioni M, Picotti GB, Bondiolotti GP, *et al.* Effects of phosphatidylserine in geriatric patients with depressive disorders. *Acta Psychiatr Scand* 1990; 81: 265–270.

3 Crook TH, Tinklenberg, Yesavage J, *et al.* Effects of phosphatidylserine in age-associated memory impairment. *Neurology* 1991; 41: 644–649.

4 Crook T, Petrie W, Wells C, *et al.* Effects of phosphatidylserine in Alzheimer's disease. *Psychopharmacol Bull* 1992; 28: 61–66.

5 Cenacchi T, Bertoldin T, Farina C, *et al.* Cognitive decline in the elderly: A double-blind, placebo-controlled multicenter study on efficacy of phosphatidylserine administration. *Aging (Milano)* 1993; 5: 123–133.

6 Engel RR, Satzger W, Gunther W, *et al.* Double-blind, crossover study of phosphatidylserine versus placebo in patients with early dementia of the Alzheimer's type. *Eur Neuropsychopharmacol* 1992; 2: 149–155.

7 Monteleone P, Beinat L, Tanzillo C, *et al.* Effects of phosphatidylserine on the neuroendocrine response to physical stress in humans. *Neuroendocrinology* 1990; 52: 243–248.

8 Monteleone P, Maj M, Beinat L, *et al.* Blunting by chronic phosphatidylserine administration of the stress-induced activation of the hypothalamic-pituitary-adrenal axis in healthy men. *Eur J Clin Pharmacol* 1992; 42: 285–288.

Potassium

Description

Potassium is an essential mineral.

Human requirements

See Table 1 for Dietary Reference Values for potassium.

Intakes

In the UK, the average adult daily diet provides: for men, 3279 mg; for women, 2562 mg.

Action

Potassium is the principal intracellular cation, and is fundamental to the regulation of acid–base and water balance. It contributes to transmission of nerve impulses, control of skeletal muscle contractility and maintenance of blood pressure.

Dietary sources

See Table 2 for dietary sources of potassium.

Table 1 Dietary Reference Values for potassium (mg/day)

EU RDA = None

Age	UK		USA minimum requirement[1]	Europe PRI
	LNRI	RNI		
0–3 months	400	800	500	–
4–6 months	400	850	500	–
7–9 months	400	700	700	800
10–12 months	450	700	700	800
1–3 years	450	800	1000	1100
4–6 years	600	1100	1400	1100
7–10 years	950	2200	1600	2000
11–14 years	1600	3100	2000	3100
15–50+ years	2000	3500	2000	3100
Pregnancy	*	*	*	*
Lactation	*	*	*	*

*No increment.

[1]Desirable intakes may exceed these values.

Note: No EAR has been derived for potassium.

Table 2 Dietary sources of potassium

Food portion	Potassium content[1] (mg)
Breakfast cereals	
1 bowl All-Bran (45 g)	450
1 bowl Bran Flakes (45 g)	250
1 bowl Corn Flakes (30 g)	30
1 bowl Muesli (95 g)	500
2 pieces Shredded Wheat	150
2 Weetabix	150
Cereal products	
Bread, brown, 2 slices	100
white, 2 slices	70
wholemeal, 2 slices	160
1 chapati	110
Pasta, brown, boiled (150 g)	200
white, boiled (150 g)	40
Rice, brown, boiled (165 g)	150
white, boiled (165 g)	80
Milk and dairy products	
½ pint (280 ml) milk, whole, semi-skimmed or skimmed	400
1 pot yoghurt (150 g)	370
Cheese (50 g)	50
1 egg, size 2 (60 g)	50
Meat and fish	
Meat, cooked (100 g)	200–300
Liver, lamb's, cooked (90 g)	300
Kidney, lamb's, cooked (75 g)	250
White fish, cooked (150 g)	400–500
Herring or mackerel (110 g)	460
Pilchards, canned (105 g)	450
Sardines, canned (70 g)	300

Food portion	Potassium content (mg)
Vegetables	
Green vegetables, average, boiled (100g)	100–200
Potatoes, boiled (150 g)	450
baked (150 g)	*950*
1 small can baked beans (200 g)	*600*
Lentils, kidney beans or other pulses, cooked (105 g)	300
Soya beans, cooked (100 g)	500
Mixed vegetable curry (300 g)	*1250*
Fruit	
1 apple	100
8 dried apricots	*600*
1 banana	350
½ cantaloupe melon	*750*
10 dates	300
4 figs	*600*
1 orange	300
1 handful raisins	350
Nuts	
20 almonds	150
10 Brazil nuts	200
30 hazelnuts	250
30 peanuts	200
Beverages	
1 mug hot chocolate	350
1 mug Build-Up	*700*
1 mug Complan (sweet)	*600*
1 mug Horlicks	*600*
1 large glass grapefruit juice	200
1 large glass orange juice	300
1 large glass tomato juice	460

Good sources (*italics*).

Metabolism

Absorption

Absorption occurs principally in the small intestine.

Elimination

Excretion is mainly via urine (the capacity of the kidneys to conserve potassium is poor); unabsorbed and intestinally-secreted potassium is eliminated in the faeces; some is lost in saliva and sweat.

Deficiency

Potassium deficiency leads to hypokalaemia, symptoms of which include anorexia, nausea, abdominal distension, paralytic ileus; muscle weakness, reduced or absent reflexes, paralysis; listlessness, apprehension, drowsiness, irrational behaviour; respiratory failure; polydypsia, polyuria; and cardiac arrhythmias.

Possible uses

Hypertension

Potassium may lower blood pressure,[1,2] but there is evidence for a stronger relationship of the sodium to potassium ratio to blood pressure than potassium alone.[3] Several other minerals (see Calcium and Magnesium monographs) may affect blood pressure, and dietary measures to reduce blood pressure might be more effective if the intake of several minerals is changed simultaneously.

There is some evidence from double-blind, placebo-controlled trials that potassium supplementation (1500–3000 mg daily) can lower blood pressure in normotensive[4,5] and hypertensive[6] individuals, but another trial failed to show any benefit.[7]

Precautions/contraindications

Excessive doses are best avoided in patients with: chronic renal failure (particularly in the elderly); gastrointestinal obstruction or ulceration; peptic ulcer; Addison's disease; heart block; severe burns; acute dehydration.

Pregnancy and breast-feeding

No data are available on potassium supplements in pregnancy.

Adverse effects

Nausea, vomiting, diarrhoea and abdominal cramps may occur, particularly if potassium is taken on an empty stomach. Gastrointestinal ulceration may result from the use of modified-release preparations. Hyperkalaemia is almost unknown with oral administration provided that renal function is normal. Intakes exceeding 17 g daily (unlikely from oral supplements) would be required to cause toxicity.

Interactions

Drugs

Angiotensin-converting enzyme (ACE) inhibitors: increased risk of hyperkalaemia.
Carbenoxolone: reduced serum potassium levels.
Corticosteroids: increased excretion of potassium.
Cyclosporin: increased risk of hyperkalaemia.
Laxatives: chronic use reduces absorption of potassium.
Loop diuretics: increased risk of hypokalaemia (but potassium supplements seldom necessary with small dose of diuretic).
Non-steroidal anti-inflammatory drugs (NSAIDs): increased risk of hyperkalaemia.
Potassium-sparing diuretics: increased risk of hyperkalaemia.
Thiazide diuretics: increased risk of hypokalaemia (but potassium supplements seldom necessary with small dose of diuretic).

Dose

Mild deficiency, oral, 1500–4000 mg daily, with plenty of fluid (liquid preparations should be diluted well).

As a dietary supplement, no dose has been established.

References

1 Khaw KT, Thom S. Randomized double-blind crossover trial of potassium on blood pressure in normal subjects. *Lancet* 1982; 2: 1127–1129.
2 Cappuccio FP, MacGregor DA. Does potassium supplementation lower blood pressure? A meta-analysis of published trials. *J Hypertens* 1991; 9: 465–473.
3 Grobbee DE, Hofman A, Roelandt JT, *et al.* Sodium restriction and potassium supplementation in young people with mildly elevated blood pressure. *J Hypertens* 1987; 5: 115–119.

4 Sacks FM, Willett WC, Smith A, *et al.* Effect on blood pressure of potassium, calcium and magnesium in women with low habitual intake. *Hypertension* 1995; 26: 950–956.
5 Brancati FL, Appel LJ, Seidler AJ, *et al.* Effect of potassium supplementation on blood pressure in African Americans on a low-potassium diet: A randomized, double-blind, placebo-controlled trial. *Arch Intern Med* 1996; 156: 61–67.
6 Fotherby MD, Potter JF. Potassium supplementation reduces clinic and ambulatory blood pressure in elderly hypertensive patients. *J Hypertens* 1992; 10: 1403–1408.
7 Sacks FM, Brown LE, Appel L, *et al.* Combinations of potassium, calcium and magnesium supplements in hypertension. *Hypertension* 1995; 26: 950–956.

Probiotics and prebiotics

Description

A probiotic is a live microbial food supplement which beneficially affects the host animal by improving its intestinal microbial balance.[1,2] For human adult use, this includes fermented milk products and over-the-counter products, such as powders, tablets and capsules that contain lyophilised bacteria. The micro-organisms involved are usually producers of lactic acid, such as lactobacilli and bifidobacteria, which are widely used in yoghurt and dairy products. However, yeasts have also been used (see Table 1). These microbes are non-pathogenic and survive passage through the stomach and small bowel.

A prebiotic is a non-digestible food ingredient, which beneficially affects the host by selectively stimulating the growth, activity or both, of one or a limited number of bacterial species already resident in the colon.[3] Prebiotics are not digested by intestinal enzymes, instead passing through the upper gastrointestinal tract to the colon where they are used selectively as fuel by beneficial bacteria.

Although any food residue entering the colon is a potential prebiotic candidate, it is the influence of the food residue on certain specific microbes that is important. Current research tends to be directed towards foods that have the ability to enhance the growth and activity of supposed health-promoting bacteria, such as lactic acid producers (see Table 1),[4,5] although future research may well look at the possible role of prebiotics that could slow the growth of pathogenic bacteria.

Lactulose was used more than 40 years ago as a prebiotic infant formula food supplement to increase numbers of lactobacilli in infant intestine,[6] but the specificity of this substrate for enhancing these micro-organisms has not been effectively proven scientifically. In humans, consumption of fructo-oligosaccharides increases the proportion of bifidobacteria in faeces.[7] Similar effects have been observed in rats fed with galacto-oligosaccharides and colonised with human faecal flora.[8]

Possible uses

The possible benefits to health of probiotics and prebiotics are:

- Prevention and treatment of diarrhoea.
- Alleviation of lactose intolerance.
- Prevention and treatment of vaginal infections.
- Enhancement of the immune system.
- Treatment of allergic conditions.
- Lowering of serum cholesterol.
- Prevention of cancer and tumour growth.

Diarrhoea

There is a relatively large volume of literature supporting the use of probiotics in diarrhoeal conditions, but it is only recently that the scientific basis for this has started to become established, with the publication of a number of respectable clinical studies. Probiotics have been examined for their effectiveness in the prevention and treatment of several types of diarrhoea, including antibiotic-associated diarrhoea, bacterial and viral diarrhoea and travellers' diarrhoea, as well as that caused by lactose intolerance. The effects of probiotics, particularly with some bacterial strains and in some types of diarrhoea, appears promising,

Table 1 Examples of commonly used probiotics and prebiotics[4,5]

Probiotics	Prebiotics
Lactobacilli	Fructo-oligosaccharides
L. acidophilus	Galacto-oligosaccharides
L. casei	Inulin
L. delbrueckii subspc. *bulgaricus*	Lactulose
L. reuteri	Lactitol
L. brevis	
L. cellobiosus	
L. curvatus	
L. fermentium	
L. plantarum	
L. gasseri	
L. rhamnosus	
Gram-positive cocci	
Lactococcus lactis subspc. *cremoris*	
Streptococcus salivarius subspc. *thermophilus*	
Enterococcus faecium	
S. diaacetylactis	
S. intermedius	
Bifidobacteria	
B. bifidum	
B. adolescentis	
B. animalis	
B. infantis	
B. longum	
B. thermophilum	
Yeasts	
Saccharomyces boulardii	
S. cerevisiae	

but the effects of prebiotics on diarrhoea are currently unknown.

Various mechanisms by which probiotics could be of benefit in diarrhoea have been proposed and summarised in two reviews.[9,10] These include: reduction in gastrointestinal pH through stimulation of lactic-acid-producing bacteria; a direct antagonistic action on gastrointestinal pathogens; competition with pathogens for binding and receptor sites; and improved immune function and competition for limited nutrients.

A detailed review[11] of all placebo-controlled, human studies supplementing *L. acidophilus, B. longum, L. casei* GG and other selected microorganisms from 1966 to 1995 concluded that, 'these studies have shown that biotherapeutic agents have been used successfully to prevent antibiotic-associated diarrhoea, to prevent acute infantile diarrhoea, to treat recurrent *Clostridium difficile* disease, and to treat various other diarrhoeal illnesses'. The authors also noted that many of the studies included small numbers of subjects.

Evidence for a beneficial effect of probiotics in diarrhoea appears to be strongest for that caused by rotavirus. Rotavirus infection causes gastroenteritis, which is characterised by acute diarrhoea and vomiting. Gastroenteritis is a leading cause of morbidity and mortality among children world-wide. A recent review of studies that used *Lactobacillus, Bifidobacterium* and *Enterococcus* concluded that *Lactobacillus GG* (a new *Lactobacillus* strain isolated from human intestine) consistently shortened the diarrhoeal phase of rotavirus by one day,[12] but that evidence was less strong for a role of *Lactobacillus GG* and other probiotics in the prevention of diarrhoea due to bacterial or other viral infections.

Travellers' diarrhoea

The prevention of travellers' diarrhoea by lactobacilli, bifidobacteria, enterococci and streptococci has been investigated in several studies, but results have been inconsistent. In a double-blind, placebo-controlled trial, 820 Finnish travellers to two holiday resorts in Turkey were randomised to receive either *Lactobacillus GG* or placebo.[13] The overall incidence of diarrhoea was 43.8%. Of the 331 sufferers, 178 (46.5%) were in the placebo group and 153 (41%) were in the *Lactobacillus* group, but the difference was not significant. However, in one of the resorts, the treatment significantly reduced the incidence of diarrhoea from 39.5% (30 out of 76) in the placebo group to 23.9% (17 out of 71) in the treatment group. In another study involving 245 travellers to developing countries, the risk of diarrhoea on any one day in travellers who took *Lactobacillus GG* was 3.9% compared with 7.4% in the control group.[14]

In another study, the incidence of diarrhoea was reduced from 71% to 43% in travellers to Egypt who were given capsules of *S. thermophilus, L. bulgaricus, L. acidophilus and B. bifidum.*[15] However, neither *L. acidophilus* nor *Enterococcus faecium* had any beneficial effects on diarrhoea in groups of Austrian tourists.[16] In addition, no effect of *L. acidophilus* or *L. fermentum* was observed in soldiers who were sent to Belize in Central America,[17] and it seems that the effect of probiotics on travellers' diarrhoea depends on the bacterial strain used, and also the destination of the traveller.[12]

Antibiotic-associated diarrhoea

Diarrhoea due to the growth of pathogenic bacteria is the most common side-effect of antibiotic use, and *in-vitro* studies have shown that some bacterial strains can inhibit this growth. One study has shown that *Lactobacillus GG* (in yoghurt) reduced the incidence and duration of diarrhoea in healthy men receiving erythromycin for seven days.[18] *Lactobacillus GG* successfully eradicated *Clostridium difficile* in five patients with relapsing colitis,[19] *Enterococcus* SF68 reduced the incidence of diarrhoea caused by antibiotics,[20] whereas studies with *L. acidophilus*[21,22] have provided no conclusive evidence of benefit with this strain in prevention of diarrhoea caused by antibiotics.

Lactose intolerance

Lactose intolerance is a problem for a large proportion of the world's population for whom lactose acts like an osmotic non-digestible carbohydrate because they have a low amount of intestinal lactase. During fermentation of yoghurt and acidophilus milk, *Lactobacilli* produce lactase that hydrolyses lactose to glucose and galactose. This predigestion of lactose could potentially reduce the symptoms associated with lactose intolerance in susceptible individuals, and probiotics have been shown to improve lactose digestion and reduce intolerance in some studies[23,24] but not others.[25] The effects of prebiotics on lactose intolerance is unknown, although their influence on colonic bacterial adaptation may mean that they are beneficial.

Vaginal infections

One of the claims frequently made for probiotics, specifically for *L. acidophilus* is that it can prevent vaginal infections. The conclusions of a review were that there was evidence – albeit limited – for *L. acidophilus* in the prevention of candidal vaginitis.[11]

In a double-blind, controlled, cross-over trial of 46 women with a history of vaginal infections, participants were randomised to receive either *L. acidophilus* yoghurt (150 ml daily) containing live organisms or pasteurised yoghurt (150 ml daily) for two months each with a two-month washout period between interventions. However, only seven subjects completed the whole study, and the reason for the high dropout rate was not explained. The yoghurt containing live organisms was associated with a significant reduction in episodes of bacterial vaginosis. Both yoghurts were associated with a decrease in candidal vaginitis, but there was no significant difference between the treatments.[26] There is no evidence from controlled trials to show that *L. acidophilus* used intravaginally can prevent or treat vaginal infections.

Immunity

The colonic microflora affects systemic and mucosal immunity in the host. Probiotics are claimed to stimulate the immune system, and preliminary evidence suggests that these substances could increase the immune response.[27,28] However, several studies have used fermented milk enriched with probiotics and it is unclear whether observed effects are due to the probiotics or the fermented milk, or both.

Allergic conditions

Recent research interest has focused on the potential role of probiotics in various conditions known to have an allergic component. There is preliminary evidence that *Lactobacillus GG*[29,30] and *Bifidobacterium Bb-12*[30] could improve symptoms in infants with atopic eczema.

Cholesterol

The influence of probiotics on serum cholesterol levels is the subject of controversy. Studies in the 1970s and 1980s frequently reported significant reductions in serum cholesterol with daily consumption of fermented milk, but these studies have been criticised on methodological grounds, including the fact that in most of the studies showing positive results, large volumes of yoghurt (0.5–8.4 l) were consumed.[31] Two fairly recent controlled trials have shown that yoghurt (200 ml daily) containing live cultures of *L. acidophilus*[32] or yoghurt (375 ml daily) fermented with *L. acidophilus* with added fructo-oligosaccharides[33] (prebiotic) reduced serum cholesterol by 2.9 and 4.4%, respectively. Another study indicated that inulin (a prebiotic) may also lower serum cholesterol levels.[34]

Cancer

Observational data suggest that consumption of fermented dairy products is associated with lower prevalence of colon cancer.[35] In addition, there is preliminary evidence from animal studies that both probiotics[36] and prebiotics[37] could be anti-mutagenic. Two studies in Japanese patients[38,39] showed that daily intake of *L. casei* postponed recurrence of bladder tumours, but this finding awaits confirmation. There is currently no conclusive evidence in humans that these products can prevent cancer.

Osteoporosis

There is some evidence that prebiotics (inulin and oligofructose) can improve calcium absorption,[40,41] and this effect could enhance bone mineral density with a consequent reduction in the risk of osteoporosis. However, there are no human studies with prebiotics assessing the risk of osteoporosis.

Conclusion

The colonic microflora is important to health, and modification of the bacterial species inhabiting the large bowel – using probiotics and prebiotics – has been suggested to produce potential heath benefits. There are a growing number of reports on the use of both probiotics and prebiotics, and although they show ability to alter the colonic microflora, evidence that they can reduce the risk of diseases is more limited. This may in part be because of differences in methodology, particularly the large number of different strains that have been used. The evidence for an effect of probiotics in diarrhoea, particularly *Lactobacillus GG* in rotavirus infection, is among the best. There is also some evidence that probiotics can reduce lactose intolerance, boost immunity, prevent vaginal infections and lower serum cholesterol levels, but further research is required. Moreover, there is (as yet) no conclusive evidence that either prebiotics or probiotics can prevent cancer in humans.

Precautions/contraindications

None known.

Pregnancy and breast-feeding

No known problems.

Adverse effects

No known toxicity or side-effects.

Interactions

None reported.

Dose

Probiotics are available in the form of tablets and capsules of *L. acidophilus*, often with other bacteria. They are also available in the form of yoghurts and various fermented milks. Many probiotics require refrigeration to maintain viability and, like any other product, should be used before the expiry date. Commercial products have not always been found to contain the bacterial strain listed on the label, and in some cases, the bacteria may not be viable.[42]

Prebiotics are available in the form of tablets, capsules and powders of fructo-oligosaccharides and inulin.

There is no established dose for any of these products.

References

1 Fuller R, ed. *Probiotics: The Scientific Basis*. London: Chapman & Hall, 1992.
2 Fuller R. A review: Probiotics in man and animals. *J Appl Bacteriol* 1989; 66: 365–378.
3 Gibson GR, Roberfroid MB. Dietary modulation of the human colonic microbiota: Introducing the concept of prebiotics. *J Nutr* 1995; 125: 1401–1412.
4 Sadler MJ, Saltmarsh M, eds. *Functional Foods*. Cambridge: Royal Society of Chemistry, 1998: 4–5.
5 Macfarlane GT, Cummings JH. Probiotics and prebiotics: Can regulating the activities of intestinal bacteria benefit health? *Br Med J* 1999; 318: 999–1003.
6 MacGillivray PC, Finlay HVL, Binns TB. Use of lactulose to create a preponderance of lactobacilli in the intestine of bottle-fed infants. *Scott Med J* 1959; 4: 182–189.
7 Gibson GR, Beatty EB, Wang X, Cummings JH. Selective stimulation of bifidobacteria in the human colon by oligofructose and inulin. *Gastroenterology* 1995; 108: 975–982.
8 Rowland IR, Tanaka R. The effects of transgalactosylated oligosaccharides on gut flora metabolism in rats associated with human faecal microflora. *J Appl Bacteriol* 1993; 74: 667–674.
9 Collins MD, Gibson GR. Probiotics, prebiotics, and synbiotics: Approaches for modulating the microbial ecology of the gut. *Am J Clin Nutr* 1999; 69: 1052S–1057S.
10 Rolfe RD. The role of probiotic cultures in the control of gastrointestinal health. *J Nutr* 2000; 130: 396S–402S.
11 Elmer GW, Surawicz CM, MacFarland LV. Biotherapeutic agents. A neglected modality for the treatment and prevention of selected intestinal and vaginal infections. *JAMA* 1996; 275: 870–876.
12 de Roos NM, Katan MB. Effects of probiotic bacteria on diarrhea, lipid metabolism, and carcinogenesis: A review of papers published between 1988 and 1998. *Am J Clin Nutr* 2000; 71: 405–411.
13 Oksanen PJ, Salminen S, Saxelin M, *et al*. Prevention of travellers' diarrhoea by *Lactobacillus GG*. *Ann Med* 1990; 22: 53–56.
14 Hilton E, Kolakowski P, Singer C, Smith M. Efficacy of *Lactobacillus GG* as a diarrheal preventive in travellers. *J Travel Med* 1997; 4: 41–43.
15 Black FT, Andersen PL, Orskov J, *et al*. Prophylactic efficacy of lactobacilli on travellers' diarrhoea. In: Steffen R, ed. *Travel Medicine. Conference on International Travel Medicine 1, Zurich, Switzerland*. Berlin: Springer, 1989: 333–335.
16 Kollaritsch H, Wiedermann G. Travellers' diarrhoea among Austrian tourists: Epidemiology, clinical features and attempts at non-antibiotic drug prophylaxis. In: Pasini W, ed. *Proceedings of the Second International Conference on Tourist Health*. Rimini: World Health Organization, 1990: 74–82.
17 Katelaris PH, Salam I, Farthing MJG. Lactobacilli to prevent travellers' diarrhea? *N Engl J Med* 1995; 333: 1360–1361.
18 Siitonen S, Vapaatalo H, Salminen S, *et al*. Effect of *Lactobacillus GG* yoghurt in prevention of antibiotic associated diarrhoea. *Ann Med* 1990; 22: 57–59.
19 Gorbach SL, Chang TW, Goldin B. Successful treatment of relapsing *Clostridium difficile* colitis with *Lactobacillus GG*. *Lancet* 1987; 2: 1519 (letter).
20 Wunderlich PF, Braun L, Fumagalli I, *et al*. Double-blind report on the efficacy of lactic acid producing *Enterococcus* SF68 in the prevention of antibiotic-associated diarrhoea in the treatment of acute diarrhoea. *J Int Med Res* 1989; 17: 333–338.
21 Tankanow RM, Ross MB, Ertel IJ, *et al*. A double-blind, placebo-controlled study of the efficacy of Lactinex in the prophylaxis of amoxicillin-induced diarrhoea. *Ann Pharmacol* 1990; 24: 382–384.
22 Black F, Einarsson K, Lidbeck A, *et al*. Effect of lactic acid producing bacteria on the human intestinal microflora during ampicillin treatment. *Scand J Infect Dis* 1991; 23: 247–254.

23 Sanders ME. Summary of the conclusions from a consensus panel of experts on health attributes on lactic cultures: significance to fluid milk products containing cultures. *J Dairy Sci* 1993; 76: 1819–1828.
24 Mustapha A, Jiang T, Savaino DA. Improvement of lactose digestion by humans following ingestion of unfermented acidophilus milk: influence of bile sensitivity, lactose transport, and acid tolerance of *Lactobacillus acidophilus*. *J Dairy Sci* 1997; 80: 1537–1545.
25 Saltzman JR, Russell RM, Golner B, *et al*. A randomized trial of *Lactobacillus acidophilus* BG2F04 to treat lactose intolerance. *Am J Clin Nutr* 1999; 69: 140–146.
26 Shalev E, Battino S, Weiner E, *et al*. Ingestion of yogurt containing *Lactobacillus acidophilus* compared with pasteurized yoghurt as prophylaxis for recurrent candidal vaginitis and bacterial vaginosis. *Arch Fam Med* 1996; 5: 593–596.
27 De Simone C, Ciardi A, Grassi A, *et al*. Effect of *Bifidobacterium bifidum* and *Lactobacillus acidophilus* on gut mucosa and peripheral blood B lymphocytes. *Immunopharmacol Immunotoxicol* 1992; 14: 331–340.
28 Schiffrin EJ, Rochat F, Link-Amster H, *et al*. Immunomodulation of human blood cells following the ingestion of lactic acid bacteria. *J Dairy Sci* 1995; 78: 491–497.
29 Majaama M, Isolauri E. Probiotics: a novel approach in the management of food allergy. *J Allergy Clin Immunol* 1997; 99: 179–185.
30 Isolauri E, Arvola T, Sutas Y, *et al*. Probiotics in the management of atopic eczema. *Clin Exp Allergy* 2000; 30: 1605–1610.
31 Jackson TG, Taylor GRJ, Clohessy AM, Williams CM. The effects of the daily intake of inulin on fasting lipid, insulin and glucose concentrations in middle-aged men and women. *Br J Nutr* 1999; 89: 23–30.
32 Anderson JW, Gilliland SE. Effect of fermented milk (yogurt) containing *Lactobacillus acidophilus* L1 on serum cholesterol by hypercholesterolemic humans. *J Am Coll Nutr* 1999; 18: 43–50.
33 Schaafsma G, Meuling WJ, van Dokkum W, Bouley C. Effects of a milk product, fermented by *Lactobacillus acidophilus* and with fructo-oligosaccharides added, on blood lipids in male volunteers. *Eur J Clin Nutr* 1998; 52: 436–440.
34 Davidson MH, Maki KC, Synecki C. Evaluation of the influence of dietary inulin on serum lipids in adults with hypercholesterolemia. *Nutrition* 1998; 18: 503–517.
35 Mital BK, Garg SK. Anticarcinogenic, hypocholesterolemic and antagonistic activities of *Lactobacillus acidophilus*. *Crit Rev Microbiol* 1995; 21: 175–214.
36 Reddy BS, Rivenson A. Inhibitory effect of *Bifidobacterium longum* on colon, mammary and liver carcinogenesis induced by 2-amino-3-methylimidazo [4,5-*f*] quinoline, a food mutagen. *Cancer Res* 1993; 53: 3914–3918.
37 Taper HS, Delzenne NM, Roberfroid MB. Growth inhibition of transplantable mouse tumours by nondigestible carbohydrates. *Int J Cancer* 1997; 71: 1109–1112.
38 Aso Y, Akazan H, BLP Study Group. Prophylactic effect of a *Lactobacillus casei* preparation on the recurrence of superficial bladder cancer. *Urol Int* 1992; 49: 125–129.
39 Aso Y, Akazan H, Kotake T, *et al*. Preventive effect of a *Lactobacillus casei* preparation on the recurrence of superficial bladder cancer in a double-blind trial. *Eur Urol* 1995; 27: 104–109.
40 Coudray C, Bellanger J, Catiglia-Delavaud C, *et al*. Effect of soluble and partly soluble dietary fibres supplementation on absorption and balance of calcium, magnesium, iron and zinc in healthy young men. *Eur J Clin Nutr* 1997; 51: 375–380.
41 van den Heuvel EGHM, Muys T, van Dokkum W, Schaafsma G. Oligofructose stimulates calcium absorption in adolescents. *Am J Clin Nutr* 1999; 69: 544–548.
42 Canganella F, Paganini S, Ovidi M, *et al*. A microbiology investigation on probiotic pharmaceutical products used for human health. *Microbiol Res* 1997; 152: 171–179.

Riboflavin

Description

Riboflavin is a water-soluble vitamin of the vitamin B complex.

Nomenclature

Riboflavin is the British Approved Name for use on pharmaceutical labels. It is known also as vitamin B_2.

Human requirements

See Table 1 for Dietary Reference Values for riboflavin.

Table 1 Dietary Reference Values for riboflavin (mg/day)

EU RDA = 1.6 mg

Age	UK			USA	WHO	Europe
	LNRI	EAR	RNI	RDA	RNI	PRI
0–6 months	0.2	0.3	0.4	0.3	0.5	–
7–12 months	0.2	0.3	0.4	0.4	0.5	0.4
1–3 years	0.3	0.5	0.6	0.5	0.8	0.8
4–6 years	0.4	0.6	0.8	–	1.1	1.0
4–8 years	–	–	–	0.6	–	–
7–10 years	0.5	0.8	1.0	1.2	1.3	1.2
9–13 years	–	–	–	0.9	–	–
Males						
11–14 years	0.8	1.0	1.2	–	1.7	1.4
15–18 years	0.8	1.0	1.3	–	1.8	1.6
19–50+years	0.8	1.0	1.3	–	1.8	1.6
14–70+ years	–	–	–	1.3	–	–
Females						
11–14 years	0.8	0.9	1.1	–	1.5	1.2
14–18 years	–	–	–	1.0	–	–
15–50+years	0.8	0.9	1.1	–	1.3	1.3
19–70+ years	–	–	–	1.1	–	–
Pregnancy	*	*	+0.3	1.4	+0.2	1.6
Lactation	–	–	+0.5	1.6	+0.4	1.7

*No increment

Intakes

In the UK, the average adult daily diet provides: for men, 2.24 mg; for women, 1.98 mg.

Action

Riboflavin functions as a component of two flavin co-enzymes – flavin mononucleotide (FMN) and flavin adenine dinucleotide (FAD). It participates in oxidation–reduction reactions in numerous metabolic pathways and in energy production. Examples include: the oxidation of glucose, certain amino acids and fatty acids; reactions with several intermediaries of the Krebs cycle; conversion of pyridoxine to its active co-enzyme; and conversion of tryptophan to niacin.

Riboflavin has a role as an antioxidant. It may be involved in maintaining the integrity of erythrocytes.

Dietary sources

See Table 2 for dietary sources of riboflavin.

Table 2 Dietary sources of riboflavin

Food portion	Riboflavin content (mg)
Breakfast cereals	
1 bowl All-Bran (45 g)	*0.5*
1 bowl Bran Flakes (45 g)	*0.6*
1 bowl Corn Flakes (30 g)	*0.4*
1 bowl Muesli (95 g)	*0.6*
1 bowl Shreddies (50 g)	**1.1**
1 bowl Start (40 g)	**0.8**
2 Weetabix	*0.6*
Milk and dairy products	
½ pint (280 ml) milk, whole, semi-skimmed or skimmed	*0.5*
½ pint (280 ml) soya milk	**0.7**
1 pot yoghurt (150 g)	*0.4*
Cheese (50 g)	*0.2*
1 egg, size 2 (60 g)	*0.3*
Meat and fish	
Beef, roast (85 g)	*0.2*
Lamb, roast (85 g)	*0.3*
Pork, roast (85 g)	*0.2*
1 chicken leg portion	*0.2*
Liver, lamb's, cooked (90 g)	**3.0**
Kidney, lamb's, cooked (75 g)	**1.6**
Fish, cooked (150 g)	*0.2*
Yeast	
Brewer's yeast (10 g)	*0.4*
Marmite, spread on 1 slice bread	*0.5*

Excellent sources (**bold**); good sources (*italics*).

Metabolism

Absorption

Riboflavin is readily absorbed by a saturable active transport system (principally in the duodenum).

Distribution

Some circulating riboflavin is loosely associated with plasma albumin, but significant amounts complex with other proteins. Conversion of riboflavin to its co-enzymes occurs in most tissues (particularly in the liver, heart and kidney).

Elimination

Riboflavin is excreted primarily in the urine (mostly as metabolites); excess amounts are excreted unchanged. Riboflavin crosses the placenta and is excreted in breast milk.

Bioavailability

Riboflavin is remarkably stable during processing that involves heat, such as canning, dehydration, evaporation and pasteurisation. Boiling in water results in leaching of the vitamin into the water, which should be used for soups and sauces. Considerable losses occur if food is exposed to light; exposure of milk in glass bottles will result in loss of riboflavin. Animal sources of riboflavin are better absorbed and hence more available than vegetable sources.

Deficiency

Deficiency of riboflavin isolated from other B vitamin deficiencies is rare. Early symptoms include soreness of the mouth and throat, burning and itching of the eyes, and personality deterioration. Advanced deficiency may lead to cheilosis, angular stomatitis, glossitis (red, beefy tongue), corneal vascularisation, seborrhoeic dermatitis (of the face, trunk and extremities), normochromic normocytic anaemia, leukopenia and thrombocytopenia.

Possible uses

Supplements may be required by vegans (strict vegetarians who consume no milk or dairy produce).

Migraine

Riboflavin has been investigated for a possible role in migraine. In an open pilot study in 49 migraine patients, 26 patients were given oral riboflavin 400 mg daily or the same plus aspirin 75 mg daily for three to five months. The number of migraine days reduced from 8.7 ± 1.5 to 2.9 ± 1.2. There were no significant differences between the two groups.[1]

In a randomised, double-blind, placebo-controlled trial, 55 patients with a history of migraine for at least one year (with two to eight attacks monthly) were randomised to receive riboflavin 400 mg or placebo daily. Migraine attack frequency and duration was significantly reduced in the riboflavin group compared with placebo.[2]

Miscellaneous

A case report demonstrated successful therapy with riboflavin 50 mg daily in a patient with documented riboflavin deficiency and carpal tunnel syndrome.[3] Riboflavin has also been used successfully in the treatment of lactic acidosis induced by antiretroviral therapy in patients with AIDS.[4,5] However, riboflavin is of unproven value for acne, mouth ulcers or muscle cramps. At present, there are no convincing scientific data which support its use in human cancer.

Precautions/contraindications

None.

Pregnancy and breast-feeding

No problems reported.

Conclusion

At normal doses there is no good evidence for the use of riboflavin for any indication other than riboflavin deficiency. Preliminary evidence exists that higher doses may be useful in migraine and in lactic acidosis induced by antiretroviral therapy.

Adverse effects

Riboflavin toxicity is unknown in humans. Large doses may cause yellow discoloration of the urine.

Interactions

Drugs

Alcohol: excessive alcohol intake induces riboflavin deficiency.
Barbiturates: prolonged use may induce riboflavin deficiency.
Oral contraceptives: prolonged use may induce riboflavin deficiency.
Phenothiazines: may increase the requirement for riboflavin.
Probenecid: reduces gastrointestinal absorption and urinary excretion of riboflavin.
Tricyclic antidepressants: may increase the requirement for riboflavin.

Nutrients

Adequate amounts of all B vitamins are required for optimal functioning; deficiency or excess of one B vitamin may lead to abnormalities in the metabolism of another.
Iron: deficiency of riboflavin may impair iron metabolism and produce anaemia.

Dose

Riboflavin is available in the form of tablets and capsules, but mainly as a constituent of multivitamin and mineral preparations.

Dietary supplements provide 1–3 mg daily.

References

1 Schoenen J, Lenaerts M, Bastings E. High-dose riboflavin as a prophylactic treatment of migraine:

Results of an open pilot study. *Cephalagia* 1994; 14: 328–329.

2 Schoenen J, Jacquy J, Lenaerts M. Effectiveness of high-dose riboflavin in migraine prophylaxis: A randomized controlled trial. *Neurology* 1998; 50: 466–470.

3 Folkers K, Wolaniuk A, Vadhanavikit S. Enzymology of the response of the carpal tunnel syndrome to riboflavin and to combined riboflavin and pyridoxine. *Proc Natl Acad Sci USA* 1984; 81: 7076–7078.

4 Fouty B, Frerman F, Reves R. Riboflavin to treat nucleoside analogue-induced lactic acidosis. *Lancet* 1998; 352: 291–292.

5 Luzzati R, DelBravo P, DiPerri G, *et al*. Riboflavine and severe lactic acidosis. *Lancet* 1999; 353: 901–902.

Royal jelly

Description

Royal jelly is a yellow-white liquid secreted by the hypopharyngeal glands of 'nurse' worker bees from the 6th–12th day of their adult life. It is an essential food for the queen bee.

Constituents

See Table 1 for the claimed nutrient composition of royal jelly.

Table 1 Claimed nutrient composition in a typical daily dose (500 mg) of royal jelly

Nutrient	Amount	% RNI[1]
Water (mg)	350	–
Carbohydrate (mg)	60	–
Protein (mg)	60	–
Lipids (mg)	25	–
Thiamine (μg)	2	0.2
Riboflavin (μg)	7	0.6
Niacin (μg)	20	0.1
Vitamin B_6 (μg)	3	0.2
Folic acid (ng)	15	0.08
Biotin (μg)	1	–
Pantothenic acid (μg)	3	–
Calcium (μg)	130	0.02
Magnesium (μg)	150	0.07
Potassium (mg)	2.5	0.07
Iron (μg)	25	0.2
Zinc (μg)	15	0.2

[1]Reference Nutrient Intake for men aged 19–50 years.

Action

Royal jelly may have some pharmacological effects, but the only available evidence comes from *in-vitro* studies and animal studies. It appears to: have anti-tumour effects;[1] improve the efficiency of insulin;[2] have vasodilator activity;[3] and exhibit anti-microbial activity.[4]

Possible uses

Published reports on the effects of royal jelly in humans are relatively few, and many of these are single case histories and not clinical trials.

Royal jelly has been claimed to be beneficial in the following circumstances: anorexia, fatigue and headaches;[5] and hypercholesterolaemia.[6,7]

A systematic review and meta-analysis[7] examined the effect of royal jelly in 17 animal studies and nine human studies. In the animal studies, royal jelly significantly reduced serum cholesterol and total lipid levels in rats and rabbits, and slowed the progress of atheromas in rabbits fed a high fat diet. Meta-analysis of the controlled human trials showed that royal jelly (30–100 mg daily for three to six weeks) resulted in a significant reduction in total serum lipids and cholesterol and normalisation of low-density lipoprotein (LDL) and high-density lipoprotein (HDL) in subjects with hyperlipidaemia.

Claims for the value of royal jelly in arthritis, depression, diabetes mellitus, dysmenorrhoea, eczema, morning sickness, multiple sclerosis, muscular dystrophy, myalgic encephalomyelitis (ME) and premenstrual syndrome (PMS) are purely anecdotal, and there is no evidence for any of these claims.

Precautions/contraindications

Royal jelly should be avoided by people with asthma (adverse effects reported).

Conclusion
Anecdotally, royal jelly is thought to be beneficial in a wide range of conditions. However, there is no sound evidence to support its use.

Pregnancy and breast-feeding

No problems reported, but there have not been sufficient studies to guarantee the safety of royal jelly in pregnancy and breast-feeding. Royal jelly is probably best avoided.

Adverse effects

Allergic reactions. These can be severe. Life-threatening bronchospasm has occurred in patients with asthma after ingestion of royal jelly.[8–11] Royal jelly has been responsible for IgE-mediated anaphylaxis,[12] leading to death in at least one individual.[13] One report of haemorrhagic colitis occurred in a 53-year-old woman after taking royal jelly for 25 days.[14]

Interactions

None reported.

Dose

Royal jelly is available in the form of tablets and capsules.

The dose is not established. Dietary supplements provide 250–500 mg daily.

References

1 Tamura T, Fujii A, Kuboyama N. Antitumour effects of royal jelly. *Nippon Yakurigaku Zasshi* 1987; 89: 73–80.
2 Kramer KJ, Tager HS, Childs CN, Spiers RD. Insulin-like hypoglycaemic and immunological activities in honey bee royal jelly. *J Insect Physiol* 1977; 23: 293–296.
3 Shinoda M, Nakajin S, Oikawa T, *et al.* Biochemical studies on vasodilator factor of royal jelly. *Yakugaku Zasshi* 1978; 98: 139–135.
4 Fujiwara S, Imaj J, Fujiwara M, *et al.* A potent anti-bacterial protein in royal jelly: Purification and determination of the primary structure of royalisin. *J Biol Chem* 1990; 265: 11333–11337.
5 Tamura T. Royal jelly from the standpoint of clinical pharmacology. *Honeybee Sci* 1985; 6: 117–124.
6 Cho YT. Studies on royal jelly and abnormal cholesterol and triglycerides. *Am Bee J* 1977; 117: 36–38.
7 Vittek J. Effect of royal jelly on serum lipids in experimental animals and humans with atherosclerosis. *Experientia* 1995; 51: 927–935.
8 Leung R, Thien FCK, Baldo BA, *et al.* Royal jelly induced asthma and anaphylaxis: Clinical characteristics and immunologic correlations. *J Allergy Clin Immunol* 1995; 96: 1004–1007.
9 Peacock S, Murray V, Turton C. Respiratory distress and royal jelly. *Br Med J* 1995; 311: 1472.
10 Larporte JR, Ibaanez L, Vendrell L, *et al.* Bronchospasm induced by royal jelly. *Allergy* 1996; 51: 440.
11 Harwood M, Harding S, Beasley R, *et al.* Asthma following royal jelly. *NZ Med J* 1996; 109: 325.
12 Thien FC, Leung R, Baldo BA, *et al.* Asthma and anaphylaxis induced by royal jelly. *Clin Exp Allergy* 1996; 26: 216–222.
13 Bullock RJ, Rohan A, Straatmans JA. Fatal royal jelly induced asthma. *Med J Aust* 1994; 160: 44.
14 Yonei Y, Shibagaki K, Tsukada N, *et al.* Case report: Hemorrhagic colitis associated with royal jelly intake. *J Gastroenterol Hepatol* 1997; 12: 495–499.

S-Adenosylmethionine

Description

S-Adenosylmethionine (SAMe) is synthesised in the body from the essential amino acid methionine.

Action

SAMe is involved in several biochemical pathways. It functions mainly as a methyl donor in synthetic pathways, which lead to the production of DNA and RNA, neurotransmitters and phospholipids. Its involvement in phospholipid synthesis may mean that it has a role in membrane fluidity. SAMe is also involved in transulphuration reactions, regulating the formation of sulphur-containing amino acids, cysteine, glutathione (GSH) and taurine. GSH is an antioxidant, so SAMe is proposed to have antioxidant activity.

Possible uses

SAMe is being investigated for its effects on a number of conditions, such as depression, osteoarthritis, fibromyalgia and cardiovascular disease.

Depression

In the early 1990s, SAMe was suggested to be of potential use as an antidepressant. Its mechanism of action for this indication is still a matter of speculation, although there is some evidence that it may raise dopamine levels.[1] Initially it was used for this purpose by parenteral administration. However, in an uncontrolled study[2] in 20 out-patients with major depression, the group as a whole improved with oral SAMe.

In a randomised, double-blind, placebo-controlled trial involving 15 in-patients with major depression, oral SAMe was found to improve symptoms of depression. However, it induced mania in one patient with no history of the condition.[3]

The efficacy of oral SAMe was assessed in the treatment of 80 depressed postmenopausal women (aged 45–59 years). The 30-day, double-blind, placebo-controlled, randomised trial found a significantly greater improvement in depressive symptoms in the group treated with 1600 mg daily of SAMe from day 10 of the study.[4]

A meta-analysis of the effect of SAMe on depression compared with placebo or tricyclic antidepressants showed a greater response rate with SAMe than placebo and an antidepressant effect comparable with tricyclic antidepressants.[5]

Osteoarthritis

SAMe appears to possess analgesic activity, and in joints there is some evidence that it stimulates the synthesis of proteoglycans by the articular chondrocytes.[6]

In a range of double-blind, randomised trials, all reported in one issue of one journal, oral SAMe was found to exert the same analgesic activity as a range of non-steroidal anti-inflammatory drugs (NSAIDs). In one study with 734 subjects, SAMe 1200 mg daily was as effective as naproxen 750 mg daily.[7] Another study in 45 patients, showed that SAMe 1200 mg daily was as effective as piroxicam (20 mg daily) in osteoarthritis of the knee.[8] Two further studies in each of 36 patients over four weeks, showed that SAMe 1200 mg daily was as effective as indometacin (150 mg daily)[9] or ibuprofen

(1200 mg daily).[10] In an uncontrolled study of 24 months' duration, 108 patients received 600 mg SAMe daily for two weeks, then 400 mg daily thereafter. Clinical symptoms, such as morning stiffness, pain at rest and pain on movement, improved during the period of SAMe administration.[11]

Fibromyalgia

Intravenous SAMe has been shown to reduce pain in patients with fibromyalgia.[12] In a double-blind, placebo-controlled trial of six weeks' duration, involving 44 patients, oral SAMe (800 mg) produced significant improvement in clinical disease activity, pain suffered during the last week, and fatigue. SAMe was associated with an improvement in mood on the Face Scale, but not on the Beck Depression Inventory.[13]

Cardiovascular disease

Elevation of homocysteine is an independent risk factor for cardiovascular disease, and SAMe controls enzymes in homocysteine metabolism. Whole-blood SAMe has been found to be lower in patients with coronary heart disease (CHD) than in controls, suggesting that low levels of SAMe might be a risk factor for the development of CHD.[14] A study with oral SAMe (400 mg in a single dose) in healthy subjects showed that SAMe did not inhibit the enzyme 5,10-methylene tetrahydrofolate reductase that catalyses the formation of 5-methyltetrahydrofolate, the active form of folate involved in the remethylation of homocysteine to methionine. However, there were no changes in plasma homocysteine levels.[15]

> **Conclusion**
>
> Preliminary research suggests there is some evidence that SAMe has antidepressant and analgesic activity, and may also have an influence on the metabolism of homocysteine. However, few trials have been conducted and there is inadequate evidence to recommend SAMe for these purposes.

Precautions/contraindications

Use with caution in individuals with a history of bleeding or haemostatic disorders. SAMe has been reported to block platelet aggregation *in vitro*.[16]

Pregnancy and breast-feeding

No problems reported, but there have not been sufficient studies to guarantee the safety of SAMe in pregnancy and breast-feeding. SAMe is best avoided.

Adverse reactions

Minor side-effects, including nausea, dry mouth and restlessness have been occasionally reported.

Interactions

None documented, but in theory SAMe could potentiate the activity of antidepressants, anticoagulants and antiplatelet drugs.

Dose

SAMe is available in the form of tablets and capsules. A review of 13 US products found that six did not pass testing for content. Among those not passing, the amount of SAMe was, on average, less than half of that declared on the labels.[17]

The dose is not established. Studies have used doses of 400–1600 mg daily.

References

1 Fava M, Rosenbaum JF, MacLaughlin JR, *et al.* Neuroendocrine effects of S-adenosyl-L-methionine, a novel putative antidepressant. *J Psychiatr Res* 1990; 24: 177–184.
2 Rosenbaum JF, Fava M, Falk WE, *et al.* The antidepressant potential of oral S-adenosylmethionine. *Acta Psychiatr Scand* 1990; 81: 432–436.
3 Kagan BL, Sultzer DL, Rosenlicht N, *et al.* Oral S-adenosyl methionine in depression: A randomised, double-blind, placebo-controlled trial. *Am J Psychiatry* 1990; 147: 591–595.
4 Salmaggi P, Bressa GM, Nicchia G, *et al.* Double-blind, placebo-controlled study of S-adenosyl-L-methionine in depressed postmenopausal women. *Psychother Psychosom* 1993; 59: 34–40.
5 Bressa GM. S-adenosyl-L-methionine (SAMe) as antidepressant: Meta-analysis of clinical studies. *Acta Neurol Scand Suppl* 1994; 154: 7–14.

6 di Padova C. S-Adenosylmethionine in the treatment of osteoarthritis: Review of clinical studies. *Am J Med* 1987; 83(5A): 60–65.
7 Caruso I, Pietrogrande V. Italian double-blind multicenter study comparing S-adenosylmethionine, naproxen, and placebo in the treatment of degenerative joint disease. *Am J Med* 1987; 83(5A): 66–71.
8 Maccagno A, Di Giorgio EE, Caston OL, *et al.* Double-blind controlled clinical trial of oral S-adenosylmethionine versus piroxicam in knee osteoarthritis. *Am J Med* 1987; 83(5A): 72–77.
9 Vetter G. Double-blind comparative clinical trial with S-adenosylmethionine and indomethacin in the treatment of osteoarthritis. *Am J Med* 1987; 83(5A): 78–80.
10 Muller-Fassbender H. Double-blind clinical trial of S-adenosylmethionine versus ibuprofen in the treatment of osteoarthritis. *Am J Med* 1987; 83(5A): 81–83.
11 Konig B. A long-term (two years) clinical trial with S-adenosylmethionine for the treatment of osteoarthritis. *Am J Med* 1987; 83(5A): 89–94.
12 Volkmann H, Norregaard J, Jacobsen S, *et al.* Double-blind, placebo-controlled cross-over study of intravenous S-adenosyl-L-methionine in patients with fibromyalgia. *Scand J Rheumatol* 1997; 26: 206–211.
13 Jacobsen S, Danneskiold-Samsoe B, Andersen RB. Oral S-adenosylmethionine in primary fibromyalgia: Double-blind clinical evaluation. *Scand J Rheumatol* 1991; 20: 294–302.
14 Loehrer FM, Angst CP, Haefeli WE, *et al.* Low whole-blood S-adenosylmethionine and correlation between 5-methyltetrahydrofolate and homocysteine in coronary artery disease. *Arterioscler Thromb Vasc Biol* 1996; 16: 727–733.
15 Loehrer FM, Schwab R, Angst CP, *et al.* Influence of oral S-adenosylmethionine on plasma 5-methyltetrahydrofolate, S-adenosylhomocysteine, homocysteine and methionine in healthy humans. *J Pharmacol Exp Ther* 1997; 282: 845–850.
16 De La Cruz JP, Merida M, Gonzalez-Correa JA, *et al.* Effects of S-adenosyl-L-methionine on platelet thromboxane and vascular prostacyclin. *Biochem Pharmacol* 1997; 53: 1761–1763.
17 Consumerlab. Product review. SAMe. http://www. consumerlab.com (accessed 7 December 2000).

Selenium

Description

Selenium is an essential trace element.

Human requirements

See Table 1 for Dietary Reference Values for selenium.

Intakes

In the UK, the average adult diet provides 25 to 129 μg daily. Selenium enters the food chain through plants, which take it up from the soil. Selenium intake is low in parts of the world where the soil content is low, and human dietary intakes therefore vary from high to low

Table 1 Dietary Reference Values of selenium (μg/day)

EU RDA = None

Age	UK			USA		WHO	Europe PRI
	LRNI	RNI	RDA	RDA	UL		
0–3 months	4	10	10	15[1]	45	6	–
4–6 months	5	13	10	15[1]	45	9	–
7–9 months	5	10	15	20[1]	45	12	8
10–12 months	6	10	15	20[1]	45	12	8
1–3 years	7	15	20	20	90	20	15
4–6 years	10	20	20	–	–	24	15
4–8 years	–	–	–	30	150	–	–
7–10 years	16	30	30	–	–	25	25
9–13 years	–	–	–	40	280	–	–
19–70+ years	–	–	–	55	400	–	–
Males							
11–14 years	25	45	40	–	–	36	35
15–18 years	40	70	50	–	–	40	45
19–50+ years	40	75	70	–	–	40	55
Females							
11–14 years	25	45	45	–	–	30	35
15–18 years	40	60	50	–	–	30	45
19–50+ years	40	60	55	–	–	30	55
Pregnancy	*	*	65	–	400	35	*
Lactation	+15	+15	75	–	400	40	+15

*No increment.

[1]Adequate Intake.

UL = Tolerable Upper Intake Level from diet and supplements.

according to geography. Selenium intakes in most parts of Europe (including the UK) are considerably lower than in the USA, European soils being a poorer source of selenium. Current UK intakes are about half the RNI, having declined considerably over the past 25 years, and this may have implications for disease risk.

Action

Selenium functions as an integral part of the enzyme glutathione peroxidase and other selenoproteins. Glutathione peroxidase prevents the generation of oxygen free radicals that cause the destruction of polyunsaturated fatty acids in cell membranes. Selenium spares the requirement for vitamin E and vice-versa. Selenium has additional effects, particularly in relation to the immune response and cancer prevention, which are not entirely due to these enzymic functions

Dietary sources

See Table 2 for dietary sources of selenium.

Metabolism

Absorption

Little is known about the intestinal absorption of selenium, but it seems to be easily absorbed.

Distribution

Selenium is stored in red cells, liver, spleen, heart, nails, tooth enamel, testes and spermatozoa. It is incorporated into the enzyme glutathione peroxidase, the metabolically active form of selenium.

Elimination

Selenium is excreted mainly in the urine.

Deficiency

Deficiency has been associated with muscle pain and tenderness; some cases of cardiomyopathy have occurred in patients on total parenteral nutrition with low selenium status. Keshan disease (seen mainly in China) is a syndrome of endemic cardiomyopathy which is alleviated by selenium supplementation.

There is evidence that less overt selenium deficiency can have adverse consequences for health. Low selenium status has been linked to loss of immunocompetence,[1] the development, virulence and progression of some viral infections,[2] miscarriage,[3] male infertility,[4] depressed mood,[5] senility and Alzheimer's disease[5] and poor thyroid function.[6]

Table 2 Dietary sources of selenium

Food portion	Selenium content (μg)
Cereals[1]	
2 slices bread	**30**
Milk and dairy products	
½ pint (280 ml) milk	3–30
1 egg	3–25
Meat and fish	
Beef, cooked (100 g)	3
Lamb, cooked (100 g)	1
Pork, cooked (100 g)	*15*
Chicken, cooked (100 g)	8
Liver (90 g)	*20*
Fish, cooked (150 g)	**30–50**
Vegetables	
1 small can baked beans (200 g)	4
Lentils, red kidney beans or other pulses, cooked (105 g)	5
Green vegetables, average, boiled (100g)	1–3
Fruit	
1 banana	2
1 orange	2
Nuts	
20 almonds	1
10 Brazil nuts	**200**
30 peanuts	1

[1]Cereals are important sources of selenium, but the content reflects the selenium content of the soils in which they are grown and is therefore highly variable.

Excellent sources (**bold**); good sources (*italics*).

Selenium deficiency has also been associated with cardiovascular disease, although results from epidemiological studies have been mixed. Thus, a two- to three-fold increase in cardiovascular mortality was found in individuals with serum selenium concentrations below 45 μg/l compared with individuals above that concentration at baseline.[7] A Danish study[8] showed that middle-aged and elderly men with serum selenium below 70 μg/l had a significantly increased risk of ischaemic heart disease. The 10-centre EURAMIC study[9] found an inverse relationship between toenail selenium levels and risk of myocardial infarction, but only in the centre with the lowest selenium (Germany). However, other studies have shown no such links.

Low selenium intake has been linked to cancer mortality. In one study[10] dietary intake of selenium in 27 countries was found to correlate inversely with total age-adjusted cancer mortality, and low selenium status has been linked with an increased risk of cancer incidence and mortality.[11,12] A nested case control study within a cohort of 9000 Finnish individuals showed the adjusted relative risk of lung cancer between the highest and lowest tertiles of serum selenium to be 0.41.[13] In a study looking at the association between selenium intake and prostate cancer involving 34 000 men, those in the lowest quintile of selenium status were found to have three times the likelihood of developing advanced prostate cancer as those in the highest quintile.[14]

Possible uses

Cancer (prevention)

Studies have shown that selenium supplementation may reduce the risk of certain cancers (e.g. colon, gastric, lung and prostate), but not others (breast, oesophageal and skin).

The US Nutritional Prevention of Cancer (NPC) trial[15] was the first double-blind, placebo-controlled trial in a western population, designed to test the hypothesis that selenium supplementation could reduce the risk of cancer. Altogether, 1312 individuals with a history of non-melanoma skin cancer were randomised to placebo or 200 μg selenium a day (as selenium yeast) for an average treatment period of 4.5 years with a total follow-up of 6.4 years. There were no statistically significant differences in incidence of basal cell carcinoma or squamous cell carcinoma. However, total cancer incidence was 37% lower in the selenium group, with 63% fewer cancers of the prostate, 58% fewer cancers of the colon, and 46% fewer cancers of the lung. There were more cases of breast cancer and leukaemia-lymphoma in the selenium group, but these differences were not statistically significant.

Supplements of dietary antioxidants (including selenium) reduced the incidence of oesophageal and gastric cancer and total cancer in a study in 30 000 adults in Linxian, China,[16] an area where the incidence of oesophageal and stomach cancer is high, and the intake of certain nutrients is low.

Cardiovascular disease

Selenium may have a role in the prevention of cardiovascular disease, but evidence for the benefit of supplementation is limited. In a double-blind, placebo-controlled study,[17] 81 patients received either selenium-rich yeast (100 μg daily) or placebo for a six-month period. During the study period there were four cardiac deaths in the placebo group but none in the selenium group. There were two non-fatal reinfarctions in the placebo group, and one in the selenium group.

Infertility

Selenium supplementation (selenomethionine 100 μg daily) increased sperm motility in a study involving 64 subfertile men.[18] Sperm count was unchanged after supplementation for three months, but sperm motility increased in 56% of the men. By the time of publication, 11% of the selenium-supplemented men had confirmed paternity, but none of the placebo group had.

Rheumatoid arthritis

Selenium may be useful as an adjunct in the treatment of recent onset rheumatoid arthritis. In one study, 15 women with rheumatoid arthritis of less than five years' duration who had been treated with non-steroidal anti-inflammatory drugs (NSAIDs) and/or with other anti-rheumatic drugs received selenium

(200 µg daily from selenium-rich yeast) supplementation for three months.[19] This led to improvement in subjective pain and clinical assessment of joint involvement in six out of eight of the treated subjects, but in none of the controls. Improvements disappeared three months after therapy was withdrawn, even though indicators of selenium status remained elevated. However, selenium (256 µg daily from selenium-rich yeast) was not effective in a trial of 40 men and women with an average arthritis duration of 13.5 years.[20]

Conclusion
Epidemiological research and evidence from a large controlled intervention trial suggest that selenium may reduce cancer risk. The role of selenium in heart disease is unclear, and controlled clinical trials are required to identify any benefits of supplementation. Results from studies of selenium in rheumatoid arthritis are conflicting.

Precautions/contraindications

Selenium products containing yeast should be avoided by patients taking monoamine oxidase inhibitors.

Pregnancy and breast-feeding

No problems with normal intakes.

Adverse effects

There is a narrow margin of safety for selenium. Adverse effects include hair loss, nail changes, skin lesions, nausea, diarrhoea, irritability, metallic taste, garlic-smelling breath, fatigue and peripheral neuropathy.

Interactions

None reported.

Dose

Selenium is available mainly in 'antioxidant' supplements with vitamin E and vitamin A, and is also an ingredient in multivitamin supplements.

The dose is not established; 50–100 µg daily is considered to be safe. Doses from supplements should not exceed 200 µg daily; intake from all sources (food and supplements) should not exceed 450 µg daily.

The bioavailability of selenium depends on the form in which it is ingested and supplements tend to contain selenomethionine, selenite or selenate. Selenomethionine is more effective in increasing apparent selenium status because it is incorporated non-specifically into proteins instead of methionine. However, it has no catalytic activity and must be catabolised to an inorganic precursor before entering the selenium pool. Selenomethionine is therefore a less bioavailable form of selenium than selenite and selenate, since these need only be reduced to selenide to provide selenophosphate, the precursor of selenocysteine, the active form of selenium in selenoproteins.[21]

References

1 Spallholz JE, Boylan LM, Larsen HS, *et al.* Advances in understanding selenium's role in the immune system. *Ann NY Acad Sci* 1990; 587: 129–139.
2 Taylor EW, Nadimpalli RG, Ramanathan CS, *et al.* Genomic structures of viral agents in relation to the biosynthesis of selenoproteins. *Biol Trace Elem Res* 1997; 56: 63–91.
3 Barrington JW, Taylor M, Smith S, Bowen-Simpkins P. Selenium and recurrent miscarriage. *J Obstet Gynaecol* 1997; 17: 199–200.
4 Oldereid NB, Thomassen Y, Purvis K, *et al.* Selenium in human male reproductive organs. *Hum Reprod* 1998; 13: 2172–2176.
5 Hawkes WC, Hornbostel L. Effects of dietary selenium on mood in healthy men living in a metabolic research unit. *Biol Psychiatry* 1996; 39: 121–128.
6 Olivieri O, Girelli D, Azzini M, *et al.* Low selenium status in the elderly influences thyroid hormones. *Clin Sci* 1995; 89: 637–642.
7 Salonen JT, Alfhthan G, Pikkarainen J, *et al.* Association between cardiovascular death and myocardial infarction and serum selenium in a matched pair longitudinal study. *Lancet* 1982; 2: 175–179.
8 Virtamo J, Valkiela E, Alfhthan G, *et al.* Serum selenium and the risk of coronary heart disease and stroke. *Am J Epidemiol* 1985; 122: 276–282.
9 Kardinaal AFM, Kok FJ, Kohlmeier L, *et al.*

Association between toenail selenium and risk of myocardial infarction in European men: The EURAMIC study. *Am J Epidemiol* 1997; 145: 373–379.

10 Schrauzer GN, White DA, Schneider CJ, *et al.* Cancer mortality correlation studies. III. Statistical association with dietary selenium intakes. *Bioinorg Chem* 1977; 7: 35–36.

11 Combs GF, Jr, Gray WP. Chemopreventive agents: Selenium. *Pharmacol Ther* 1998; 79: 179–182.

12 Kok FJ, de Bruin AM, Hofman A, *et al.* Is serum selenium a risk factor for cancer in men only? *Am J Epidemiol* 1987; 125: 12–16.

13 Knekt P, Marniemi J, Teppo L, *et al.* Is low selenium status a risk factor for lung cancer? *Am J Epidemiol* 1998; 148: 975–982.

14 Yoshizawa K, Willett WC, Morris SJ, *et al.* Study of prediagnostic selenium level in toenails and the risk of advanced prostate cancer. *J Natl Cancer Inst* 1998; 90: 1219–1224.

15 Clark LC, Combs Jr, GF, Turnbill BW. Effects of selenium supplementation for cancer prevention in patients with carcinoma of the skin: a randomized controlled trial: Nutritional Prevention of Cancer Study Group. *JAMA* 1996; 276: 1957–1963.

16 Blot WJ, Li J-Y, Taylor PR, *et al.* Nutrition intervention trial in Linxian, China: Supplementation with specific vitamin/mineral combinations, cancer incidence and disease-specific mortality in the general population. *J Natl Cancer Inst* 1993; 85: 1483–1492.

17 Korpela H, Kumpulainen J, Jussila E. Effect of selenium supplementation after acute myocardial infarction. *Res Commun Pathol Pharmacol* 1989; 65: 249–252.

18 Scott R, MacPherson A, Yates RWS, *et al.* The effect of oral selenium supplementation on human sperm motility. *Br J Urol* 1998; 82: 76–80.

19 Peretz A, Neve J, Duchateau J, *et al.* Adjuvant treatment of recent onset rheumatoid arthritis by selenium supplementation. *Br J Rheumatol* 1992; 31: 281–282.

20 Tarp U, Overvad K, Thorling EB, *et al.* Selenium treatment in rheumatoid arthritis. *Scand J Rheumatol* 1985; 14: 364–368.

21 Allan CB, Lacourciere GM, Stadtman TC, *et al.* Responsiveness of selenoproteins to dietary selenium. *Annu Rev Nutr* 1999; 19: 1–16.

Shark cartilage

Description

Cartilage obtained from various types of shark.

Constituents

Cartilage tissue contains a mixture of glycosaminoglycans, one of which is chondroitin sulphate. Shark cartilage is also thought to contain compounds known as anti-angiogenesis factors, including sphyrnastatin 1 and 2.[1] These are factors that inhibit the growth of new blood vessels, typically seen in malignant tumours, and this mechanism could, in theory, be helpful in human cancer.

Action

It has been suggested that shark cartilage may prevent tumour growth. The proposed mechanism is that the anti-angiogenesis factors prevent tumours from developing the network of blood vessels they need to supply them with nutrients. This supposedly starves tumours and causes them to shrink. The popularity of this anti-cancer theory increased as a result of a popular book, *Sharks Don't Get Cancer*.[2]

Possible uses

Shark cartilage has been proposed as a supplement for the treatment of cancer and (because of its chondroitin content) for the treatment of osteoarthritis.

Cancer

Various *in vitro*,[2–4] animal[5] and human[6] studies have shown that shark cartilage has anti-angiogeneic properties. However, there is no evidence from controlled trials that shark cartilage cures cancer in humans.

In a study of cancer patients taking shark cartilage either rectally or orally, 10 of the 20 patients reported an improved quality of life, including increased appetite and reduced pain, after eight weeks. In addition, four of the 20 patients showed partial or complete response (50–100% reduction in tumour mass). However, information on patient selection criteria, cartilage dose and concomitant cytotoxic therapy were not provided.[7]

A 12-week open clinical trial on 60 patients with advanced cancer assessed the efficacy and safety of shark cartilage at a dose of 1 g/kg daily. No complete or partial positive responses were found, and the authors concluded that shark cartilage had no anti-cancer activity and no effect on the quality of life.[8]

Conclusion

There is currently no evidence from clinical trials to show that shark cartilage helps to cure cancer in humans.

Precautions/contraindications

Avoid in patients with hepatic disease. There has been a single case report of hepatitis attributed to shark cartilage.[9]

Pregnancy and breast-feeding

There are no available data. Shark cartilage should be avoided.

Adverse effects

Hepatitis and various gastrointestinal effects (e.g. nausea, vomiting, constipation) have been reported.

Interactions

None reported.

Dose

Shark cartilage is available in the form of tablets, capsules and powder.

The dose is not established. There is no proven value of shark cartilage supplements.

References

1 McGuire TR, Kazakoff PW, Hoie EB, *et al.* Antiproliferative activity of shark cartilage with and without tumor necrosis factor-alpha in human umbilical vein endothelium. *Pharmacotherapy* 1996; 16: 237–244.
2 Lane IW. *Sharks Don't Get Cancer*. Garden City Park, New York: Avery Publishing Group, 1992: 107–118.
3 Sheu JR, Fu CC, Tsai ML, *et al.* Effect of U-995, a potent shark cartilage-derived angiogenesis inhibitor, on anti-angiogenesis and anti-tumour activities. *Anticancer Res* 1998; 18: 4435–4441.
4 Dupont E, Savard PE, Jourdain C, *et al.* Antiangiogenic properties of a novel shark cartilage extract: Potential role in the treatment of psoriasis. *J Cutan Med Surg* 1998; 2: 146–152.
5 Horsman MR, Alsner J, Overgaard J. The effect of shark cartilage extracts on the growth and metastatic spread of the SCCVII carcinoma. *Acta Oncol* 1998; 37: 441–445.
6 Berbari P, Thibodeau A, Germain L, *et al.* Antiangiogenic effect of the oral administration of liquid cartilage extract in humans. *J Surg Res* 1999; 87: 108–113.
7 Mathews J. Media feeds frenzy over shark cartilage as cancer treatment. *J Natl Cancer Inst* 1993; 85: 1190–1191.
8 Miller DR, Anderson GT, Stark JJ, *et al.* Phase I/II trial of the safety and efficacy of shark cartilage in the treatment of advanced cancer. *J Clin Oncol* 1998; 16: 3649–3655.
9 Ahsar B, Vargo E. Shark-cartilage induced hepatitis. *Ann Intern Med* 1996; 125: 780–781.

Spirulina

Description

Spirulina is a blue-green microscopic alga; it grows in fresh-water ponds and lakes, thriving in warm and alkaline environments.

Constituents

See Table 1 for the claimed nutrient content of spirulina.

Action

Spirulina consists of approximately 65–70% crude protein, high concentrations of B vitamins, phenylalanine, iron and other minerals. However, all the B vitamins (including B_{12}) are thought to be in the form of analogues and nutritionally insignificant. The iron is believed to be highly bioavailable, with 1.5–2 mg being absorbed from a 10-g dose of spirulina.

Possible uses

Lipid lowering

Various pilot studies have shown that spirulina may have lipid-lowering and hypoglycaemic effects in patients with non-insulin-dependent diabetes mellitus (NIDDM). One study[1] examined the long-term effect of spirulina supplementation (2 g daily) on blood sugar levels, serum lipid profile and glycated serum protein levels in 15 NIDDM patients. Supplementation for two months resulted in a significant reduction in triglycerides and total cholesterol, as well as a reduction in blood sugar and glycated serum protein levels. Levels of high-density lipoprotein (HDL) increased, while those of low-density lipoprotein (LDL) fell.

Miscellaneous

Spirulina has been shown *in vitro* to have antiviral activity.[2,3] It is claimed to act as a tonic and be beneficial in: allergies; Alzheimer's disease; peptic ulcer; increasing stamina in athletes; and retarding ageing. There is no evidence for any of these claims. When spirulina was introduced into the USA in 1979 as a slimming aid, the Food and Drug Administration could find no evidence to support these claimed benefits.

> **Conclusion**
> There is preliminary evidence that spirulina could lower lipids and have an antiviral effect. However, controlled trials are required to confirm these effects.

Precautions/contraindications

Spirulina may be contaminated with mercury.

Pregnancy and breast-feeding

Avoid (contaminants – see Precautions).

Adverse effects

Effects not known (contaminants – see Precautions).

Interactions

None known.

Dose

Spirulina is available in the form of tablets, capsules and powders.

Table 1 Claimed[1] nutrient content of spirulina

Nutrient	per 100 g	per typical dose	%RNI[2] (10 g)
Protein (g)	70	7	–
Fat (g)	7	0.7	–
Carbohydrate (g)	15	1.5	–
Betacarotene (mg)	170	17	–
Thiamine (mg)	5.5	0.5	55
Riboflavin (mg)	4.0	0.4	33
Niacin (mg)	11.8	1.2	8
Pyridoxine (mg)	0.3	0.03	2.5
Vitamin B_{12} (μg)	200	20	1333
Folic acid (μg)	50	5	2.5
Pantothenic acid (mg)	1.1	0.1	–
Biotin (μg)	40	4	–
Vitamin E (mg)	19	0.2	–
Inositol (mg)	35	3.5	–
Calcium (mg)	132	13	2
Magnesium (mg)	192	19	6
Potassium (mg)	1540	154	4
Phosphorus (mg)	894	89	16
Iron (mg)	58	5.8	48
Zinc (mg)	4	0.4	6
Manganese (mg)	2.5	0.2	–
Selenium (μg)	40	4	2

[1]Reported on a product label.

[2]Reference Nutrient Intake for males aged 19–50 years.

The dose is not established. There is no proven benefit of spirulina. Dietary supplements provide 6–10 g per daily dose.

References

1 Mani UV, Desai S, Iyer U. Studies on the long term effect of spirulina supplementation on serum lipid profile and glycated proteins in NIDDM patients. *J Nutraceut Funct Med Foods* 2000; 2: 25–32.

2 Hayashi K, Hayashi T, Kojima I. A natural sulfated polysaccharide, calcium spirulan, isolated from *Spirulina platensis*: In vitro and ex vivo evaluation of anti-herpes simplex virus and anti-human immunodeficiency virus activities. *AIDS Res Hum Retroviruses* 1996; 12: 1463–1471.

3 Hayashi T, Hayashi K, Maeda M, *et al.* Calcium spirulan, an inhibitor of enveloped virus replication, from blue-green algae *Spirulina platensis*. *J Nat Prod* 1996; 59: 83–87.

Superoxide dismutase

Description

Superoxide dismutase (SOD) is a group of enzymes which is widely distributed in the body; several different forms exist which vary in their metal content. Copper-containing SOD is extracellular and present in high concentrations in the lungs, thyroid and uterus and in small amounts in plasma. SOD containing copper and zinc is present within the cells and found in high concentrations in brain, erythrocytes, kidney, liver, pituitary and thyroid.

Action

SOD enzymes act as scavengers of superoxide radicals, and protect against oxidative damage (by catalysing conversion of superoxide radicals to peroxide).

Possible uses

SOD is claimed to be useful for: prevention of cardiovascular disease, cancer and retardation of ageing. Such claims are partly based on studies which have used SOD by injection in clinical management. SOD is not absorbed from an oral dose, and dietary supplements are therefore likely to be ineffective.

Precautions/contraindications

None known.

Pregnancy and breast-feeding

No problems reported, but there have been insufficient studies to guarantee the safety of SOD in pregnancy and breast-feeding.

Adverse effects

None reported from oral doses.

Interactions

None reported.

Dose

SOD is available in the form of tablets and capsules. However, products may not have any of the stated activity because they are acid-labile and break down before absorption.

The dose is not established. Not recommended as a dietary supplement (probably ineffective).

Thiamine

Description

Thiamine is a water-soluble vitamin of the vitamin B complex.

Nomenclature

Thiamine is the British Approved Name for use on pharmaceutical labels. It is also known as vitamin B_1 and aneurine.

Human requirements

Thiamine requirements depend on energy intake; values are therefore often given as mg/1000 kcal and also as total values based on estimated average energy requirements for the majority of people in the UK (Table 1).

Intakes

In the UK, the average adult daily diet provides: for men, 1.95 mg; for women, 1.56 mg.

Action

Thiamine functions as a co-enzyme in the oxidative decarboxylation of alpha ketoacids (involved in energy production) and in the transketolase reaction of the pentose phosphate pathway (involved in carbohydrate metabolism). Thiamine is also important in nerve transmission (independently of co-enzyme function).

Dietary sources

See Table 2 for dietary sources of thiamine.

Metabolism

Absorption

Absorption occurs mainly in the jejunum and ileum by both active transport and passive diffusion.

Distribution

Thiamine is transported in the plasma bound to albumin and stored in the heart, liver, muscle, kidneys and brain. Only small amounts are stored and turnover is relatively high, so continuous intake is necessary. Thiamine is rapidly converted to its biologically active form, thiamine pyrophosphate (TPP).

Elimination

Thiamine is eliminated mainly in the urine (as metabolites). Excess beyond requirements is excreted as free thiamine. Thiamine crosses the placenta and is excreted in breast milk.

Bioavailability

Bioavailability may be reduced by alcohol. Requirements are increased by increasing carbohydrate intake. Thiamine is unstable above pH 7, and the addition of sodium bicarbonate to peas or green beans (to retain the green colour) can lead to large losses of thiamine. It is also destroyed by heat and by processing foods at alkaline pHs, high temperature and in the presence of oxygen or other oxidants. Freezing does not affect thiamine.

Thiamine antagonists (thiaminases) in coffee, tea, raw fish, betel nuts and some vegetables can lead to thiamine destruction in foods during food processing or in the gut after ingestion.

Table 1 Dietary Reference Values for thiamine

EU RDA = 1.4 mg

Age	UK				USA	WHO	Europe
	LNRI[1]	EAR[1]	RNI[1]	RNI[2]	RDA[2]	RNI[2]	PRI[2]
0–6 months	0.2	0.23	0.3	0.2	0.2	0.3	0.3
7–12 months	0.2	0.23	0.3	0.3	0.3	0.3	0.5
1–3 years	0.23	0.3	0.4	0.5	0.5	0.5	0.5
4–6 years	0.23	0.3	0.4	0.7	–	0.7	0.7
4–8 years	–	–	–	–	0.6	–	–
7–10 years	0.23	0.3	0.4	0.7	–	0.9	0.8
9–13 years	–	–	–	–	0.9	–	–
Males							
11–14 years	0.23	0.3	0.4	0.9	–	1.2	1.0
15–50 years	0.23	0.3	0.4	0.9	–	1.2	1.1
14–70+ years	–	–	–	–	1.2	–	–
Females							
11–14 years	0.23	0.3	0.4	0.7	–	1.0	0.8
14–18 years	–	–	–	–	1.0	–	–
15–50+ years	0.23	0.3	0.4	0.8	–	0.9	0.9
19–70+ years	–	–	–	–	1.1	–	–
Pregnancy	0.23	0.3	0.4	+0.1[3]	1.4	+0.1	1.0
Lactation	0.23	0.3	0.4	+0.2	1.5	+0.2	1.1

[1] mg/1000 kcal.
[2] mg/day.
[3] Last trimester only.

Deficiency

Thiamine deficiency may lead to beri-beri (rare in the UK). Deficiency is associated with abnormalities of carbohydrate metabolism. Early signs of deficiency (including subclinical deficiency) are anorexia, irritability, and weight loss; later features include headache, weakness, tachycardia and peripheral neuropathy.

Advanced deficiency is characterised by involvement of two major organ systems: the cardiovascular system (wet beri-beri) and the nervous system (dry beri-beri, Wernicke's encephalopathy and Korsakoff's psychosis). The Wernicke–Korsakoff syndrome may be associated with a genetic variant of transketolase, which requires a higher than normal concentration of thiamine diphosphate for activity.[1] This would suggest that there may be a group in the population who have a higher than average requirement for thiamine, but the evidence is not convincing. Signs of wet beri-beri include enlarged heart with normal sinus rhythm (usually tachycardia) and peripheral oedema. Signs of dry beri-beri include mental confusion, anorexia, muscle weakness and wasting, ataxia and ophthalmoplegia.

Thiamine deficiency has been observed in HIV-positive patients,[2] those with chronic fatigue syndrome,[3] hospitalised elderly patients[4] and patients on emergency admission to hospital.[5]

Possible uses

Supplementary thiamine may be beneficial in older people (aged >65 years), people who

Table 2 Dietary sources of thiamine

Food portion	Thiamine content (mg)	Food portion	Thiamine content (mg)
Breakfast cereals		Lamb, roast (85 g)	0.12
1 bowl All-Bran (45 g)	**0.4**	**Pork, roast (85 g)**	**0.55**
1 bowl Bran Flakes (45 g)	**0.5**	**1 pork chop, grilled (135 g)**	**0.7**
1 bowl Corn Flakes (30 g)	**0.3**	**2 slices ham**	**0.3**
1 bowl Muesli (95 g)	**0.4**	**1 gammon rasher, grilled (120 g)**	**1.1**
1 bowl porridge (160 g)	0.1	1 chicken leg portion	0.1
2 pieces Shredded Wheat	*0.15*	*Liver, lamb's, cooked (90 g)*	*0.2*
1 bowl Shreddies (50 g)	**0.6**	**Kidney, lamb's, cooked (75 g)**	**0.4**
1 bowl Start (40 g)	**0.6**	*Fish, cooked (150 g)*	*0.15*
2 Weetabix	**0.4**		
		Vegetables	
Cereal products		**Peas, boiled (100 g)**	**0.3**
Bread, brown, 2 slices	*0.2*	**Potatoes, boiled (150 g)**	**0.3**
white, 2 slices	*0.15*	*1 small can baked beans (200 g)*	*0.2*
wholemeal, 2 slices	*0.2*	Chickpeas, cooked (105 g)	0.1
1 chapati	*0.15*	*Red kidney beans (105 g)*	*0.2*
1 naan	**0.3**	Dahl, lentil (150 g)	0.1
1 white pitta bread	*0.15*		
Pasta, brown, boiled (150 g)	**0.3**	**Fruit**	
white, boiled (150 g)	0.01	1 apple, bannana, or pear	0.04
Rice, brown, boiled (160 g)	*0.2*	*1 orange*	*0.2*
white, boiled (160 g)	0.01		
2 heaped tablespoons wheatgerm	**0.3**	**Nuts/seeds**	
		10 Brazil nuts	**0.3**
Milk and dairy products		30 hazelnuts	0.1
½ pint (280 ml) milk, whole,		**30 peanuts**	**0.3**
semi-skimmed or skimmed	0.1	1 tablespoon sunflower seeds	0.1
½ pint (280 ml) soya milk	*0.15*		
Cheese (50 g)	*0.15*	**Yeast**	
		Brewers yeast (10 g)	**1.6**
Meat and fish		*Marmite, spread on 1 slice bread*	*0.15*
3 rashers bacon, back, grilled	**0.3**		
Beef, roast (85 g)	0.07		

Excellent sources (**bold**); good sources (*italics*).

consume quantities of alcohol in excess of two units daily, smokers and in HIV-positive patients. However, deficiency of one B vitamin is often associated with deficiencies of other B vitamins, and a multiple vitamin supplement is often more appropriate.

A double-blind, placebo-controlled trial in 76 elderly people found that thiamine 10 mg daily for three months significantly improved quality of life, and reduced blood pressure and weight in comparison with placebo, but only in subjects with low thiamine status. There was also a non-significant trend to improvement in sleep and energy levels with supplementary thiamine, and the authors concluded that older people could benefit from increasing thiamine intake from supplements or diet.[6]

Thiamine has been thought to be of value in various conditions such as Alzheimer's disease and mouth ulcers.

Alzheimer's disease

One double-blind, placebo-controlled trial found that 3000 mg thiamine daily improved global cognitive scores compared with a niacinamide placebo, but had no effect on behavioural ratings or clinician's subjective judgement of symptoms.[7] Another small double-blind, placebo-controlled trial using 3000 mg thiamine found no benefits of thiamine over placebo in slowing the development of Alzheimer's disease.[8] A more complex placebo-controlled trial in patients with Alzheimer's disease, designed with two phases, used doses of 3000 mg thiamine in the first phase which lasted one month, and then doses of 4000–8000 mg daily over five to 13 months. In the second phase, high-dose thiamine improved scores on various neuropsychological tests, but the authors advised caution in interpretation of the results, lest hopes were unrealistically raised.[9]

Mouth ulcers

Low erythrocyte thiamine has been found in people with recurrent mouth ulcers,[10] and replacement of B vitamins (thiamine, riboflavin and pyridoxine) led to improvement in clinical symptoms in individuals who were deficient in one or more of these vitamins.[11]

Insect repellent

Anecdotally, thiamine has been found to be of value as an insect repellent, but further research is required to confirm these effects.

Miscellaneous

Higher doses of thiamine (25 mg daily) have been found to be beneficial in diabetic neuropathy,[12] HIV[13] and erectile dysfunction,[14] but usually only in those with poor thiamine status. Studies have sometimes used other B vitamins as well, so it is difficult to attribute any benefits to thiamine supplementation alone.

Conclusion

There is some evidence that the elderly could benefit from increased thiamine intake, but evidence for a benefit of thiamine supplementation in Alzheimer's disease is equivocal, and studies have used very high doses (3000–7000 mg daily). Preliminary evidence suggests that thiamine deficiency could be associated with mouth ulcers, but further research is required to determine whether supplements can improve the condition.

Precautions/contraindications

Known hypersensitivity to thiamine.

Pregnancy and breast-feeding

No problems reported.

Adverse effects

There appear to be no toxic effects (except possibly gastric upset) with high oral doses. Large parenteral doses are generally well tolerated, but there have been rare reports of anaphylactic reactions (coughing, difficulty in breathing and swallowing, flushing, skin rash, swelling of face, lips and eyelids).

Interactions

Drugs

Alcohol: excessive alcohol intake induces thiamine deficiency.

Frusemide: may increase urinary loss of thiamine;[15] prolonged frusemide therapy may induce thiamine deficiency;[16,17] thiamine supplementation (200 mg daily) has been shown to improve left ventricular function in patients with congestive heart failure receiving frusemide therapy.[18]

Nutrients

Adequate amounts of all B vitamins are required for optimal functioning; deficiency or excess of one B vitamin may lead to abnormalities in the metabolism of another.

Dose

Thiamine is available in the form of tablets and capsules. It is also found in multivitamins and in brewer's yeast supplements.

No benefit of a dose beyond the RDA has been established.

References

1 Bender DA. Optimum nutrition: Thiamin, biotin and pantothenate. *Proc Nutr Soc* 1999; 58: 427–433.
2 Muri RM, Von Overbeck J, Furrer J, Ballmer PE. Thiamin deficiency in HIV-positive patients: Evaluation by erythrocyte transketolase activity and thiamin pyrophosphate effect. *Clin Nutr* 1999; 18: 375–378.
3 Heap LC, Peters TJ, Wessely S. Vitamin B status in patients with chronic fatigue syndrome. *J R Soc Med* 1999; 92: 183–185.
4 Pepersack T, Garbusinski J, Robberecht, J *et al.* Clinical relevance of thiamine status amongst hospitalized elderly patients. *Gerontology* 1999; 45: 96–101.
5 Jamieson CP, Obeid OA, Powell Tuck J. The thiamin, riboflavin and pyridoxine status of patients on emergency admission to hospital. *Clin Nutr* 1999; 18: 87–91.
6 Wilkinson TJ, Hanger HC, Elmslie J, *et al.* The response to treatment of subclinical thiamine deficiency in the elderly. *Am J Clin Nutr* 1997; 66: 925–928.
7 Blass JP, Gleason P, Brush D, *et al.* Thiamine and Alzheimer's disease: A pilot study. *Arch Neurol* 1988; 45: 833–835.
8 Nolan KA, Black RS, Sheu KF, *et al.* A trial of thiamine in Alzheimer's disease. *Arch Neurol* 1991; 48: 81–83.
9 Meador K, Loring D, Nichols M, *et al.* Preliminary findings of high-dose thiamine in dementia of Alzheimer's type. *J Geriatr Psychiatry Neurol* 1993; 6: 222–229.
10 Haisreili-Shalish M, Livneh A, Katz J, *et al.* Recurrent aphthous stomatitis and thiamine deficiency. *Oral Surg Oral Med Oral Pathol Oral Radiol Endod* 1996; 82: 634–636.
11 Nolan A, McIntosh WB, Allam BF, *et al.* Recurrent aphthous ulceration: Vitamin B1, B2 and B6 status and response to replacement therapy. *J Oral Pathol Med* 1991; 20: 389–391.
12 Abbas ZG, Swai ABM. Evaluation of the efficacy of thiamine and pyridoxine in the treatment of diabetic peripheral neuropathy. *East Afr Med J* 1997; 74: 803–808.
13 Tang AM, Graham NMH, Saah AJ. Effects of multinutrient intake on survival in human immunodeficiency type 1 infection. *Am J Epidemiol* 1996; 143: 1244–1256.
14 Tjandra BS, Jangknegt RA. Neurogenic impotence and lower urinary tract symptoms due to vitamin B1 deficiency in chronic alcoholism. *J Urol* 1997; 157: 954–955.
15 Rieck J, Halkin H, Almog S, *et al.* Urinary loss of thiamine is increased by low doses of furosemide in healthy volunteers. *J Lab Clin Med* 1999; 134: 238–243.
16 Brady JA, Rock CL, Horneffer MR. Thiamin status, diuretic medications, and the management of congestive heart failure. *J Am Dietet Assoc* 1995; 95: 541–544.
17 Seligmann H, Halkin H, Rauchfleish S, *et al.* Thiamin deficiency in patients with congestive heart failure receiving long-term furosemide therapy: A pilot study. *Am J Med* 1991; 91: 151–155.
18 Shimon I, Almog S, Vered Z, *et al.* Improved ventricular function after thiamine supplementation in patients with congestive heart failure receiving long-term furosemide therapy. *Am J Med* 1995; 98: 485–490.

Vitamin A

Description

Vitamin A is a fat-soluble vitamin.

Nomenclature

Vitamin A is a generic term used to describe the compounds that exhibit the biological activity of retinol. The two main components of vitamin A in foods are retinol and the carotenoids (see Carotenoids monograph).

The term 'retinoid' refers to the chemical entity retinol or other closely related naturally occurring derivatives. These include:

- retinal (retinaldehyde);
- retinoic acid; and
- retinyl esters (e.g. retinyl acetate, retinyl palmitate, retinyl propionate).

Retinoids also include structurally related synthetic analogues which may or may not have retinol-like (vitamin A) activity.

Units

The UK Dietary Reference Values express the requirement for vitamin A in terms of retinol equivalents.

$$\text{Retinol equivalents } (\mu g) = \text{retinol } (\mu g) + \frac{\text{betacarotene equivalents } (\mu g)}{6}$$

The system of International Units for vitamin A was discontinued in 1954, but continues to be widely used (particularly on dietary supplement labels): 1 retinol equivalent (μg) = 3.3 units

One unit is equal to:

- 0.3 retinol equivalents (μg)
- 0.3 μg retinol
- 0.3 μg retinol acetate
- 0.5 μg retinol palmitate
- 0.4 μg retinol propionate

Human requirements

See Table 1 for Dietary Reference Values for vitamin A.

Intakes

In the UK, the average adult daily diet provides (retinol equivalents): for men, 1834 μg (6052 units); for women, 1606 μg (5300 units).

Action

Vitamin A (in the form of retinal) is essential for normal function of the retina, and particularly for visual adaptation to darkness. Other forms (retinol, retinoic acid) are necessary for maintenance of the structural and functional integrity of epithelial tissue and the immune system, cellular differentiation and proliferation, bone growth, testicular and ovarian function and embryonic development. Vitamin A may act also as a co-factor in biochemical reactions.

Dietary sources

See Table 2 for dietary sources of retinol.

Table 1 Dietary Reference Values for vitamin A (μg retinol equivalent/day)

EU RDA (for labelling purposes) = 800 μg

Age	UK			USA		WHO Safe level	Europe PRI
	LNRI	EAR	RNI	RDA	UL		
0–6 months	150	250	350	400[1]	600	350	–
7–12 months	150	250	350	500[1]	600	350	–
1–3 years	200	300	400	300	600	400	400
4–6 years	200	300	400	–	–	400	400
4–8 years	–	–	–	400	900	–	–
7–10 years	250	350	500	–	–	400	500
9–13 years	–	–	–	600	1700	–	–
Males							
11–14 years	250	400	600	–	–	550	600
14–18 years	–	–	–	900	2800	–	–
15–50+ years	300	500	700	1000	–	600	700
19–70+ years	–	–	–	900	3000	–	–
Females							
11–50+ years	250	400	600	–	–	500	600
14–18 years	–	–	–	700	2800	–	–
19–70+ years	–	–	–	700	3000	–	–
Pregnancy	–	–	+100	770[2]	3000[3]	600	*
Lactation	–	–	+350	1300[4]	3000[4]	850	*

*No increment.

[1]Adequate Intakes (AIs).

[2]aged <18 years, 750 μg.

[3]aged <18 years, 2800 μg.

[4]aged <18 years, 1200 μg.

UL = Tolerable Upper Intake Level.

Metabolism

Absorption

Vitamin A is readily absorbed from the upper gastrointestinal tract (duodenum and jejunum) by a carrier-mediated process. Absorption requires the presence of gastric juice, bile salts, pancreatic and intestinal lipase, protein and dietary fat.

Distribution

The liver contains at least 90% of body stores (approximately two years' adult requirements). Small amounts are stored in the kidney and lungs. Vitamin A is transported in the blood in association with a carrier, retinol binding protein (RBP).

Elimination

Vitamin A is eliminated in the bile or urine (as metabolites). It appears in the breast milk.

Bioavailability

Absorption is markedly reduced if the intake of dietary fat is <5 g daily (extremely rare) and by the presence of peroxidised fat and other oxidising agents in food. Deficiencies of protein (extremely rare in the UK), vitamin E, and zinc, and excessive amounts of alcohol adversely affect vitamin A transport, storage and utilisation.

Table 2 Dietary sources of retinol

Food portion	Retinol (µg)	Food portion	Retinol (µg)
Cereals		**Fats and oils**	
Breads, grains, cereals	0	Butter, on 1 slice bread (10 g)	80
		Margarine on 1 slice bread (10 g)	80
Milk and dairy products		Low-fat spread on 1 slice bread (10 g)	92
½ pint (280 ml) whole milk	*150*	*2 tablespoons ghee (30 g)*	*210*
½ pint (280 ml) semi-skimmed milk	55	2 teaspoons cod liver oil (10 ml)	1800
½ pint (280 ml) skimmed milk	2		
½ pint (280 ml) skimmed milk, fortified	100–150 (various brands)	**Meat and fish**	
2 tablespoons dried skimmed milk, fortified (30 g)	120	Bacon, beef, lamb, pork, poultry	Trace
Single cream (35 g)	100	Kidney, lamb's, cooked (75 g)	80
Whipping cream (35 g)	*190*	**Liver, lamb's, cooked (90 g)**	**20 000**
Double cream (35 g)	*200*	**Liver, calf, cooked (90 g)**	**36 000**
Hard cheese (e.g. cheddar) (50 g)	*160*	**Liver, ox, cooked (90 g)**	**18 000**
Hard cheese, reduced fat (50 g)	80	**Liver, pig, cooked (90 g)**	**21 000**
Brie cheese (50 g)	*140*	**Liver paté (60 g)**	**4400**
Cream cheese (30 g)	*130*	**4 slices liver sausage (35 g)**	**870**
1 carton yoghurt, low fat (150 g)	10	White fish	Trace
1 carton yoghurt, whole milk (150 g)	45	2 fillets herring, cooked (110 g)	60
Ice cream, dairy (75 g)	90	2 fillets kipper, cooked (130 g)	40
Ice cream, non-dairy (75 g)	1	2 fillets mackerel, cooked (110 g)	55
1 egg, size 2 (60 g)	*110*		

Excellent sources (**bold**); good sources (*italics*).

Note: For dietary sources of betacarotene, see Carotenoids monograph.

Deficiency

Vitamin A deficiency is widespread in young children in developing countries and is associated with general malnutrition in these countries. In the UK, deficiency is relatively rare, (especially in adults), but marginal intakes may occur in children.

Symptoms of deficiency include: night blindness (due to decreased sensitivity of rod receptors in the retina); xerophthalmia (can be irreversible), characterised by conjunctival and corneal xerosis, ulceration and liquefaction; ultimately severe visual impairment and blindness; dryness of the skin and papular eruptions (not a unique indicator of vitamin A deficiency because other nutrient deficiencies cause similar disorders); metaplasia and keratinisation of the cells of the respiratory tract and other organs; increased susceptibility to respiratory and urinary tract infections; occasionally diarrhoea and loss of appetite.

Possible uses

Children

The Department of Health[1] advises that most children from the age of six months to five years should receive supplements of vitamins A and D, unless the adequacy of their diet can be assured.

Cancer

A large number of studies have assessed the association between vitamin A and cancer, but not all of them distinguish between retinol (preformed vitamin A) and carotenoids. Some case-control studies reporting on the association between preformed vitamin A and breast cancer have found modest decreases in risk with higher intake,[2–4] but others[5,6] have found no association. Prospective data are compatible with a modest protective effect of preformed vitamin A.[7–9]

There is some preliminary evidence that preformed vitamin A may be modestly protective against colon cancer in both men[10] and women.[11] In a nested, case-control study,[12] subjects in the highest quintile of serum retinol were at reduced risk of colon cancer for up to nine years of follow-up. However, another study[13] failed to find any association between colon cancer and vitamin A intake.

Most data suggest that preformed vitamin A does not protect against prostate cancer, and an initial study[14] suggesting an adverse effect has not been confirmed. However, the possibility that higher intakes of vitamin A increase the risk of prostate cancer requires further investigation.

The risk of lung cancer may be related to dietary carotene intake rather than retinol, and studies have shown no benefit of vitamin A in prevention of lung cancer.[15–17]

There is some evidence that people taking vitamin A-containing supplements have a lower risk of gastric cancer than non-users.[18]

Miscellaneous

There is no evidence of any value of vitamin A in eye problems, or prevention and treatment of infections unrelated to vitamin A deficiency. Vitamin A supplements in normal safe doses have no proven benefits in skin problems (e.g. acne), but synthetic retinoids may be prescribed for this purpose.

Single case studies have appeared periodically in the literature indicating that vitamin A may be beneficial in premenstrual syndrome, but these effects have not been confirmed in randomised trials.

Conclusion

The Department of Health recommends a supplement containing vitamin A (and vitamin D) in children aged six months to five years, unless a good diet can be assured. There is very little evidence for any benefit of vitamin A supplements except for cases of deficiency. Evidence for a role of preformed vitamin A in cancer is limited. Such evidence as exists relates more to carotenoids.

Pregnancy and breast-feeding

Excessive doses of vitamin A have been shown to be teratogenic,[19,20] though the level at which this occurs has not been firmly established. No teratogenic effects were observed in 1203 women receiving 6000 units daily at least from one month prior to conception until the 12th week of pregnancy,[21] and an apparent threshold of 10 000 units daily has been identified.[22] Other studies[23,24] suggest low risk with intakes up to 30 000 units daily.

The Department of Health has recommended that women who are (or may become) pregnant should not take dietary supplements which contain vitamin A (including fish liver oil), except on the advice of a doctor or antenatal clinic, and should also avoid liver and products containing liver (e.g. liver paté and liver sausage).

Adverse effects

Acute toxicity

Acute toxicity may be induced by single doses of 300 mg retinol (1 million units) in adults, 60 mg retinol (200 000 units) in children or 30 mg retinol (100 000 units) in infants.

Signs and symptoms are usually transient (most often occurring about 6 h after ingestion of acute dose and disappearing after 36 h) and include: severe headache (due to raised intracranial pressure), sore mouth, bleeding gums, dizziness, vomiting, blurred vision, hepatomegaly, irritability and (in infants) bulging of the fontanelle.

Chronic toxicity

Signs of chronic toxicity may appear when daily intake is >15 mg retinol (50 000 units) in adults and 6 mg (20 000 units) in infants and young children.

Signs may include: dryness of the skin, pruritus, dermatitis, skin desquamation, skin erythema, skin rash, skin scaliness, papilloedema, disturbed hair growth, fissure of the lips, bone and joint pain, hyperostosis, headache, fatigue, irritability, insomnia, anorexia, nausea, vomiting, diarrhoea, weight loss, hepatomegaly, hepatotoxicity, raised intracranial pressure, bulging fontanelle (in infants), hypercalcaemia (due to increase in activity of alkaline phosphatase activity).

Not all signs appear in all patients, and relative severity varies widely among different individuals. Most signs and symptoms disappear within a week, but skin and bone changes may remain evident for several months.

Interactions

Drugs

Anticoagulants: large doses of vitamin A (>750 µg; 2500 units) may induce a hypoprothrombinaemic response.
Cholestyramine and colestipol: may reduce intestinal absorption of vitamin A.
Colchicine: may reduce intestinal absorption of vitamin A.
Liquid paraffin: may reduce intestinal absorption of vitamin A.
Neomycin: may reduce intestinal absorption of vitamin A.
Retinoids (acitrecin, etreninate, isotretinoin, tretinoin): concurrent administration of vitamin A may result in additive toxic effects.
Statins: prolonged therapy with statins may increase serum vitamin A levels.
Sucralfate: may reduce intestinal absorption of vitamin A.

Nutrients

Iron: in vitamin A deficiency, plasma iron levels fall.
Vitamin C: under conditions of hypervitaminosis A, tissue levels of vitamin C may be reduced and urinary excretion of vitamin C increased; vitamin C may ameliorate the toxic effects of vitamin A.
Vitamin E: large doses of vitamin A increase the need for vitamin E; vitamin E protects against the oxidative destruction of vitamin A.
Vitamin K: under conditions of hypervitaminosis A, hypothrombinaemia may occur; it can be corrected by administration of vitamin K.

Dose

In the absence of malabsorption or gastrointestinal disease, the following regular daily intakes (from food and supplements) should *not* be exceeded:

- adult women 7500 µg (25 000 units);
- pregnant women 2400 µg (8000 units);
- adult men 9000 µg (29 700 units);
- infants 900 µg (2970 units);
- children aged 1–3 years 1800 µg (5940 units);
- children aged 4–6 years 3000 µg (9900 units);
- children aged 6–12 years 4500 µg (14 850 units); and
- adolescents 6000 µg (19 800 units).

Therapeutic doses may exceed these limits, but only under medical supervision. For example, in cystic fibrosis, doses of 1200–3300 µg (4000–10 000 units) daily may be given.

References

1 Department of Health. Weaning and the weaning diet: Report of the Working Group on the Weaning Diet of the Committee on Medical Aspects of Food Policy. Report on Health and Social Subjects No 45. London: HMSO, 1994.
2 London SJ, Stein EA, Henderson IC. Carotenoids, retinol and vitamin E and risk of proliferative benign breast disease and breast cancer. *Cancer Causes Control* 1992; 3: 503–512.
3 Longnecker M, Newcomb P, Mittendorf PR, *et al.* Intake of carrots, spinach and supplements containing vitamin A in relation to the risk of breast cancer. *Cancer Epidemiol Biomarkers Prev* 1997; 6: 887–892.
4 Zaridze D, Lifanova Y, Maximovitch D, *et al.* Diet, alcohol consumption and reproductive factors in a case-control study of breast cancer in Moscow. *Int J Cancer* 1991; 48: 493–501.

5 Ingram DM, Nottage E, Roberts T. The role of diet in the development of breast cancer: A case-control study of patients with breast cancer, benign epithelial hyperplasia and fibrocystic disease of the breast. *Br J Cancer* 1991; 64: 187–191.
6 La Vecchia C, Decarli A, Franceschi S, *et al.* Dietary factors and the risk of breast cancer. *Nutr Cancer* 1987; 10: 205–214.
7 Graham S, Zielezny M, Marshall J. Diet in the epidemiology of breast cancer in the New York state cohort. *Am J Epidemiol* 1992; 136: 1327–1337.
8 Hunter DJ, Mason JE, Colditz GA. A prospective study of the intake of vitamins C, E and A and risk of breast cancer. *N Engl J Med* 1993; 329: 324–340.
9 Rohan TE, Howe GR, Friedenreich CM, *et al.* Dietary fiber, vitamins A, C and E, and risk of breast cancer: A cohort study. *Cancer Causes Control* 1993; 4: 29–37.
10 Graham S, Marshall B, Haughey B. Dietary epidemiology of cancer of colon in western New York. *Am J Epidemiol* 1986; 128: 490–503.
11 Heilbrun LK, Nomura A, Hankin JH, Stemmerman GN. Diet and colorectal cancer with special reference to fiber intake. *Int J Cancer* 1989; 44: 1–6.
12 Comstock GW, Helzlsouer KJ, Bush TL. Prediagnostic serum levels of carotenoids and vitamin E as related to subsequent cancer in Washington County, Maryland. *Am J Clin Nutr* 1991; 53: 260S–264S.
13 Potter JD, McMichael AJ. Diet and cancer of the colon and rectum: a case-control study. *J Natl Cancer Inst* 1986; 76: 557–569.
14 Graham S, Haughey B, Marshall J. Diet in the epidemiology of carcinoma of the prostate gland. *J Natl Cancer Inst* 1983: 70: 687–692.
15 Omenn GS, Goodman GE, Thornquist MD, *et al.* Effects of a combination of betacarotene and vitamin A on lung cancer and cardiovascular disease. *N Engl J Med* 1996; 334: 1150–1155.
16 De Klerk N, Musk W, Ambrosini G, *et al.* Vitamin A and cancer prevention II: Comparison of the effects of vitamin A and betacarotene. *Int J Cancer* 1998; 75: 362–367.
17 Musk W, De Klerk N, Ambrosini G, *et al.* Vitamin A and cancer prevention I: Observations in workers previously exposed to asbestos at Wittnoom, Western Australia. *Int J Cancer* 1998; 75: 355–361.
18 Botterweck AA, van Den Brandt PA, Goldbohm RA. Vitamins, carotenoids, dietary fiber, and the risk of gastric carcinoma: Results from a prospective study after 6.3 years of follow-up. *Cancer* 2000; 88: 737–748.
19 Pinnock CB, Alderman CP. The potential for teratogenicity of vitamin A and its cogeners. *Med J Aust* 1992; 157: 804–809.
20 Underwood BA. Teratogenicity of vitamin A. *Int J Vit Nutr Res* 1989; 30 (suppl.): 42–55.
21 Dudas I, Czeizel AE. Use of 6,000 IU vitamin A during early pregnancy without teratogenic effect (letter). *Teratology* 1992; 45: 335–336.
22 Rothman KJ, Moore LL, Singer MR, *et al.* Teratogenicity of high vitamin A intake. *N Engl J Med* 1995; 333: 1369–1373.
23 Mastroiacovo P, Mazzone T, Addis A, *et al.* High vitamin A intake in early pregnancy and major malformations: A multicenter prospective controlled study. *Teratology* 1999; 59: 7–11.
24 Miller RK, Hendricks AG, Mils JL, *et al.* Periconceptual vitamin A use: How much is teratogenic? *Reprod Toxicol* 1998; 12: 75–88.

Vitamin B_6

Description

Vitamin B_6 is a water-soluble member of the vitamin B complex.

Nomenclature

Vitamin B_6 is a generic term used to describe the compounds that exhibit the biological activity of pyridoxine. It occurs in food as pyridoxine, pyridoxal and pyridoxamine. Thus the term 'pyridoxine' is not synonymous with the generic term 'vitamin B_6'.

Human requirements

Vitamin B_6 requirements depend on protein intake; values are therefore given as µg/g protein and also as total values (Table 1).

Intakes

In the UK, the average adult daily diet provides: for men, 2.59 mg; for women, 3.48 mg.

Action

Vitamin B_6 is converted in erythrocytes to pyridoxal phosphate and, to a lesser extent, pyridoxamine phosphate. It acts as a co-factor for enzymes which are involved in more than 100 reactions that affect protein, lipid and carbohydrate metabolism. Pyridoxal phosphate is also involved in: the synthesis of several neurotransmitters; the metabolism of several vitamins (e.g. the conversion of tryptophan to niacin); haemoglobin and sphingosine formation.

Dietary sources

See Table 2 for dietary sources of vitamin B_6.

Metabolism

Absorption

Occurs mainly by a non-saturable process (absorption is greatest in the jejunum).

Distribution

Vitamin B_6 is stored in the liver, muscle and brain. Pyridoxal phosphate is transported in the plasma (bound to albumin) and in erythrocytes (in association with haemoglobin).

Elimination

Primarily in the urine (mainly as metabolites), but excess amounts are excreted largely unchanged. It also appears in breast milk.

Bioavailability

Bioavailability of vitamin B_6 is affected by food processing and storage. The vitamin is sensitive to light, especially in acid or neutral solutions.

Deficiency

Deficiency of vitamin B_6 does not produce a characteristic syndrome, but as with deficiency of the other B vitamins, symptoms such as dermatitis, cheilosis, glossitis and angular stomatitis may occur. Advanced deficiency may produce weakness, irritability, depression, dizziness, peripheral neuropathy and seizures; diarrhoea, anaemia and seizures are particular characteristics of deficiency in infants and

Table 1 Dietary Reference Values for vitamin B_6

EU RDA = 2 mg

Age	UK				USA		Europe
	LNRI[1]	EAR[1]	RNI[1]	RNI[2]	RDA[2]	UL[2]	PRI[2]
0–6 months	3.5	6	8	0.2	0.1	–	–
7–9 months	6	8	10	0.3	0.3	–	0.4
10–12 months	8	10	13	0.4	0.3	–	0.4
1–3 years	8	10	13	0.7	0.5	–	0.7
4–6 years	8	10	13	0.9	–	–	0.9
4–8 years	–	–	–	–	0.6	40	–
7–10 years	8	10	13	1.0	–	–	1.0
9–13 years	–	–	–	–	1.0	60	–
Males							
11–14 years	11	13	15	1.2	–	–	1.3
14–18 years	–	–	–	–	1.3	80	–
15–18 years	11	13	15	1.4	–	–	1.5
19–50+ years	11	13	15	1.4	1.3	100	1.5
51–70+ years	–	–	–	–	1.7	100	–
Females							
11–14 years	11	13	15	1.0	–	–	1.1
14–18 years	–	–	–	–	1.2	80	–
15–18 years	11	13	15	1.2	–	–	1.1
19–50+ years	11	13	15	1.2	1.3	100	1.1
51–70+ years	–	–	–	–	1.5	100	–
Pregnancy	*	*	*	*	1.9	–	1.3
Lactation	*	*	*	*	2.0	–	1.3

*No increment.
[1]μg/g protein.
[2]mg/day.

children. Chronic deficiency may lead to secondary hyperoxaluria (increased risk of kidney stone formation) and to hypochromic, microcytic anaemia.

Possible uses

Vitamin B_6 has been investigated for a range of conditions, including carpal tunnel syndrome, premenstrual syndrome (PMS), asthma, diabetic neuropathy, cardiovascular disease and autism.

Carpal tunnel syndrome

Idiopathic carpal tunnel syndrome, with swelling of the synovia and compression of the median nerve by the transverse carpal ligament, has been attributed to pyridoxine deficiency.[1,2] Several uncontrolled studies in the 1980s demonstrated the efficacy of vitamin B_6 treatment.[3–5] However, another study showed no consistent improvement in patients with carpal tunnel syndrome and normal vitamin B_6 status.[6] These findings led to the suggestion[7] that clinical improvement in some patients with carpal tunnel syndrome may be due to correction of unrecognised peripheral neuropathy, which could compound symptoms of the syndrome. A review article concluded that studies have not provided sufficient evidence for the use of vitamin B_6 as the sole treatment for carpal tunnel syndrome, but that it could be of some benefit as

Table 2 Dietary sources of vitamin B_6

Food portion	Vitamin B_6 content (mg)
Breakfast cereals	
1 bowl All-Bran (45 g)	**0.6**
1 bowl Bran Flakes (45 g)	**0.8**
1 bowl Corn Flakes (30 g)	**0.6**
1 bowl Muesli (95 g)	**1.5**
1 bowl Start (40 g)	**1.1**
2 Weetabix	**0.4**
Milk and dairy products	
½ pint (280 ml) milk, whole, semi-skimmed or skimmed	0.15
½ pint (280 ml) soya milk	0.15
Meat and fish	
Beef, roast (85 g)	*0.3*
Lamb, roast (85 g)	*0.2*
Pork, roast (85 g)	*0.3*
2 slices ham	*0.3*
1 chicken leg portion	*0.3*
Liver, lamb's, cooked (90g)	**0.4**
Kidney, lamb's, cooked (75 g)	*0.2*
Fish, cooked (150 g)	**0.5**
Vegetables	
Potatoes, boiled (150 g)	**0.5**
1 small can baked beans (200 g)	*0.3*
Fruit	
½ an avocado pear	**0.4**
1 banana	*0.3*
Nuts	
30 peanuts	*0.2*
Yeast	
Brewer's yeast (10 g)	*0.2*

Excellent sources (**bold**); good sources (*italics*).

adjunct therapy because of its potential benefit on pain perception and increasing pain threshold.[8]

Premenstrual syndrome

Pyridoxine has been reported to be of benefit in PMS,[9–11] but some researchers have found no significant benefit.[12–14] Doses of pyridoxine which have shown beneficial effects have been relatively high (500 mg daily), and these high doses should not be recommended because of the risk of toxicity. However, a good response has been reported with a dose of 50 mg daily.[15] Studies are complicated by the subjective nature of symptoms in PMS, and conclusions limited by the poor quality of many of the trials. Nevertheless, a systematic review[16] of nine published trials representing 940 patients with PMS suggests that doses of vitamin B_6 up to 100 mg daily are likely to be of benefit in treating premenstrual symptoms and premenstrual depression.

Asthma

Low vitamin B_6 status has been reported in adults with asthma,[17,18] and in asthmatic children.[19] This may in part be due to use of theophylline which reduces vitamin B status.[20,21] A supplement of 15 mg of pyridoxine per day reduced side-effects of theophylline related to nervous system function.[22]

Vitamin B_6 supplementation (50 mg daily) reduced the severity and frequency of asthma attacks,[18] and pyridoxine (200 mg daily) reduced the need for asthma medication in children.[23] However, a dose of 300 mg daily failed to improve asthma in patients requiring steroids.[24]

Diabetic neuropathy

Peripheral neuropathy in patients with diabetes has been suggested to be associated with pyridoxine deficiency. Diabetics with symptoms of neuropathy and low vitamin B_6 status were given 150 mg of vitamin B_6 daily for six weeks.[25] Neuropathic symptoms were eliminated in all subjects. The same dose of pyridoxine gradually improved pain in patients with painful neuropathy.[26] In diabetic patients whose vitamin B_6 status was normal, pyridoxine supplementation resulted in no improvement in neuropathic symptoms.[27] Further studies are required to investigate the possible benefits of vitamin B_6 in diabetic neuropathy.

Coronary heart disease

A raised level of plasma homocysteine is associated with an increased risk of coronary heart disease. This in turn has been linked with low intake and low level of folic acid (see Folic acid monograph) and other B vitamins, including vitamin B_6. However, whether vitamin B_6 has an influence independent of folic acid is uncertain. In the Framingham Heart Study,[28] folic acid, vitamin B_6 and vitamin B_{12} were determinants of homocysteine levels, with folic acid showing the strongest association. In the Nurse's Health Study[29] those with the highest vitamin B_6 intake had a 33% lower risk of heart disease than those with the lowest intake, while in those with the highest intake of both vitamin B_6 and folate, the risk of heart disease was reduced by 45%. In a prospective, case-cohort study, heart disease was negatively associated with plasma vitamin B_6 in both men and women, and after correcting for a large number of risk factors, the association with pyridoxine still held, pointing to the possibility that vitamin B_6 offers independent protection.[30] However, a meta-analysis[31] concluded that although folic acid reduced plasma homocysteine levels, vitamin B_6 had no additional effect.

Miscellaneous

Pyridoxine has also been reported to be effective in treating pregnancy sickness,[32,33] depression[34,35] and hypertension.[36] Autism has also been shown to respond to vitamin therapy, including vitamin B_6, but a review of 12 studies using vitamin B_6 and magnesium concluded that although results were favourable, studies suffered from methodological problems of poor design, small numbers of subjects and failure to follow up long term.[37]

Precautions/contraindications

Hypersensitivity to pyridoxine.

Pregnancy and breast-feeding

No problems reported with normal intakes. Large doses may result in pyridoxine dependency in infants. There has been one report of amelia of the leg at the knee in an infant whose mother had taken 50 mg pyridoxine daily during pregnancy.

Conclusion

The role of vitamin B_6 supplements in carpal tunnel syndrome, premenstrual syndrome and asthma is controversial, although supplements may help some individuals. Low vitamin B_6 status has been linked with high plasma homocysteine levels and increased risk of coronary heart disease, but whether vitamin B_6 has an effect independent of folic acid and vitamin B_{12} is not yet clear. Further properly controlled clinical trials are needed to assess the benefit of vitamin B_6 supplements for all these purposes as well as for autism, depression and pregnancy sickness.

Adverse effects

Peripheral neuropathy; unsteady gait; numbness and tingling in feet and hands; loss of limb reflexes; impaired or absent tendon reflexes; photosensitivity on exposure to sun; dizziness; nausea; breast tenderness; exacerbation of acne.

Adverse effects usually occur with megadoses only. Doses of 100–150 mg daily over 5–10 years have not generally been associated with toxicity. However, doses averaging 117 mg daily have been associated with neurological symptoms (e.g. numbness, tingling, bone pain) in 60% of women taking supplements for three years, but this study has been severely criticised. Moreover, symptoms were reversed six months after patients ceased to take the supplement.[38] Another paper reported that women taking 500 to 5000 mg daily for PMS developed peripheral neuropathy over a one- to three-year period.[39]

Interactions

Drugs

Alcohol: increases turnover of pyridoxine.
Cycloserine: may cause anaemia or peripheral neuritis by acting as pyridoxine antagonist.
Hydralazine: may cause anaemia or peripheral neuritis by acting as pyridoxine antagonist.
Isoniazid: may cause anaemia or peripheral neuritis by acting as pyridoxine antagonist.
Levodopa: effects of levodopa are reversed by

pyridoxine (even doses as low as 5 mg daily); vitamin B_6 supplements should be avoided; interaction does not occur with co-beneldopa or co-careldopa.
Oestrogens (including oral contraceptives): may increase requirement for vitamin B_6.
Penicillamine: may cause anaemia or peripheral neuritis by acting as pyridoxine antagonist.
Theophylline: may increase requirement for vitamin B_6.

Nutrients

Adequate amounts of all B vitamins are required for optimal functioning; deficiency or excess of one B vitamin may lead to abnormalities in the metabolism of another.
Vitamin C: deficiency of vitamin B_6 may lead to vitamin C deficiency.

Dose

Premenstrual syndrome, 10–50 mg daily. As a dietary supplement, 2–5 mg daily.

References

1 Ellis J, Azuma J, Watanebe T, *et al.* Survey and new data on treatment with pyridoxine of patients having a clinical syndrome including carpal tunnel and other defects. *Res Commun Chem Pathol Pharmacol* 1977; 17: 165–177.
2 Fuhr JE, Farrow A, Nelson HS, Jr. Vitamin B6 levels in patients with carpal tunnel syndrome. *Arch Surg* 1989; 124: 1329–1330.
3 Driskell JA, Wesley RL, Hess IE. Effectiveness of pyridoxine hydrochloride treatment on carpal tunnel syndrome patients. *Nutr Rep Int* 1986; 34: 1031–1040.
4 Ellis J, Folkers K, Levy M, *et al.* Therapy with vitamin B6 with and without surgery for treatment of patients having the idiopathic carpal tunnel syndrome. *Res Commun Chem Pathol Pharmacol* 1981; 33: 331–344.
5 Ellis J, Folkers K, Watanebe T, *et al.* Clinical results of a crossover treatment with pyridoxine and placebo of the carpal tunnel syndrome. *Am J Clin Nutr* 1979; 32: 2040–2046.
6 Smith GP, Rudge PJ, Peters TJ. Biochemical studies of pyridoxal and pyridoxal phosphate status and therapeutic trial of pyridoxine in patients with carpal tunnel syndrome. *Ann Neurol* 1984; 15: 104–107.
7 Byers CM, DeLisa JA, Frankel DL, Kraft GH. Pyridoxine metabolism in carpal tunnel syndrome with and without peripheral neuropathy. *Arch Phys Med Rehabil* 1984; 65: 712–716.
8 Jacobson MD, Plancher KD, Kleinman WB. Vitamin B_6 (pyridoxine) therapy for carpal tunnel syndrome. *Hand Clin* 1996; 12: 253–257.
9 Barr W. Pyridoxine supplements in the premenstrual syndrome. *Practitioner* 1984; 228: 425–427.
10 Day JB. Clinical trials in the premenstrual syndrome. *Curr Med Res Opin* 1979; 6: 40–45.
11 Kerr GD. The management of premenstrual syndrome. *Curr Med Res Opin* 1977; 4: 29–34.
12 Hagen I, Neshmein BI, Tuntlund T. No effect of vitamin B6 against premenstrual tension. *Acta Obstet Gynecol Scand* 1985; 64: 667–670.
13 Malmgren R, Collins A, Nilsson CG. Platelet serotonin uptake and effects of vitamin B6 treatment in premenstrual tension. *Neurophysiology* 1987; 18: 83–88.
14 Smallwood J, Ah-Kye D, Taylor I. Vitamin B6 in the treatment of pre-menstrual mastalgia. *Br J Clin Pract* 1986; 40: 532–533.
15 Mattes JA, Martin D. Pyridoxine in premenstrual depression. *Hum Nutr Appl Nutr* 1982; 36A: 131–133.
16 Wyatt KM, Dimmock PW, Jones PW, *et al.* Efficacy of vitamin B6 in the treatment of premenstrual syndrome. *Br Med J* 1999; 318: 1375–1381.
17 Delport R, Ubbink JB, Serfontein WJ, *et al.* Vitamin B6 nutritional status in asthma: The effect of theophylline therapy on plasma pyridoxal-5'-phosphate and pyridoxal levels. *Int J Vit Nutr Res* 1988; 58: 67–72.
18 Reynolds RD, Natta CL. Depressed plasma pyridoxal phosphate concentrations in adult asthmatics. *Am J Clin Nutr* 1985; 41: 684–688.
19 Hall MA, Thom H, Russell G. Erythrocyte aspartate aminotransferase activity in asthmatic and non-asthmatic children and its enhancement by vitamin B6. *Ann Allergy* 1985; 47: 464–466.
20 Ubbink JB, Vermaak WJH, Delport R, *et al.* The relationship between vitamin B6 metabolism, asthma and theophylline therapy. *Ann NY Acad Sci* 1990; 585: 285–294.
21 Shimizu T, Maesda S, Arakawa H, *et al.* Relation between theophylline and circulating levels in children with asthma. *Pharmacology* 1996; 53: 384–389.
22 Bartel PR, Ubbink JB, Delport R, *et al.* Vitamin B6 supplementation and theophylline-related effects in humans. *Am J Clin Nutr* 1994; 60: 93–99.
23 Collipp PJ, Goldzier S, Weiss N, *et al.* Pyridoxine treatment in childhood bronchial asthma. *Ann Allergy* 1977; 35: 93–97.
24 Sur S, Camara M, Buchmeier A, *et al.* Double-blind trial of pyridoxine (vitamin B6) in the treatment of steroid-dependent asthma. *Ann Allergy* 1993; 70: 147–152.

25 Jones CL, Gonzalez V. Pyridoxine deficiency: A new factor in diabetic neuropathy. *J Am Podiatr Assoc* 1978; 68: 646–653.

26 Bernstein AL, Lobitz CZ. A clinical and electrophysiologic study of the treatment of painful diabetic neuropathies with pyridoxine. In Leklem JE, Reynolds RD, eds. *Clinical and Physiological Applications of Vitamin B_6*. New York: Alan R. Liss, 1988: 415–423.

27 Levin ER, Hanscomb TA, Fisher M, *et al*. The influence of pyridoxine in diabetic neuropathy. *Diabetes Care* 1981; 4: 606–609.

28 Selhub J, Jaques PF, Wilson PWF, *et al*. Vitamin status and intake as primary determinants of homocystinaemia in an elderly population. *JAMA* 1993; 270: 2693–2698.

29 Rimm EB, Willett WC, Hu FB, *et al*. Folate and vitamin B_6 from diet and supplements in relation to risk of coronary heart disease among women. *JAMA* 1998; 279: 359–364.

30 Folsom AR, Nieto FJ, McGovern PG, *et al*. Prospective study of coronary heart disease incidence in relation to fasting total homocysteine, related genetic polymorphisms, and B vitamins: The Atherosclerosis Risk in Communities (ARIC) study. *Circulation* 1998; 98: 204–210.

31 Homocysteine Lowering Trialists' Collaboration. Lowering blood homocysteine with folic acid based supplements; meta-analysis of randomised trials. *Br Med J* 1998; 316: 894–898.

32 Sahakian V, Rouse D, Sipes S. Vitamin B_6 is effective therapy for nausea and vomiting of pregnancy: A randomised, double-blind, placebo controlled study. *Obstet Gynecol* 1991; 78: 33–36.

33 Vutyavenich T, Wongra-ngan S, Ruangsvi R. Pyridoxine for nausea and vomiting of pregnancy: A randomised, double-blind, placebo-controlled trial. *Am J Obstet Gynecol* 1995; 173: 881–884.

34 Bell IR, Edman JS, Marrow FD. B complex vitamin patterns in geriatric and young adult inpatients with major depression. *J Am Geriatr Soc* 1991; 39: 252–257.

35 Russ CS, Hendricks TA, Chrisley BM. Vitamin B6 status of depressed and obsessive-compulsive patients. *Nutr Rep Int* 1983; 27: 867–873.

36 Ayback M, Sermet A, Ayyildiz MO. Effect of oral pyridoxine hydrochloride supplementation on arterial blood pressure in patients with essential hypertension. *Arzneimittelforschung* 1995; 45: 1271–1273.

37 Pfeiffer SI, Norton J, Nelson L, *et al*. Efficacy of vitamin B_6 and magnesium in the treatment of autism. *J Autism Dev Disord* 1995; 25: 481–483.

38 Dalton K, Dalton MJ. Characteristics of pyridoxine overdose neuropathy syndrome. *Acta Neurol Scand* 1987; 76: 8–11.

39 Bernstein AL. Vitamin B_6 in clinical neurology. *Ann NY Acad Sci* 1990; 585: 250–260.

Vitamin B_{12}

Description

Vitamin B_{12} is a water-soluble member of the vitamin B complex.

Nomenclature

Vitamin B_{12} is the generic term used to describe the compounds that exhibit the biological activity of cyanocobalamin. It includes a range of cobalt-containing compounds, known as cobalamins. Cyanocobalamin and hydroxocobalamin are the two principal forms in clinical use.

Human requirements

See Table 1 for Dietary Reference Values for vitamin B_{12}.

Table 1 Dietary Reference Values for vitamin B_{12} (μg/day)

EU RDA = 1 μg

Age	UK			USA RDA	WHO Safe level	Europe PRI
	LNRI	EAR	RNI			
0–6 months	0.1	0.25	0.3	0.4	0.1	–
7–12 months	0.25	0.35	0.4	0.5	0.1	0.5
1–3 years	0.3	0.4	0.5	0.9	0.5	0.7
4–6 years	0.5	0.7	0.8	–	0.8	0.9
4–8 years	–	–	–	1.2	–	–
7–10 years	0.6	0.8	1.0	–	1.0	1.0
9–13 years	–	–	–	1.8	–	–
Males						
11–14 years	0.8	1.0	1.2	–	1.0	1.3
15–50+ years	1.0	1.25	1.5	–	1.0	1.4
14–70+ years	–	–	–	2.4	–	–
Females						
11–14 years	0.8	1.0	1.2	–	1.0	1.2
15–50+ years	1.0	1.25	1.5	–	1.0	1.4
14–70+ years	–	–	–	2.4	–	–
Pregnancy	–	–	*	2.6	1.4	1.6
Lactation	–	–	+0.5	2.8	1.3	1.9

*No increment.

Intakes

In the UK, the average adult daily diet provides: for men, 7.7 μg; for women, 5.9 μg.

Action

Vitamin B_{12} is involved in the recycling of folate co-enzymes and the degradation of valine. It is also required for nerve myelination, cell replication, haematopoiesis and nucleoprotein synthesis.

Dietary sources

See Table 2 for dietary sources of vitamin B_{12}.

Table 2 Dietary sources of vitamin B_{12}

Food portion	Vitamin B_{12} content (μg)
Breakfast cereals	
1 bowl All-Bran (45 g)	*0.5*
1 bowl Bran Flakes (45 g)	**0.8**
1 bowl Corn Flakes (30 g)	*0.5*
1 bowl Start (40 g)	**1.0**
Milk and dairy products	
½ pint (280 ml) milk, whole, semi-skimmed or skimmed	**1.0**
Soya milk	
Gold, ½ pint (280 ml)	**1.5**
Plamil, diluted, ½ pint (280 ml)	**3.2**
1 pot yoghurt (150 g)	*0.3*
Cheese (50 g)	**1.0**
1 egg, size 2 (60 g)	*0.4*
Fats and oils	
Butter, margarine, spreads, oils	Trace
Fortified margarine (vegetarian) (10 g)	**0.5**
Meat and fish	
Meat, roast (85 g)	**1.6**
Liver, lamb's, cooked (90g)	**70.0**
Kidney, lamb's, cooked (75 g)	**55.0**
White fish, cooked (150 g)	**1.5–4.0**
2 fillets herring, cooked (110 g)	**9.0**
2 fillets kipper, cooked (130 g)	**8.0**
2 fillets mackerel, cooked (110 g)	**15.0**
Pilchards, canned (100 g)	**12.0**
Sardines, canned (70 g)	**10.0**
Tuna, canned (95 g)	**4.0**
Vegetable protein mixes	
Protoveg Burgamix (100 g)	**3.6**
Protoveg Sosmix (100 g)	**1.8**
Yeast extracts	
Marmite, spread on 1 slice bread	*0.4*
Natex, spread on 1 slice bread	*0.4*
Vecon, spread on 1 slice bread	*0.6*

Excellent sources (**bold**); good sources (*italics*).

Note: Plant foods (unless fortified commercially) are devoid of vitamin B_{12}, except for the adventitious inclusion of microbiologically formed B_{12} from water or soil.

Metabolism

Absorption

Absorption occurs almost exclusively in the terminal ileum by an active saturable process, but large amounts (>30 μg) may also be absorbed by passive diffusion (a maximum of 1.5 μg may be absorbed from oral doses of 5–50 μg). For normal absorption, the vitamin must bind to salivary haptocorrin and then to 'intrinsic factor', a highly specific glycoprotein secreted by the parietal cells of the stomach.

Distribution

Vitamin B_{12} is stored mainly in the liver. In the blood, it is bound to specific plasma proteins (transcobalamins).

Elimination

Elimination is via the urinary, biliary and faecal routes. Enterohepatic recycling serves to conserve B_{12}. Vitamin B_{12} appears in breast milk.

Deficiency

Deficiency of vitamin B_{12} leads to macrocytic, megaloblastic anaemia. Symptoms include neurological manifestations (due to demyelination of the spinal cord, brain, and optic and peripheral nerves), and less specific symptoms such as weakness, sore tongue, constipation and postural hypotension. Neuropsychiatric manifestations of deficiency may occur in the absence of anaemia (particularly in the elderly).

Pernicious anaemia is a specific form of anaemia caused by lack of intrinsic factor (not lack of vitamin B_{12} in the diet).

Individuals with a reduced ability to absorb B_{12} develop deficiency within two to three years. Strict vegetarians (at risk of dietary deficiency, but with normal absorptive efficiency) may not show signs and symptoms for 20–30 years.

Possible uses

Vegans

Supplementary vitamin B_{12} may be required by vegans. Vitamin B_{12} is found only in animal products and certain foods fortified with the vitamin (see Table 2). If vegans do not regularly consume a source of vitamin B_{12}, they will require a supplement. This applies particularly to vegan women during pregnancy, as the infant may suffer deficiency. Breast-fed infants whose mothers do not take a source of vitamin B_{12} should be supplemented.

The elderly

Prevalence of vitamin B_{12} deficiency increases with age,[1,2] especially over the age of 65 years, and elderly people should be advised to take a supplement or obtain their requirements from fortified foods (e.g. breakfast cereals, yeast spreads). Poor vitamin B_{12} (and folate) status may be associated with age-related hearing dysfunction[3] and tinnitus.[4]

Supplementation has been used with some success in reversing impaired mental function due to low vitamin B_{12} status. Several studies have shown that the best responders are those with impaired memory of less than six months' duration. In one study in 18 subjects, only those with symptoms of less than 12 months' duration showed improvement with supplementation.[5]

In addition, vitamin B_{12} deficiency appears to be common in patients with Alzheimer's disease,[6,7] and supplements may reverse symptoms of the condition in a few people, but high doses may be needed.

Neural tube defects

One study[8] has suggested that deficiency of vitamin B_{12} may be a risk factor for neural tube defects. This study showed that in affected pregnancies both plasma B_{12} and folate influenced the maternal red cell folate concentration and were independent risk factors for neural defects. More evidence is required before a definite recommendation can be made.

Multiple sclerosis

Vitamin B_{12} has been used to treat multiple sclerosis because it was thought that vitamin B_{12} might have a role in the formation of myelin, the fatty substance which coats nerve cell axons. However, results of early studies in the 1950s and 1960s were inconclusive and interest in vitamin B_{12} as a treatment for multiple sclerosis declined. More recently, case reports have appeared[9,10] describing an association between vitamin vitamin B_{12} and multiple sclerosis, or clinical syndromes resembling multiple sclerosis, and it is possible that vitamin B_{12} deficiency may exacerbate the disease.[11] However, other researchers[12] have concluded that serum B_{12} deficiency is uncommon in multiple sclerosis. Further studies into the metabolism of vitamin B_{12} in multiple sclerosis are warranted.

Sleep disorders

Results from studies investigating vitamin B_{12} for sleep disorders have been equivocal. One study[13] showed that 3 mg vitamin B_{12} was associated with a reduction in daytime melatonin production, improved sleep quality, and improved concentration and feelings of being refreshed the next day. Another study using the same dose of vitamin B_{12} found no change in mood or daytime drowsiness or night sleep compared with placebo.[14]

Miscellaneous

Vitamin B_{12} has been used with some success in patients with diabetic neuropathy[15] and mouth ulcers.[16] Low serum levels of vitamin B_{12} have been found in patients with HIV[17] and have also been associated with a more rapid progress towards AIDS.[18] Because of its role in homocysteine metabolism, vitamin B_{12} has been suggested to play a role in reducing the risk of coronary heart disease. However, there is no evidence that B_{12} has an independent protective effect.

Conclusion
Vitamin B_{12} deficiency is a risk in elderly people and can progress to produce symptoms of dementia. The role of supplements in dementia caused by B_{12} deficiency seems to depend on the duration of the symptoms, and there is no good evidence that supplements help to delay the progress of Alzheimer's disease unrelated to vitamin B_{12} deficiency. There is some evidence that supplementation can improve symptoms of diabetic neuropathy, but the role of vitamin B_{12} in multiple sclerosis is unclear. Further research is needed to confirm the benefits of vitamin B_{12} for any indication other than deficiency or marginal deficiency.

Precautions/contraindications

Vitamin B_{12} should not be given for treatment of deficiency until the diagnosis is fully established (administration of >10 μg daily may produce a haematological response in patients with folate deficiency).

Pregnancy and breast-feeding

Supplementation may sometimes be warranted (see Vegans). No problems reported with normal intakes.

Adverse effects

Vitamin B_{12} may occasionally cause diarrhoea and itching skin. Signs of polycythaemia vera may be unmasked. Megadoses may exacerbate acne.

Interactions

Drugs

Alcohol: excessive intake may reduce absorption of vitamin B_{12}.
Aminoglycosides: may reduce absorption of vitamin B_{12}.
Aminosalicylates: may reduce absorption of vitamin B_{12}.
Antibiotics: may interfere with microbiological assay for serum and erythrocyte vitamin B_{12} (false low results).
Chloramphenicol: may reduce the absorption of vitamin B_{12}.
Colestyramine: may reduce the absorption of vitamin B_{12}.
Colchicine: may reduce the absorption of vitamin B_{12}.
Histamine H_2-receptor antagonists: may reduce the absorption of vitamin B_{12}.
Metformin: may reduce the absorption of vitamin B_{12}.
Methyldopa: may reduce the absorption of vitamin B_{12}.
Nitrous oxide: prolonged nitrous oxide anaesthesia inactivates vitamin B_{12}.
Oral contraceptives: may reduce blood levels of vitamin B_{12}.
Potassium chloride (modified release): prolonged administration may reduce absorption of vitamin B_{12}.
Proton-pump inhibitors: long-term therapy may reduce serum vitamin B_{12} levels.

Nutrients

Folic acid: large doses given continuously may reduce vitamin B_{12} in blood.
Vitamin C: may destroy vitamin B_{12} (avoid large doses of vitamin C within 1 h of oral vitamin B_{12}).

Dose

Vitamin B_{12} is available in the form of tablets and capsules, and is also found in many multivitamin supplements. Deficiency of vitamin B_{12} due to lack of intrinsic factor is generally treated with parenteral cobalamin, but one study showed that 2 mg daily given orally was as efficient as 1 mg given intramuscularly each month.[19]

In cases of deficiency, 2 to 25 μg daily are needed.

References

1 Sabler SP, Lindenbaum J, Allen RH. Vitamin B-12 deficiency in the elderly: Current dilemmas. *Am J Clin Nutr* 1997; 66: 741–749.
2 Baik HW, Russell RM. Vitamin B12 deficiency in the elderly. *Annu Rev Nutr* 1999; 19: 357–377.

3 Houston DK, Johnson MA, Nozza RJ, *et al.* Age-related hearing loss, vitamin B-12, and folate in elderly women. *Am J Clin Nutr* 1999; 69: 564–571.
4 Shemesh Z, Attias J, Ornana M, *et al.* Vitamin B_{12} deficiency in patients with chronic tinnitus and noise induced hearing loss. *Am J Otolaryngol* 1993; 14: 94–99.
5 Martin DC, Francis J, Protetch J, *et al.* Time dependency of cognitive recovery with cobalamin replacement: A report of a pilot study. *J Am Geriatr Soc* 1992; 40: 168–172.
6 Abalan F, Delile JM. B12 deficiency in presenile dementia. *Biol Psychiatr* 1985; 20: 1251.
7 Levitt AJ, Karlinsky H. Folate, vitamin B12 and cognitive impairment in patients with Alzheimer's disease. *Acta Psychiatr Scand* 1992; 86: 301–305.
8 Kirke PM, Molly AM, Daly LE, *et al.* Maternal plasma folate and vitamin B12 are independent risk factors for neural tube defects. *Q J Med* 1993; 86: 703–708.
9 Ransohoff RM, Jacobsen DW, Green R. Vitamin B12 deficiency and multiple sclerosis. *Lancet* 1990; 1: 1285–1286.
10 Reynolds EH, Linnell JC. Vitamin B12 deficiency, demyelination and multiple sclerosis. *Lancet* 1987; 2: 920.
11 Reynolds E. Multiple sclerosis and vitamin B12 metabolism. *J Neuroimmunol* 1992; 40: 225–230.
12 Sandyk R, Awerbuch G. Vitamin B12 and its relationship to age of onset to multiple sclerosis. *Int J Neurosci* 1993; 71: 93–99.
13 Mayer G, Krozer M, Meier-Ewert K. Effects of vitamin B_{12} on performance and circadian rhythm in normal subjects. *Neuropsychopharmacology* 1996; 15: 456–464.
14 Okawa M, Takahashi K, Egashira K, *et al.* Vitamin B_{12} treatment for delayed sleep phase syndrome: A multi-center double-blind study. *Psychiatry Clin Neurosci* 1997; 51: 275–279.
15 Yaqub BA, Siddique A, Sulimani R. Effects of methylcobalamin on diabetic neuropathy. *Clin Neurol Neurosurg* 1992; 94: 105–111.
16 Weusten BL, van de Wile A. Aphthous ulcers and vitamin B12 deficiency. *Neth J Med* 1998; 53: 172–175.
17 Paltiel O, Falutz J, Veilleux M, *et al.* Clinical correlates of subnormal vitamin B_{12} levels in patient infected with human immunodeficiency virus. *Am J Hematol* 1995; 49: 318–322.
18 Tang AM, Graham NM, Chandra RK, *et al.* Low serum vitamin B-12 concentrations are associated with faster human immunodeficiency virus type 1 (HIV-1) disease progression. *J Nutr* 1997; 127: 345–351.
19 Kuzminski AM, Del Giacco EJ, Allen RH, *et al.* Effective treatment of cobalamin deficiency with oral cobalamin. *Blood* 1998; 92: 1191–1198.

Vitamin C

Description

Vitamin C is a water-soluble vitamin.

Nomenclature

Vitamin C is a generic term used to describe the compounds that exhibit the biological activity of ascorbic acid. These include L-ascorbic acid (ascorbic acid) and L-dehydroascorbic acid (dehydroascorbic acid).

Human requirements

See Table 1 for Dietary Reference Values for vitamin C.

Intakes

In the UK, the average adult daily diet provides: for men, 77.9 mg; for women, 81.8 mg.

Action

The functions of vitamin C are based mainly on its properties as a reducing agent. It is required for:

- the formation of collagen and other organic constituents of the intercellular matrix in bone, teeth and capillaries; and
- the optimal activity of several enzymes – it activates certain liver-detoxifying enzyme systems (including drug-metabolising enzymes) and is involved in the synthesis of carnitine and norepinephrine (noradrenaline) and in the metabolism of folic acid, histamine, phenylalanine, tryptophan and tyrosine.

Vitamin C also acts:

- as an antioxidant (reacting directly with aqueous free radicals) – this is important in the protection of cellular function; and
- to enhance the intestinal absorption of non-haem iron.

Dietary sources

See Table 2 for dietary sources of vitamin C.

Metabolism

Absorption

Vitamin C is absorbed by passive and active transport mechanisms, predominantly in the distal portion of the small intestine (jejunum) and to a lesser extent in the mouth, stomach and proximal intestine. Some 70–90% of the dietary intake is absorbed, but absorption falls to 50% with a dose of 1.5 g.

Distribution

It is transported in the free form (higher concentrations in leukocytes and platelets than red blood cells and plasma), and is readily taken up by body tissues (highest concentration in glandular tissue, e.g. adrenals and pituitary); body stores are generally about 1.5 g.

Elimination

The urine is the main route of elimination, but very little is excreted unchanged (unless plasma concentration >1.4 mg/100 ml). Vitamin C crosses the placenta and is excreted in breast milk.

Table 1 Dietary Reference Values for vitamin C (mg/day)

EU RDA (for labelling purposes) = 60 mg

Age	UK			USA				WHO	Europe
	LRNI	EAR	RNI	EAR	RDA	AI	UL	RNI	PRI
0–6 months	6	15	25	–	–	40	–	–	–
7–12 months	6	15	25	–	–	50	–	20	20
1–3 years	8	20	30	13	–	–	400	20	25
4–6 years	8	20	30	–	–	–	–	20	25
4–8 years	–	–	–	22	25	–	650	–	–
7–10 years	8	20	30	–	–	–	–	20	30
9–13 years	–	–	–	39	45	–	1200	–	–
Males									
11–14 years	9	22	35	–	–	–	–	30	35
14–18 years	–	–	–	63	75	–	1800	–	–
15–50+ years	10	25	40	–	–	–	–	30	45
19–70+ years	–	–	–	75	90	–	2000	–	–
Females									
11–14 years	9	22	35	–	–	–	–	30	35
14–18 years	–	–	–	56	65	–	1800	–	–
15–50+ years	10	25	40	–	–	–	–	35	40
19–70+ years	–	–	–	60	75	–	2000	–	–
Pregnancy	–	–	+10	66[1]/70[2]	80[1]/85[2]	–	1800[1]/2000[2]	50	55
Lactation	–	–	+30	96[1]/100[2]	115[1]/120[2]	–	1800[1]/2000[2]	50	70

[1]Up to the age of 18 years.

[2]Age 19–50 years.

UL = Tolerable Upper Intake Level from diet and supplements.

Bioavailability

Storage and cooking lead to loss of vitamin C through oxidation, and boiling results in leaching of the vitamin into the cooking water (cooking water should be consumed in gravies and soups). Microwaving and stir-frying are the best cooking methods for preserving vitamin C.

Deficiency

Vitamin C deficiency may lead to scurvy. Subclinical deficiency has been associated with poor wound healing and ulceration. Early signs of deficiency may be non-specific and include general weakness, lethargy, fatigue, shortness of breath and aching of the limbs. As the disease progresses, petechiae are often prominent and may appear over the arms after application of a sphygmomanometer.

Signs of advanced deficiency include perifollicular haemorrhages (particularly about the hair follicles); swollen, bleeding gums; pallor and anaemia (the result of prolonged bleeding or associated folic acid deficiency); joints, muscles and subcutaneous tissue may become sites of haemorrhage. In children, disturbances of growth occur and bones, teeth and blood vessels develop abnormally; gum signs are only found in the presence of erupted teeth.

Groups at risk of low vitamin C status include smokers, the elderly, patients in hospitals and other institutions, and patients with diabetes.

Table 2 Dietary sources of vitamin C

Food portion	Vitamin C (mg)	Food portion	Vitamin C (mg)
Bread and cereals[1]	0	*Blackberries, stewed (100 g)*	*10*
Milk and dairy products	0	**Blackcurrants, stewed (100 g)**	**115**
Meat and fish[2]	0	*12 cherries*	*10*
		Fruit salad	
Vegetables		canned (130 g)	4
Broccoli, boiled (100 g)	**44**	**fresh (130 g)**	**20**
Brussels sprouts, boiled (100 g)	**60**	**½ a grapefruit**	**54**
Cabbage, raw (100 g)	**49**	Grapes (100 g)	3
Cabbage, boiled (100 g)	**20**	**Guava (100 g)**	**230**
Carrots, boiled (100 g)	2	**1 kiwi fruit**	**60**
Cauliflower, boiled (100 g)	**43**	**Lychees (100 g)**	**45**
Courgette, stir-fried (100 g)	*15*	**1 mango**	**50**
Cucumber, raw (30 g)	2	**½ melon, cantaloupe**	**60**
Kale, boiled (100 g)	**71**	*1 slice melon, honeydew*	*18*
Lettuce (30 g)	2	**1 slice watermelon**	**20**
Mange-tout peas, boiled (50 g)	*14*	**1 orange**	**90**
stir-fried (50 g)	**26**	**4 passion fruits**	**20**
Peas, boiled (100 g)	*16*	**1 slice paw-paw**	**90**
Peppers, green, raw (50 g)	**120**	**1 peach**	**30**
Peppers, red, raw (50 g)	**140**	*1 pear*	*9*
Potatoes		*1 slice pineapple*	*15*
chips (250 g)	**27**	3 plums	6
new, boiled (150 g)	*15*	**Raspberries (100 g)**	**32**
old, boiled (150 g)	*9*	**Strawberries (100 g)**	**77**
sweet, boiled (150 g)	**23**	**1 tangerine**	**22**
Spinach, boiled (100 g)	*8*		
2 tomatoes, raw 150 g	**25**	**Beverages**	
Watercress (20 g)	*12*	**1 large glass apple juice**	**28**
		1 large glass grapefruit juice	**60**
Fruit		**1 large glass orange juice**	**80**
1 apple	*15*	*1 large glass tomato juice*	*16*
1 banana	*16*	**1 large glass Ribena (diluted)**	**120**

[1]A few breakfast cereals have added vitamin C (average 10 mg/portion).

[2]Liver contains approximately 15 mg/100 g.

Excellent sources (**bold**); good sources (*italics*).

Possible uses

Many health claims have been made for megadose intakes of vitamin C (i.e. 250–10 000 mg per day), including the prevention and treatment of colds, infections, stress, cancer, hypercholesterolaemia and atherosclerosis. Few of these claims have been tested in controlled clinical intervention trials.

Colds

Since Linus Pauling's claims about the beneficial effects of vitamin C in the prevention of colds and reducing their symptoms, many studies have investigated the effects of vitamin C on the common cold. A summary of 27 trials conducted between 1970 and 1986[1] concluded that vitamin C did not prevent colds, but could have a small therapeutic effect. Of these 27 trials, five were intervention trials of vitamin C or placebo given at the start of cold symptoms and for a few days, all of which found no benefit. The other 22 were double-blind controlled trials giving daily vitamin C or placebo before and during colds. Of these trials, 12 showed no preventive effect and no reduction in duration or severity of symptoms, five showed no prevention and only slight non-significant lessening of severity, and the other five reported no prevention and a small but significant reduction in the duration of colds.

A more recent review of several studies indicated that vitamin C alleviates common cold symptoms,[2] although the magnitude of benefit appears to vary depending on the population group studied and the dose. A review of 30 trials by the Cochrane Collaboration[3] concluded that long-term daily supplementation with large doses of vitamin C does not appear to prevent colds, but there appears to be a modest benefit in terms of reducing duration of cold symptoms from ingestion of high doses. The review also concluded that the relation of dose to therapeutic benefit needs further exploration.

Cancer

It has been suggested that vitamin C may be useful in the prevention of cancer.[4] Possible mechanisms for this protective effect may be that vitamin C acts as an antioxidant, blocks formation of nitrosamines and faecal mutagens, enhances immune system response and accelerates detoxifying liver enzymes.

Many epidemiological studies have shown an inverse correlation between vitamin C intake and cancer incidence, but the evidence is largely indirect since it is based on the consumption of fruits and vegetables known to contain vitamin C and other nutrients such as betacarotene and folate. The strongest evidence for a protective effect seems to be for stomach cancer.[5–8] The evidence for oesophageal cancer is not as strong. Findings are contradictory for cancers of the lung, breast, colon and rectum.

There is some evidence that vitamin C supplements may help to prevent stomach cancer,[7] reduce pre-cancerous changes in colon cancer[9] and help to manage prostate cancer.[10] However, subjects with advanced colorectal cancer responded no better than placebo to vitamin C supplementation.[11] Vitamin C may also benefit cancer patients who are undergoing radiation treatment by enabling them to withstand larger doses of radiation, with fewer side-effects.[12]

Coronary heart disease

Epidemiological studies have shown associations between low vitamin C intakes and cardiovascular disease risk.[13] However, two other epidemiological studies of about 87 000 female nurses and 4000 male health professionals found no effect of vitamin C intakes from diets or supplements on cardiovascular risk.[14,15]

An association between vitamin C and atherosclerosis has been suggested in studies investigating the relationship between vitamin C and cholesterol. When 1 g of vitamin C was given to healthy young people, cholesterol levels tended to fall[16] but in older people no significant pattern of serum cholesterol change was found. Leukocyte levels were found to be lower in patients with coronary heart disease (CHD) than those in patients without CHD.[17] Vitamin C may also have beneficial effects on blood pressure[18] and on stroke.[19]

Cataracts

Patients with cataracts have been found to have lower levels of vitamin C in the lens than patients with no cataracts[20] and as cataracts develop, the vitamin C content of the lens declines.[21] In a retrospective study, a lower incidence of cataract was found in subjects whose ascorbic acid intake was in the highest quintile compared with those in the lowest quintile.[22] There is some evidence that long-term supplementation of vitamin C (>10 years) may reduce the development of age-related opacities.[23,24]

Wound healing

Reductions in blood ascorbic acid levels have been reported in postoperative patients.[25,26] Some researchers suggest that this reduction represents increased need, while others suggest that ascorbic acid is redistributed to the tissues. Tissue ascorbic acid concentration at the site of a wound has been found to increase.[27] Studies have shown accelerated wound healing with vitamin C supplements.[27,28]

Periodontal disease

There is evidence that vitamin C status is related to periodontal disease. Vitamin C depletion in humans has been associated with significantly increased gum bleeding even though no clinical symptoms of scurvy were observed in any subject.[29] The degree of gingival inflammation was directly related to ascorbic acid status, and a reduction in bleeding was observed with vitamin C supplementation.

Smoking

Vitamin C requirements are higher in smokers than non-smokers,[30] and supplemental vitamin C may help to restore plasma vitamin C concentration in smokers. Vitamin C supplements may also protect against smoking-related damage, such as build-up of atherosclerotic plaque.[31]

Conclusion

Various groups of the population are at risk of vitamin C deficiency, particularly the elderly and smokers. Vitamin C may reduce the duration of the common cold and also the severity of symptoms such as sneezing and coughing, particularly if it is taken immediately the symptoms start. Preventive effects of vitamin C supplementation appear to be limited mainly to people with low dietary intake, while therapeutic effects may occur in wider population groups. Epidemiological studies have shown a link between low blood vitamin C concentrations and cardiovascular disease, cancer and cataracts. However, further controlled clinical trials are needed to confirm the value of vitamin C supplements for these conditions.

Precautions/contraindications

Vitamin C supplements should be used with caution in: diabetes mellitus (interference with glucose determinations); glucose-6-phosphate dehydrogenase (G6PD) deficiency (risk of haemolytic anaemia); haemochromatosis; renal failure (risk of oxalate stones); sickle cell anaemia (risk of precipitating a crisis); sideroblastic anaemia; thalassaemia. Prolonged administration of large doses (>1 g daily) of vitamin C in pregnancy may result in increased requirements and scurvy in the neonate.

Because ascorbic acid is a strong reducing agent it interferes with all diagnostic tests based on oxidation–reduction reactions. Vitamin C administration (megadoses only: >1 g daily) may interfere with tests for:

- blood glucose (false negative); and
- urinary glucose (false positive with analyses using cupric sulphate, e.g. Clinitest; false negative with analyses using glucose oxidase, e.g. Clinistix).

Adverse effects

Vitamin C is considered to be one of the safest of all the vitamins. There appear to be no serious health risks with doses up to 10 g daily, but doses of >1 g daily are associated with osmotic diarrhoea (due to large amounts of unabsorbed ascorbic acid in the intestine), gastric discomfort and mild increase in urination.

Oxalic acid is a major metabolite of vitamin C, and there has been concern about an increased risk of renal oxalate stones with high doses. However, oxalate formation is saturable and there is unlikely to be a risk in healthy people; doses of vitamin C in renal failure should not exceed 100–200 mg daily.

There have been occasional reports that vitamin C destroys vitamin B_{12} in the tissues and of rebound scurvy after administration of vitamin C is stopped, but these remain unsubstantiated.

Prolonged use of chewable vitamin C products may cause dental erosion and increased incidence of caries.

Interactions

Drugs

Vitamin C is important for the optimal activity of some of the drug-metabolising enzymes, including the hepatic cytochrome P450 mixed-function oxidase system. Large doses (>1 g daily) of ascorbic acid (but not ascorbates) may

lower urinary pH, leading to increased renal tubular reabsorption of acidic drugs and increased excretion of alkaline drugs.
Aspirin: prolonged administration may reduce blood levels of ascorbic acid.
Anticoagulants: occasional reports that vitamin C reduces the activity of warfarin.
Anticonvulsants: administration of barbiturates or primidone may increase urinary excretion of ascorbic acid.
Desferrioxamine: iron excretion induced by desferrioxamine is enhanced by administration of vitamin C.
Disulfiram: prolonged administration of large doses (>1 g daily) of vitamin C may interfere with the alcohol-disulfiram reaction.
Mexiletine: large doses (>1 g daily) of ascorbic acid may accelerate excretion of mexiletine.
Oral contraceptives (containing oestrogens): may reduce blood levels of ascorbic acid; large doses (>1 g) of vitamin C may increase plasma oestrogen levels (possibly converting low-dose oral contraceptive to high-dose oral contraceptive); possibly breakthrough bleeding associated with withdrawal of high-dose vitamin C.
Tetracyclines: prolonged administration may reduce blood levels of ascorbic acid.

Nutrients

Copper: high doses of vitamin C (>1 g daily) may reduce copper retention.
Iron: vitamin C increases absorption of non-haem iron, but not haem iron. For maximal iron absorption from a non-meat meal, a source of vitamin C providing 50–100 mg should be ingested. Vitamin C supplements appear to have no deleterious effect on iron status in patients with iron overload. Iron administration reduces blood levels of ascorbic acid (ascorbic acid is oxidised).
Vitamin A: vitamin C may reduce the toxic effects of vitamin A.
Vitamin B_6: deficiency of vitamin C may increase urinary excretion of pyridoxine.
Vitamin B_{12}: excess vitamin C has been claimed to destroy vitamin B_{12}, but this does not appear to occur under physiological conditions.
Vitamin E: vitamin C can spare vitamin E, and vice-versa.

Heavy metals

Vitamin C may reduce tissue and plasma levels of cadmium, lead, mercury, nickel and vanadium.

Dose

Vitamin C is available in the form of tablets, chewable tablets, capsules and powders. It is found in most multivitamin preparations. A review of 26 US vitamin C products found that three failed to pass the tests for labelled content of vitamin C, and one product failed on disintegration.[32]

Dietary supplements contain between 25 and 1500 mg per daily dose.

References

1 Truswell AS. Ascorbic acid (letter). *N Engl J Med* 1986; 315: 709.
2 Hemila H. Vitamin C supplementation and common cold symptoms: Factors affecting the magnitude of benefit. *Med Hypotheses* 1999; 52: 171–178.
3 Douglas RM, Chalker EB, Treacy B. Vitamin C for preventing and treating the common cold (Cochrane Review). In: The Cochrane Library, Issue 2, 2000. Oxford Update Software. Available in The Cochrane Library (ISSN 1464-780X).
4 Blocke G, Menkes M. Ascorbic acid in cancer prevention. In: Moon TE, Micozzi MS, eds. *Nutrition and Cancer Prevention. Investigating the Role of Micronutrients*. New York: Marcel Dekker, 1989: 341–348.
5 Bjelke E. Dietary factors and the epidemiology of cancer of the stomach and the large bowel. *Klin Prax Suppl* 1978; 2: 10–17.
6 Correa P, Malcom E, Schmidt B, *et al*. Antioxidant micronutrients and gastric cancer. *Aliment Pharmacol Ther* 1998; 12 (suppl. 1): 73–82.
7 Risch HA, Jain M, Choi NW, *et al*. Dietary factors and the incidence of cancer of the stomach. *Am J Epidemiol* 1985; 122: 947–949.
8 You WC, Blot WJ, Chang YS, *et al*. Diet and high risk of stomach cancer in Shandong, China. *Cancer Res* 1988; 48: 3518–3523.
9 Waring AJ, Drake IM, Schorah CJ, *et al*. Ascorbic acid and total vitamin C concentrations in plasma, gastric juice and gastrointestinal mucosa: Effects of gastritis and oral supplementation. *Gut* 1996; 38: 171–176.
10 Paganelli GM, Biasco G, Brandi G, *et al*. Effect of vitamin A, C, and E supplementation on rectal cell

proliferation in patients with colorectal adenomas. *J Natl Cancer Inst* 1992; 84: 47–51.

11 Moertal CG, Fleming TR, Geegen ET. High dose vitamin C versus placebo in the treatment of patients with advanced cancer who have had no prior chemotherapy: A randomised double-blind comparison. *N Engl J Med* 1985; 312: 137–141.

12 Okunieff P. Interactions between ascorbic acid and the radiation of bone marrow, skin and tumour. *Am J Clin Nutr* 1991; 54: 1281S–1283S.

13 Gaby SK, Singh VN. Vitamin C. In: Gaby SK, Bendich A, Sing VN, Machlin LJ, eds. *Vitamin Intake and Health: A Scientific Review*. New York: Marcel Dekker, 1991: 103–161.

14 Rimm EB, Stampfer MJ, Ascherio A, *et al.* Vitamin E consumption and the risk of coronary heart disease in men. *N Engl J Med* 1993; 328: 1450–1456.

15 Stampfer MJ, Hennekens CH, Manson JE, *et al.* Vitamin E consumption and the risk of coronary heart disease in women. *N Engl J Med* 1993; 328: 1444–1449.

16 Spittle CR. Atherosclerosis and vitamin C. *Lancet*, 1972; 1: 798.

17 Ramirez J, Flowers NC. Leucocyte ascorbic acid and its relationship to coronary artery disease in man. *Am J Clin Nutr* 1980; 33: 2079–2087.

18 Ness AR, Chee D, Elliot P, *et al.* Vitamin C and blood pressure – an overview. *J Hum Hypertens* 1997; 11: 343–350.

19 Gale CR, Martyn CN, Winter PD, *et al.* Vitamin C and risk of death from stroke and coronary heart disease in cohorts of elderly people. *Br Med J* 1995; 310: 1563–1566.

20 Chandra DB, Varma R, Ahmad S, Varma SD. Vitamin C in the human aqueous humour and cataracts. *Int J Vit Nutr Res* 1986; 56: 165–168.

21 Lohmann W. Ascorbic acid and cataract. *Ann NY Acad Sci* 1987; 498: 307–311.

22 Jaques PF, Phillips J, Chylack LT, *et al.* Vitamin intake and senile cataract. *J Am Coll Nutr* 1987; 6: 435.

23 Chasan-Taber L, Willett WC, Seddon JM, *et al.* A prospective study of vitamin supplement intake and cataract extraction among US women. *Epidemiology* 1999; 10: 679–684.

24 Jaques PF, Taylor A, Hankinson SE, *et al.* Long-term vitamin C supplement use and prevalence of early age-related lens opacities. *Am J Clin Nutr* 1997; 66: 911–916.

25 Irvin TT, Chattopadhyay DK, Smythe A. Ascorbic acid requirements in postoperative patients. *Surg Gynaecol Obstet* 1978; 147: 49–55.

26 Shukla SP. Plasma and urinary ascorbic acid levels in the post-operative period. *Experientia* 1969; 25: 704.

27 Crandon JH, Lennihan R Jr, Mikal S, Reif AE. Ascorbic acid economy in surgical patients. *Ann NY Acad Sci* 1961; 92: 246–267.

28 Ringsdorf WM, Jr, Cheraskin E. Vitamin C and human wound healing. *Oral Surg* 1982; 53: 231–236.

29 Leggott PJ, Robertson PB, Rothman DL, *et al.* The effect of controlled ascorbic acid depletion and supplementation on periodontal health. *J Periodontol* 1986; 57: 480–485.

30 Lykkesfeldt J, Christen S, Wallock LM, *et al.* Ascorbate is depleted by smoking and repleted by moderate supplementation: A study in male smokers and nonsmokers with matched dietary antioxidant intakes. *Am J Clin Nutr* 2000; 71: 530–536.

31 Weber C, Erl W, Weber K, Weber PC. Increased adhesiveness of isolated monocytes to endothelium is prevented by vitamin C intake in smokers. *Circulation* 1996; 93: 1488–1492.

32 Consumerlab. Product review. Vitamin C. http://www.consumerlab.com (accessed 7 December 2000).

Vitamin D

Description

Vitamin D is a fat-soluble vitamin.

Nomenclature

Vitamin D is a generic term used to describe all sterols that exhibit the biological activity of cholecalciferol. These include:

- vitamin D_1 (calciferol)
- vitamin D_2 (ergocalciferol)
- vitamin D_3 (cholecalciferol)
- 1 $(OH)D_3$
  (1 Hydroxycholecalciferol; alfacalcidol)
- $25(OH)D_3$
  (25 Hydroxycholecalciferol; calcifediol)
- $1,25(OH)_2D_3$
  (1,25, Dihydroxycholecalciferol; calcitriol)
- $24,25(OH)_2D_3$
  (24,25, Dihydroxycholecalciferol)
- dihydrotachysterol.

Vitamin D_2 is the form most commonly added to foods and dietary supplements.

Units

One International Unit of vitamin D is defined as the activity of 0.025 µg of cholecalciferol.
Thus: 1 µg vitamin D = 40 units vitamin D
and: 1 unit vitamin D = 0.025 µg vitamin D.

Human requirements

See Table 1 for Dietary Reference Values for vitamin D.

Intakes

In the UK, the average adult diet provides 2.96 µg daily.

Cutaneous synthesis

Exposure of the skin to ultraviolet (UV) rays results in the synthesis of cholecalciferol (vitamin D_3); this is the major source of vitamin D. The amount obtained depends on length of exposure, area of skin exposed, wavelength of UV light, pollution, skin pigmentation (higher melanin concentration requires longer exposure to achieve same degree of synthesis) and age (the elderly may have approximately half the capacity for synthesis of younger people).

Brief, casual exposure of face, arms and hands to sunlight is thought to be equivalent to the ingestion of 5 µg (200 units) of vitamin D.[1] The use of sunscreens may affect vitamin D production; application of a sunscreen with a sun protection factor of 8 can completely prevent the cutaneous production of cholecalciferol. However, this should not discourage the use of sunscreens.

Action

Vitamin D is essential for promoting the absorption and utilisation of calcium and phosphorus, and normal calcification of the skeleton. Along with parathyroid hormone and calcitonin, it regulates serum calcium concentration by altering serum calcium and phosphate blood levels as needed, and mobilising calcium from bone. It maintains neuromuscular function and various other cellular processes, including the immune system.

Table 1 Dietary Reference values for vitamin D (μg/day)

EU RDA = 5 μg

Age	UK RNI	USA		WHO RNI	Europe PRI
		AI[2]	UL[3]		
Males and females					
0–6 months	8.5	5	–	10	10–25
7 months–3 years	7.0	5	–	10	10
4–6 years	0[1]	5	–	10	0–10
7–10 years	0[1]	5	–	2.5	0–10
11–24 years	0[1]	5	–	2.5	0–15
25–50+ years	0[1]	–	–	2.5	0–10
65+ years	10	–	–	2.5	10
51–70+ years	–	10	50	–	–
>70 years	–	15	50	–	–
Pregnancy and lactation	10	5	–	10	10

[1]If skin is exposed to adequate sunlight.
[2]Adequate Intake (1997).
[3]Tolerable Upper Intake Level.

Dietary sources

See Table 2 for dietary sources of vitamin D.

Metabolism

Absorption (dietary source)

Vitamin D is absorbed with the aid of bile salts from the small intestine via the lymphatic system and its associated chylomicrons. The efficiency of absorption is estimated to be about 50%.

Distribution

Vitamin D is converted by hydroxylation (predominantly in the liver) to $25(OH)D_3$; this is the major circulating form of vitamin D. From the liver, $25(OH)D_3$ is transported to the kidney and converted by further hydroxylation to $1,25(OH)_2D_3$, the metabolically active form.

Synthesis is regulated mainly by circulating levels of the metabolite $1,25(OH)_2D_3$. When levels of this metabolite are high, synthesis is low and vice-versa. Synthesis is also stimulated by hypocalcaemia, hypophosphataemia and parathyroid hormone (PTH) and inhibited by hypercalcaemia. A second metabolite of vitamin D is produced in the kidney, $24,25(OH)_2D_3$. Both $1,25(OH)_2D_3$ and $24,25(OH)_2D_3$ may be required for the biological activity of vitamin D.

Vitamin D is transported in the plasma bound to a specific vitamin D-binding protein and is stored mainly in the liver, adipose tissue and muscle. Some vitamin D derivatives are excreted in breast milk.

Deficiency

Deficiency of vitamin D results in: inadequate intestinal absorption of calcium and phosphate; hypocalcaemia, hypophosphataemia and increase in serum alkaline phosphatase activity; hyperparathyroidism. Demineralisation of bone leads to rickets in children and osteomalacia in adults. Infants may develop convulsions and tetany.

Possible uses

Requirements may be increased and/or supplements necessary in:

Table 2 Dietary sources of vitamin D

Food portion	Vitamin D content (μg)
Breakfast cereals	
1 bowl All-Bran (45 g)	0.8
1 bowl Bran Flakes (45 g)	1.0
1 bowl Corn Flakes (25 g)	0.5
1 bowl Frosties (45 g)	1.0
1 bowl Rice Krispies (35 g)	0.7
1 bowl Special K (35 g)	0.9
Muesli, porridge, Shredded Wheat, Sugar Puffs, Weetabix	0
Bread	0
Milk and dairy products	
½ pint (280 ml) whole milk	0.1
½ pint (280 ml) semi-skimmed milk	0.03
½ pint (280 ml) skimmed milk	0
½ pint (280 ml) skimmed milk, fortified	0.2–0.5 (various brands)
2 tablespoons dried skimmed milk, fortified (30 g)	1.0
Hard cheese (50 g)	0.1
Feta cheese (50 g)	0.25
1 carton whole-milk yoghurt (150 g)	0.06
1 carton low-fat yoghurt (150 g)	0.01
1 egg, size 2 (60 g)	1.0
Fats and oils	
Butter on 1 slice bread (10 g)	0.25
Margarine on 1 slice bread (10 g)	*2.5*
Low-fat spread on 1 slice bread (10 g)	*2.5*
2 tablespoons ghee (30 g)	0.6
2 teaspoons cod liver oil (10 ml)	**21.0**
Meat and fish	
Liver, lamb's, cooked (90 g)	0.5
Liver, calf, cooked (90 g)	0.3
Liver, ox, cooked (90 g)	1.0
Liver, pig, cooked (90 g)	1.0
White fish	Trace
Sardines (70 g)	**5.6**
Tinned salmon (100 g)	**12.5**
Tinned pilchards (100 g)	**8.0**
Tinned tuna (100 g)	**5.0**
2 fillets herring, cooked (110 g)	**20.0**
2 fillets kipper, cooked (130 g)	**20.0**
2 fillets mackerel, cooked (110 g)	**21.0**
Beverages	
1 mug Ovaltine[1] (300 ml)	0.7
1 mug Horlicks[1] (300 ml)	0.7
1 mug Build-Up[1] (300 ml)	*3.0*
1 mug Complan[2] (300 ml)	*1.5*

[1]Made with milk (whole or skimmed).
[2]Made with water.
Excellent sources (>5 μg/portion) (**bold**); good sources (>1.5 μg/portion) (*italics*).

- infants who are breast-fed without supplemental vitamin D or who have minimal exposure to sunlight;
- pregnancy;
- breast-feeding (particularly with babies born in the autumn);
- the elderly, whose exposure to sunlight may be reduced because of poor mobility;
- individuals with dark skins;
- strict vegetarians; and
- those who do not get much exposure to sunlight.

The Department of Health[2] advises that all children from the age of 1–5 years should receive supplements of vitamins A and D.

Vitamin D has been investigated for a potential role in osteoporosis, cancer and hypertension.

Osteoporosis

Vitamin D (independently of calcium) may be useful in the prevention of osteoporosis. Some research has shown that women with hip fractures have lower levels of plasma vitamin D.[3] People with a certain type of vitamin D receptor may be more susceptible to osteoporosis, and women with different types of vitamin D receptor seem to respond differently to vitamin D supplements.[4]

There is some evidence that vitamin D supplementation helps to reduce bone loss[5-7] and fracture risk[8,9] and, in combination with calcium,[10] may enhance the effect of hormone replacement therapy. However, other studies have not shown any reduction in rates of fracture with vitamin D supplementation. A Dutch study involving 2500 healthy men and women over the age of 70 years, showed that a daily dose of 400 units daily of vitamin D had no effect on fracture rates.[11] Differences in effects may be due to differences in the types of vitamin D compounds used. With regard to postmenopausal osteoporosis, there is evidence that vitamin D analogues – rather than plain vitamin D – may have bone-sparing actions. This may be because the type of vitamin D deficiency is a reflection of $1,25(OH)_2D_3$ deficiency or resistance, and plain vitamin D will have no effect. Thus, a vitamin D analogue (e.g. calcitriol) could reduce bone loss as a result of a pharmacological action rather than replenishing a deficiency.

Cancer

There is suggestive evidence that low levels of vitamin D are linked to various cancers, including those of the colon, prostate and breast. Prospective data from a 19-year dietary survey[12] showed that risk of mortality from colorectal cancer was inversely correlated with both vitamin D and calcium consumption. In another prospective study,[13] serum concentrations of 20 mg/ml or more were associated with one-third of the risk of developing colon cancer that was associated with lower levels of 25-hydroxy vitamin D. More recent studies have also demonstrated a link between low intakes of vitamin D and colon cancer,[14,15] and breast cancer[16] and low plasma vitamin D levels with prostate cancer.[17]

Hypertension

Vitamin D, presumably via a mechanism affecting calcium metabolism, appears to play some role in regulating blood pressure. Vitamin D analogues have been found to reduce blood pressure in intervention trials.[18–20] It remains to be seen whether a beneficial effect on blood pressure can be derived from an increase in dietary or supplemental vitamin D.

Miscellaneous

There is some evidence that low plasma levels of vitamin D are linked to osteoarthritis[21] and rheumatoid arthritis[22] and risk of diabetes.[23] Whether supplements of vitamin D have any benefit in preventing these conditions is unknown.

> **Conclusion**
> Vitamin D is important for bone health, and some research has shown that supplementation with vitamin D may reduce the risk of osteoporosis and fracture. It is unclear whether most benefit is achieved from vitamin D alone or from vitamin D with calcium, and what the appropriate doses are. Epidemiological studies have found a link between colon cancer and low vitamin D, but whether supplements can reduce the risk of cancer is unknown.

Precautions/contraindications

Vitamin D should be avoided in: hypercalcaemia; renal osteodystrophy with hyperphosphataemia (risk of metastatic calcification).

Vegetarians

Supplements containing vitamin D_3 (cholecalciferol) are obtained from animal sources (usually as a by-product of wool fat) and are not suitable for strict vegetarians (vegans). Vitamin D_2 (ergocalciferol) is obtained from plant sources and can be recommended.

Pregnancy and breast-feeding

No problems reported with normal intakes. There is a risk of hypercalcaemic tetany in breast-fed infants whose mothers take excessive doses of vitamin D.

Adverse effects

Vitamin D is the most likely of all the vitamins to cause toxicity; the margin of safety is very narrow. There is a wide variation in tolerance to vitamin D, but doses of 250 µg (50 000 units) daily for six months may result in toxicity. Infants and children are generally more susceptible than adults; prolonged administration of 45 µg (1800 units) daily may arrest growth in children. Some infants seem to be hyper-reactive to small doses. There is no risk of vitamin D toxicity from prolonged exposure to sunlight.

Excessive intake leads to hypercalcaemia and its associated effects. These include: apathy, anorexia, constipation, diarrhoea, dry mouth, fatigue, headache, nausea and vomiting, thirst and weakness.

Later symptoms are often associated with calcification of soft tissues and include: bone pain, cardiac arrhythmias, hypertension, renal damage (increased urinary frequency, decreased urinary concentrating ability; nocturia, proteinuria), psychosis (rare) and weight loss.

Interactions

Drugs

Anticonvulsants (phenytoin, barbiturates or primidone): may reduce effect of vitamin D by accelerating its metabolism; patients on long-term anticonvulsant therapy may require vitamin D supplementation to prevent osteomalacia.
Calcitonin: effect of calcitonin may be antagonised by vitamin D.
Colestyramine, colestipol: may reduce intestinal absorption of vitamin D.
Digoxin: caution because hypercalcaemia caused by vitamin D may potentiate effects of digoxin, resulting in cardiac arrhythmias.
Liquid paraffin: may reduce intestinal absorption of vitamin D (avoid long-term administration of liquid paraffin).
Sucralfate: may reduce intestinal absorption of vitamin D.
Thiazide diuretics: may increase risk of hypercalcaemia.
Vitamin D analogues (alfacalcidol, calcitriol, dihydrotachysterol): increased risk of toxicity with vitamin D supplements.

Nutrients

Calcium: may increase risk of hypercalcaemia.

Dose

Vitamin D is available in the form of tablets and capsules, as well as in multivitamin preparations and fish oils.

A suitable dose of vitamin D in most cases is 10 µg daily.

References

1 Haddad J. Vitamin D – solar rays, the milky way, or both? *N Engl J Med* 1992; 326: 1213–1215.
2 Department of Health. Weaning and the weaning diet: Report of the Working Group on the Weaning Diet of the Committee on Medical Aspects of Food Policy. Report on Health and Social Subjects No 45. London: Her Majesty's Stationery Office, 1994.
3 LeBoff MS, Kohlmeier L, Hurwitz S, *et al.* Occult vitamin D deficiency in postmenopausal US women with acute hip fracture. *JAMA* 1999; 281: 1505–1511.
4 Graafmans WC, Lips P, Ooms ME, *et al.* The effect of vitamin D supplementation on the bone mineral density of the femoral neck is associated with vitamin D receptor genotype. *J Bone Miner Res* 1997; 12: 1241–1245.
5 Dawson-Hughes B, Dallal GE, Kraal EA, *et al.* Effect of vitamin D supplementation on wintertime and overall bone loss in healthy postmenopausal women. *Ann Intern Med* 1991; 115: 505–512.
6 Ooms ME, Roos JC, Bezemer PD, *et al.* Prevention of bone loss by vitamin D supplementation in elderly women: A randomised double-blind trial. *J Clin Endocrinol Metab* 1995; 80: 1052–1058.
7 Dawson-Hughes B, Harris SS, Kraal EA, *et al.* Rates of bone loss in postmenopausal women randomly assigned to one of two dosages of vitamin D. *Am J Clin Nutr* 1995; 61: 1140–1145.
8 Chapuy MC, Arlot ME, Duboeuf F, *et al.* Vitamin D and calcium to prevent hip fractures in elderly women. *N Engl J Med* 1992; 327: 1637–1642.
9 Dawson-Hughes B, Harris SS, Krall EA, Dallal GE. Effect of calcium and vitamin D supplementation on bone density in men and women 65 years of age or older. *N Engl J Med* 1997; 337: 670–676.
10 Recker RR, Davies KM, Dowd RM, Heaney RP. The effect of low-dose continuous estrogen and progesterone therapy with calcium and vitamin D on bone in elderly women: A randomized, controlled trial. *Ann Intern Med* 1999; 130: 897–904.
11 Lips P, Graafmans WC, Ooms ME, *et al.* Vitamin D supplementation and fracture incidence in elderly

persons: A randomized, placebo-controlled clinical trial. *Ann Intern Med* 1996; 124: 400–406.

12 Garland C, Barrett-Connor E, Rossoff AH, *et al.* Dietary vitamin D and calcium and risk of colorectal cancer: A 19-year prospective study in men. *Lancet* 1985; 1: 307–309.

13 Garland CF, Garland FC, Shaw EK, *et al.* Serum 25-hydroxyvitamin D and colon cancer: Eight-year prospective study. *Lancet* 1989; i: 176–178.

14 Pritchard RS, Baron JA, Gerhardsson de Verdier M. Dietary calcium, vitamin D and the risk of colorectal cancer in Stockholm, Sweden. *Cancer Epidemiol Biomarkers Prev* 1996; 5: 897–900.

15 Martinez ME, Giovannucci EL, Colditz GA, *et al.* Calcium, vitamin D and the occurrence of colorectal cancer among women. *J Natl Cancer Inst* 1996; 88: 1375–1382.

16 Janowsky EC, Lester GE, Weinberg CR, *et al.* Association between low levels of 1,25-dihydroxyvitamin D and breast cancer risk. *Public Health Nutrition* 1999; 2: 283–291.

17 Gann PH, Ma J, Hennekens CH, *et al.* Circulating vitamin D metabolites in relation to subsequent development of prostate cancer. *Cancer Epidemiol Biomarkers Prev* 1996; 5: 121–126.

18 Lind L, Lithell H, Skarfors E, *et al.* Reduction of blood pressure by treatment with alphacalcidol: a double-blind, placebo-controlled study in patients with impaired glucose tolerance. *Acta Med Scand* 1988; 223: 211–217.

19 Lind L, Wengle B, Ljunghall S. Reduction of blood pressure during long-term treatment with active vitamin D (alphacalcidol) is dependent on plasma renin activity and calcium status: A double-blind, placebo-controlled study. *Am J Hypertens* 1989; 2: 20–25.

20 Ott SM, Chesnut CH, III. Calcitriol treatment is not effective in postmenopausal osteoporosis. *Ann Intern Med* 1989; 110: 267–274.

21 McAlindon TE, Felson DT, Zhang Y, *et al.* Relation of dietary intake and serum levels of vitamin D to progression of arthritis of the knee among participants in the Framingham study. *Ann Intern Med* 1996; 125: 353–359.

22 Oelzer P, Muller A, Deschner F, *et al.* Relationship between disease activity and serum levels of vitamin D metabolites and PTH in rheumatoid arthritis. *Calcif Tissue Int* 1998; 62: 193–198.

23 Baynes KC, Boucher BJ, Feskens EJ, Kromhout D. Vitamin D, glucose tolerance and insulinaemia in elderly men. *Diabetologia* 1997; 40: 344–347.

Vitamin E

Description

Vitamin E is a fat-soluble vitamin.

Nomenclature

Vitamin E is a generic term used to describe all tocopherol and tocotrienol derivatives that exhibit the biological activity of alpha tocopherol. Those used commercially with their differing biological activities are shown in Table 1.

Table 1 Biological activity of commercially used vitamin E substances

Name	Biological activity (%)
d-alpha tocopherol[1]	100
d-alpha tocopherol acetate	91
d-alpha tocopherol succinate	81
d,l-alpha tocopherol[2]	74
d,l-alpha tocopherol acetate	67
d,l-alpha tocopherol succinate	60

[1]Natural vitamin E.
[2]Synthetic vitamin E.

Units

The UK Dietary Reference Values express the requirement for vitamin E in terms of milligrams (mg). The system of International Units for Vitamin E was discontinued in 1956, but continues to be widely used (particularly on dietary supplement labels).

1 unit = 1 mg of a standard synthetic preparation of alpha tocopheryl acetate and is equivalent to:

- 1 unit *dl*-alpha tocopheryl acetate
- 1.36 units *d*-alpha tocopheryl acetate
- 1.10 units *dl*-alpha tocopherol
- 1.49 units *d*-alpha tocopherol
- 0.89 units *dl*-alpha tocopheryl acid succinate
- 1.21 units *d*-alpha tocopheryl acid succinate

Vitamin-E activity can also be expressed in terms of alpha tocopherol activity and:

1 alpha tocopherol equivalent = 1 mg
natural *d*-alpha tocopherol = 0.67 units

Human requirements

See Table 2 for Dietary Reference Values for vitamin E.

There is an increased requirement for vitamin E with diets high in polyunsaturated fatty acids (PUFA), but many items high in PUFA (e.g. vegetable oils and fish oils) are also high in vitamin E (see Table 3). In general, the requirement for vitamin E appears to be: 0.4 mg/g of linoleic acid; 3–4 mg/g of eicosapentaenoic and docosahexaenoic acid combined.

Intakes

In the UK, the average adult diet provides 8.3 mg daily.

Action

Vitamin E is an antioxidant, protecting polyunsaturated fatty acids in membranes and other critical cellular structures from free radicals and products of oxidation. It works in conjunction with dietary selenium (a co-factor for glutathione peroxidase), and also with

Table 2 Dietary Reference Values for vitamin E (mg/day)

EU RDA (for labelling purposes) = 10 mg

Age	UK Safe Intake	USA				European PRI
		EAR	RDA	AI	UL	
0–6 months	0.4 mg/g PUFA	–	–	4	–	0.4 mg/g PUFA
7–12 months	0.4 mg/g PUFA	–	–	5	–	0.4 mg/g PUFA
1–3 years	0.4 mg/g PUFA	5	6	–	200	0.4 mg/g PUFA
4–8 years	–	6	7	–	300	–
9–13 years	–	9	11	–	600	–
14–70+ years	–	12	15	–	1000[1]	–
Males						
11–50+ years	>4	–	–	–	–	>4
Females						
11–50+ years	>3	–	–	–	–	>3
Pregnancy	–	16	19	–	800[2]/1000[3]	–
Lactation	–	16	19	–	800[2]/1000[3]	–

[1]Age 14–18 years, 800 mg.
[2]Age up to 18 years.
[3]Age 19–50 years.
PUFA = polyunsaturated fatty acid.
UL = Tolerable Upper Intake Levels from supplements.

vitamin C and other enzymes, including superoxide dismutase and catalase.

Dietary sources

See Table 3 for dietary sources of vitamin E.

Metabolism

Absorption

Absorption of vitamin E is relatively inefficient (20–80%); the efficiency of absorption falls as the dose increases. Normal bile and pancreatic secretion are essential for maximal absorption. Absorption is maximal in the median part of the intestine; it is not absorbed in the large intestine to any great extent.

Distribution

Vitamin E is taken up principally via the lymphatic system and is transported in the blood bound to lipoproteins. More than 90% is carried by the low-density lipoproteins (LDL) fraction. There is some evidence that a greater proportion is transported by the high-density lipoproteins (HDL) fraction in females than in males. Vitamin E is stored in all fatty tissues, in particular adipose tissue, liver and muscle.

Elimination

The major route of elimination is the faeces; usually less than 1% of orally administered vitamin E is excreted in the urine. Vitamin E appears in breast milk.

Bioavailability

Absorption is enhanced by dietary fat; medium-chain triglycerides enhance absorption, whereas polyunsaturated fats are inhibitory.

Vitamin E is not very stable; significant losses from food may occur during storage and cooking. Losses also occur during food processing, particularly if there is significant

Table 3 Dietary sources of vitamin E

Food portion	Vitamin E content (mg)	Food portion	Vitamin E content (mg)
Breakfast cereals		Kidney (75 g)	0.3
1 bowl All-Bran (45 g)	1.0	Sardines (70 g)	0.3
1 bowl Muesli (95 g)	**3.0**	*Tinned salmon (100 g)*	*1.5*
2 pieces Shredded Wheat	0.5	Tinned pilchards (100 g)	0.7
1 bowl Start (35 g)	**6.2**	Tinned tuna (100 g)	0.5
2 Weetabix	0.5	2 fillets herring, cooked (110 g)	0.3
		2 fillets kipper, cooked (130 g)	0.4
Cereal products			
Brown rice, boiled (160 g)	0.5	**Vegetables**	
Brown pasta	0	Broccoli, boiled (100 g)	1.3
Wholemeal bread, 2 slices	*1.5*	Brussels sprouts, boiled (100 g)	0.9
2 heaped tablespoons wheatgerm	**3.6**	**Sweet potatoes, boiled (150 g)**	**6.5**
		2 tomatoes	*1.8*
Milk and dairy products		1 small can baked beans (200 g)	0.75
½ pint (280 ml) whole milk	0.08	*Chick peas, cooked (105 g)*	*1.6*
½ pint (280 ml) soya milk	*1.7*	Red kidney beans, cooked (105 g)	0.2
Hard cheese (50 g)	0.25		
1 egg, size 2 (60 g)	0.6	**Fruit**	
		1 apple	0.4
Fats and oils		**½ an avocado pear**	**3.0**
Butter on 1 slice bread (10 g)	0.2	1 banana	0.3
Margarine on 1 slice bread (10 g)	0.8	*Blackberries, stewed (100 g)*	*2.0*
Low-fat spread on 1 slice bread (10 g)	0.6	1 orange	0.3
2 tablespoons ghee (30 g)	1.0	3 plums	0.6
1 tablespoon olive oil	1.0		
1 tablespoon sunflowerseed oil	**10**	**Nuts/seeds**	
1 tablespoon wheatgerm oil	**27**	**20 almonds**	**4.8**
2 teaspoons cod liver oil	*2.0*	*10 Brazil nuts*	*2.5*
		30 hazelnuts	**6.2**
Meat and fish		**30 peanuts**	**3.3**
Liver, lamb's, cooked (90 g)	0.3	Peanut butter on 1 slice bread (10 g)	0.5
Liver, calf, cooked (90 g)	0.4	**1 tablespoon sunflower seeds**	**7.5**
Liver, ox, cooked (90 g)	0.3		

Excellent sources (>3.0 mg/portion) (**bold**); good sources (>1.5 mg/portion) (*italics*).

exposure to heat and oxygen. There can be appreciable losses of vitamin E from vegetable oils during cooking.

Water-miscible preparations are superior to fat-soluble preparations in oral treatment of patients with fat malabsorption syndromes. The bioavailability of natural vitamin E is greater than that of synthetic vitamin E (see Table 1). However, several studies indicate that these differences may be even greater than originally thought.[1–4]

Deficiency

Deficiency of vitamin E is not generally recognised as a clearly definable syndrome. In premature infants, deficiency is associated with haemolytic anaemia, thrombocytosis, increased platelet aggregation, intraventricular haemorrhage and increased risk of retinopathy (but prophylaxis is controversial; see Possible uses).

The only children and adults who show

clinical signs of vitamin E deficiency are those with severe malabsorption (i.e. in abetalipoproteinaemia, chronic cholestasis, biliary atresia and cystic fibrosis), or those with familial isolated vitamin E deficiency (rare inborn error of vitamin E metabolism). Clinical signs of deficiency include axonal dystrophy, reduced red blood cell half-life and neuromuscular disturbances.

Possible uses

A large number of claims for vitamin E have been made, but they are generally difficult to evaluate since they are often anecdotal or deduced from poorly designed trials.

Cancer

Vitamin E has been suggested to be protective against cancer, and several epidemiological studies have found either low dietary intakes of vitamin E and/or lower serum levels of vitamin E in patients who have cancer than in those people without cancer. However, not all studies have shown protective effects.

The prospective Iowa Womens' Health Study[5] showed that a reduced risk of colon cancer was associated with high intakes of supplemental vitamin E in women under 65 years of age. Further data from this study showed that higher intakes of vitamin E are linked to lower risk of gastric, oesophageal, oral and pharyngeal cancers.[6] High dietary intake of vitamin E has been associated with reduced risk of breast cancer,[7] but another study showed no protective effect.[8] There is some evidence that high plasma vitamin E levels protect against cervical cancer,[9] lung cancer[10] and prostate cancer.[11]

A large Finnish study involving 29 133 male smokers showed that vitamin E supplementation (50 mg daily) reduced the risk of prostate cancer deaths by 41% compared with those who took no vitamin E.[12]

Cardiovascular disease

Epidemiological studies have shown that low dietary intakes are associated with an increased risk of cardiovascular disease in both men[13] and women.[14] Plasma vitamin E levels have also been found to be low in patients with variant angina.[15]

Several randomised, placebo-controlled trials have looked at the effects of vitamin E supplementation in cardiovascular disease. The Cambridge Heart Antioxidant Study (CHAOS)[16] which involved a total of 2002 subjects with angiographically proven cardiovascular disease showed that those who received vitamin E (400 or 800 units daily had a 47% reduction in death from cardiovascular death and non-fatal myocardial infarction (MI). This effect was due to a significant reduction (77%) in the risk of non-fatal MI.

However, there was no effect on death from cardiovascular disease alone. A non-significant increase in cardiovascular disease (CVD) death was found in the supplemented group. However, a subsequent analysis of the CVD-related deaths[17] showed of the 59 deaths due to ischaemic heart disease, six were in the group of patients that complied with vitamin E supplementation, 21 were in the non-compliant group, and 32 in the placebo group. This subsequent analysis has reduced concern about the possible adverse effects of vitamin E in this group of patients with established CVD.

An Italian trial – the Gruppo Italiano per lo Studio Della Sopravvivenza nell'Infarto Miocardio (GISSI)[18] – involved 11 324 patients who had survived an MI within the three-month period before enrolment. The four arms of the study included vitamin E, n-3 PUFA, a mixture of the two or placebo, and the primary end-points were death, non-fatal MI and stroke. Vitamin E reduced the risk for the primary end points by 11%, and the n-3 PUFA by 15%, with only the latter reaching statistical significance. Possible explanations for the differences in the results between CHAOS and GISSI have been suggested and include the fact that 50% of the GISSI subjects were on lipid-lowering drugs and that they presumably ate a Mediterranean diet with a high intake of fruit and vegetables.

The Alpha Tocopherol Beta Carotene (ATBC) trial, which involved 27 271 men, was designed to investigate the influence of antioxidant supplements on cancer in Finnish smokers. However, an analysis of heart disease[19] in this trial showed that vitamin E (50 mg) reduced the risk of primary major coronary events by 4% and the incidence of fatal coronary heart disease by 8%. Neither of these benefits was found to be statistically significant, but the trial used a small dose of a synthetic vitamin E supplement. A further analysis of the prevention of recurrence of angina for subjects in the ATBC trial[20] showed no significant protective effect of vitamin E.

The Heart Outcomes Prevention Evaluation (HOPE) study[21] enrolled a total of 2545 women and 6996 men aged 55 years or more who were at high risk of cardiovascular events, because they had either CVD or diabetes in addition to one other risk factor. They were assigned to natural vitamin E (400 units daily), an angiotensin-converting enzyme (ACE) inhibitor or placebo for a mean of 4.5 years. In comparison with placebo, there were no significant differences in the number of deaths from cardiovascular causes, MI and stroke with vitamin E.

Cataract

Epidemiological evidence suggests an association between cataract incidence and antioxidant status. Subjects with a low to moderate intake of vitamin E from foods had a higher risk of cataract relative to subjects with higher intakes,[22] and low serum levels of vitamin E and betacarotene were related to increased risk of cataract in a Finnish study,[23] a French study[24] and a US study.[25] However, an analysis of the ATBC study showed that vitamin E (50 mg daily) had no effect on cataract prevalence in middle-aged smoking men.[26] Another study in 750 elderly people with cataracts[27] showed that those who took vitamin E supplements halved the risk of their cataracts progressing over a four-and-a-half-year period.

Diabetes

In a double-blind, placebo controlled, crossover study, 25 elderly patients with type 2 diabetes were randomised to receive 900 mg vitamin E or placebo daily for three months. Vitamin E supplementation was associated with a significant reduction in plasma glucose, haemoglobin A_{1c}, triglycerides, free fatty acids, total and LDL cholesterol and apoprotein B levels. The authors concluded that daily vitamin E supplementation produces a small but significant improvement in metabolic control in type 2 diabetes, but that more studies are needed to draw conclusions about the safety of long-term supplementation.[28]

Neuropsychiatric disorders

Vitamin E supplementation has been associated with some success in tardive dyskinesia.[29,30]

In a double-blind, placebo-controlled study, 341 patients with Alzheimer's disease were randomised to receive 2000 units alpha tocopherol, 10 mg selegiline, selegiline plus alpha tocopherol, or placebo. There was no significant difference in outcomes between the groups, but after adjustment for confounding factors, there were significant improvements in outcome with all three treatment groups compared with placebo. Vitamin E led to the greatest improvement followed by selegiline, followed by the combination.[31]

Miscellaneous

Vitamin E supplementation (1200 units for three months) may have an anti-inflammatory effect. In the first study to show this effect,[32] 75 subjects were recruited who were diabetic, or diabetic with vascular disease, or age- and sex-matched healthy controls. Vitamin E treatment reduced the oxidation of low-density lipoprotein (LDL) cholesterol, and reduced free radical levels and other markers of inflammation. Vitamin E could therefore help to decrease the development of vascular disease in diabetes. However, in this study, the diabetics with or without vascular disease were not distinguishable by any of the markers of inflammation. Much larger, longer-term studies are needed to show that vitamin E has an anti-inflammatory effect in patients with vascular disease.

Some studies have shown that vitamin E reduces oxidative damage during exercise,[33] improves lung function[34] and improves immune function in the elderly.[35]

Vitamin E has been suggested to be of benefit in a vast range of conditions including arthritis, asthma, infertility and Parkinson's disease. Preliminary trials have shown some positive benefits, but larger trials are required to confirm these findings. There is some evidence that vitamin E (together with vitamin C) may raise the tolerance to ultraviolet rays and therefore reduce the risk of sunburn.

Conclusion

Several epidemiological studies have shown a link between low vitamin E intakes and coronary heart disease (CHD). There is some evidence that supplements (>100 units daily) reduce the risk of CHD, but some studies do not demonstrate a benefit. Evidence therefore remains promising but inconclusive. There is little evidence of benefit with vitamin E supplements in cancer prevention. There is preliminary evidence that vitamin E supplements improve immune function and lung function, and reduce oxidative damage during exercise. They may also improve glucose ultilisation in diabetes, reduce the risk of cataract, delay the progress of Alzheimer's disease and improve symptomatology in tardive dyskinesia. However, further research is required before vitamin E can be recommended as a supplement for these purposes.

Precautions/contraindications

Vitamin E supplements should be avoided: by patients taking oral anticoagulants (increased bleeding tendency); in iron-deficiency anaemia (vitamin E may impair haematological response to iron) and hyperthyroidism.

Pregnancy and breast-feeding

No problems reported at normal intakes.

Adverse effects

Vitamin E is relatively non-toxic (fractional absorption declines rapidly with increasing intake, thereby preventing the accumulation of toxic concentrations of vitamin E in the tissues). Most adults can tolerate 100–800 mg daily, and even doses of 3200 mg daily do not appear to lead to consistent adverse effects.

Large doses (>1000 mg daily for prolonged periods) have occasionally been associated with the following side-effects: increased bleeding tendency in vitamin K-deficient patients; altered endocrine function (thyroid, adrenal and pituitary); rarely, blurred vision, diarrhoea, dizziness, fatigue and weakness, gynaecomastia, headache and nausea.

Interactions

Drugs

Anticoagulants: large doses of vitamin E may increase the anticoagulant effect.
Anticonvulsants (phenobarbitone, phenytoin, carbamazepine): may reduce plasma levels of vitamin E.
Colestyramine or colestipol: may reduce intestinal absorption of vitamin E.
Digoxin: requirement for digoxin may be reduced with vitamin E (monitoring recommended).
Insulin: requirement for insulin may be reduced by vitamin E (monitoring recommended).
Liquid paraffin: may reduce intestinal absorption of vitamin E (avoid long-term use of liquid paraffin).
Oral contraceptives: may reduce plasma vitamin E levels.
Sucralfate: may reduce intestinal absorption of vitamin E.

Nutrients

Copper: large doses of copper may increase requirement for vitamin E.
Iron: large doses of iron may increase requirements for vitamin E; vitamin E may impair the haematological response in iron-deficiency anaemia.
Polyunsaturated fatty acids (PUFA): the dietary requirement for vitamin E increases when the intake of PUFA increases.
Vitamin A: vitamin E spares vitamin A and protects against some signs of vitamin A toxicity; very high levels of vitamin A may increase requirement for vitamin E; excessive doses of vitamin E may deplete vitamin A.
Vitamin C: vitamin C can spare vitamin E; vitamin E can spare vitamin C.
Vitamin K: large doses of vitamin E (1200 mg

daily) increase the vitamin K requirement in patients taking anticoagulants.
Zinc: zinc deficiency may result in reduced plasma vitamin E levels.

Dose

Vitamin E is available in the form of tablets and capsules and is an ingredient of multivitamin preparations. Dietary supplements provide between 10 and 1000 mg per daily dose.

References

1 Ferslew KE, Acuff RV, Daigneault EA, *et al.* Pharmacokinetics and bioavailability of the RRR and all racemic stereoisomers of alpha-tocopherol in humans after single oral administration. *J Clin Pharmacol* 1993; 33: 84–88.
2 Acuff RV, Thedford SS, Hidiroglou NN, *et al.* Relative bioavailability of RRR- and all-rac-alpha-tocopherol acetate in humans: Studies using deuterated compounds. *Am J Clin Nutr* 1994; 60: 397–402.
3 Kiyose C, Muramtsu R, Kameyana Y, *et al.* Biodiscrimination of alpha-tocopherol stereoisomers in humans after oral administration. *Am J Clin Nutr* 1997; 65: 785–789.
4 Burton GW, Traber MG, Acuff RV, *et al.* Human plasma and tissue alpha-tocopherol concentrations in response to supplementation with deuterated natural and synthetic vitamin E. *Am J Clin Nutr* 1998; 67: 669–684.
5 Bostick RM, Potter JD, McKenzie DR, *et al.* Reduced risk of colon cancer with high intake of vitamin E: The Iowa Women's health study. *Cancer Res* 1993; 53: 4230–4237.
6 Zheng W, Sellers TA, Doyle TJ, *et al.* Retinol, antioxidant vitamins and cancers of the upper digestive tract in a prospective cohort study of postmenopausal women. *Am J Epidemiol* 1995; 142: 955–960.
7 London SJ, Stein EA, Henderson IC, *et al.* Carotenoids, retinol and vitamin E and risk of proliferative benign breast disease and breast cancer. *Cancer Causes Control* 1992; 3: 503–512.
8 Hunter DJ, Manson JE, Colditz GA, *et al.* A prospective study of the intake of vitamins C, E and A and the risk of breast cancer. *N Engl J Med* 1993; 329: 234–240.
9 Palan PR, Mikhail MS, Basu J, Romney SL. Plasma levels of antioxidant bet-carotene and alpha-tocopherol in uterine cervix dysplasias and cancer. *Nutr Cancer* 1991; 15: 13–20.
10 Comstock GW, Helzlouser KJ, Bush TL. Prediagnostic serum levels of carotenoids and vitamin E as related to subsequent cancer in Washington County, Maryland. *Am J Clin Nutr* 1991; 53 (suppl. 1): 260S–264S.
11 Eichholzer M, Stahelin HB, Ludin E, Bernasconi F. Smoking, plasma vitamins C, E, retinol and carotene and fatal prostate cancer: Seventeen year follow up of the prospective Basel study. *Prostate* 1999; 38: 189–198.
12 Heinonen OP, Albanes D, Virtamo J, *et al.* Prostate cancer and supplementation with alpha-tocopherol and beta-carotene; incidence and mortality in a controlled trial. *J Natl Cancer Inst* 1998; 90: 440–446.
13 Rimm BE. Vitamin E consumption and the risk of coronary heart disease in men. *N Engl J Med* 1993; 328: 1450–1456.
14 Kushi LH, Fee RM, Sellers TA, *et al.* Intake of vitamins A, C and E and postmenopausal breast cancer: The Iowa Women's Health Study. *Am J Epidemiol* 1996; 144: 165–174.
15 Miwa K, Miyagi Y, Igawa A, *et al.* Vitamin E deficiency in variant angina. *Circulation* 1996; 94: 14–18.
16 Stephens NG, Parsons A, Schofield PM, *et al.* Randomised controlled trial of vitamin E in patients with coronary disease: Cambridge heart antioxidant study (CHAOS). *Lancet* 1996; 347: 781–786.
17 Mitchinson MJ, Stephens NG, Parsons A, *et al.* Mortality in the CHAOS trial. *Lancet* 1999; 353: 381–382.
18 Marchioli R: GISSI-Prevenzione Investigators. Dietary supplementation with n-3 polyunsaturated fatty acids and vitamin E after myocardial infarction: Results of the GISSI-Prevenzione trial. *Lancet* 1999; 354: 447–455.
19 Virtamo J, Rapola JM, Ripatti S, *et al.* Effects of vitamin E and beta carotene on the incidence of primary non-fatal myocardial infarction and fatal coronary heart disease. *Arch Intern Med* 1998; 158: 668–675.
20 Rapola JM, Virtamo J, Ripatti S, *et al.* Effects of alpha tocopherol and beta carotene supplements on symptoms, progression and prognosis of angina pectoris. *Heart* 1998; 79: 454–458.
21 The Heart Outcomes Prevention Evaluation Study Investigators. Vitamin E supplementation and cardiovascular events in high risk patients. *N Engl J Med* 2000; 342: 145–153.
22 Jacques PF, Chylack LT. Epidemiologic evidence of a role for the antioxidant vitamins and carotenoids in cataract prevention. *Am J Clin Nutr* 1991; 53: 352S–355S.
23 Knekt P, Heliovaara M, Rissanen A, *et al.* Serum antioxidant vitamins and risk of cataract. *Br Med J* 1992; 305: 1392–1394.
24 Delcourt C, Cristol JP, Tessier F, *et al.* Age-related macular degeneration and antioxidant status in the POLA study. POLA Study Group. Pathologies

Oculaires Liees a l'Age. *Arch Ophthalmol* 1999; 117: 1384–1390.

25 Lyle BJ, Mares-Perlman JA, Klein BE, *et al.* Serum carotenoids and tocopherols and incidence of age-related cataract. *Am J Clin Nutr* 1999; 69: 272–277.

26 Teikari JM, Virtamo J, Rautalahti M, *et al.* Long-term supplementation with alpha-tocopherol and beta-carotene and age-related cataract. *Acta Ophthalmol Scand* 1997; 75: 634–640.

27 Leske MC, Chylack LT, He Q, *et al.* Antioxidant vitamins and nuclear opacities: the longitudinal study of cataract. *Ophthalmology* 1998; 105: 831–836.

28 Paolisso G, D'Amore A, Galzerano D, *et al.* Daily vitamin E supplements improve metabolic control but not insulin secretion in elderly type II diabetic patients. *Diabetes Care* 1993; 16: 1433–1437.

29 Lohr JB, Caliguiri MP. A double-blind, placebo-controlled study of vitamin E treatment of tardive dyskinesia. *J Clin Psychiatr* 1996; 57: 167–173.

30 Adler LA, Edson R, Lavori P, *et al.* Long-term treatment effects of vitamin E treatment of tardive dyskinesia. *Biol Psychiatr* 1998; 43: 868–872.

31 Sano M, Ernesto C, Thomas RG, *et al.* A controlled trial of selegiline, alpha-tocopherol, or both, as treatment for Alzheimer's disease: The Alzheimer's Disease Co-operative Study. *N Engl J Med* 1997; 336: 1216–1222.

32 Devaraj S, Jialal I. Low-density lipoprotein post-secretory modification, monocyte function, and circulating adhesion molecules in type 2 diabetic patients with and without macrovascular complications. *Circulation* 2000; 102: 191–196.

33 Meydani M, Evans WJ, Handelman G, *et al.* Protective effect of vitamin E on exercise-induced oxidative damage in young and older adults. *Am J Physiol* 1993; 264 (5 pt2): R992–R998.

34 Dow L, Tracey M, Villar A, *et al.* Does dietary intake of vitamin C and E influence lung function in older people? *Am J Respir Crit Care Med* 1996; 154: 1401–1404.

35 Meydani SN, Meydani M, Blumberg JB, *et al.* Vitamin E supplementation and in vivo immune response in healthy elderly subjects: A randomized controlled trial. *JAMA* 1997; 277: 1380–1386.

Vitamin K

Description

Vitamin K is a fat-soluble vitamin.

Nomenclature

Vitamin K is a generic term for 2-methyl-1,4-naphthaquinone and all derivatives that exhibit qualitatively the biological activity of phytomenadione. The form of vitamin K present in foods is phytomenadione (vitamin K_1). The substances synthesised by bacteria are known as menaquinones (vitamin K_2). The parent compound of the vitamin K series is known as menadione (vitamin K_3); it is not a natural substance and is not used in humans. Menadiol sodium phosphate is a water-soluble derivative of menadione.

Human requirements

See Table 1 for Dietary Reference Values for vitamin K.

Action

Vitamin K is an essential co-factor for the hepatic synthesis of proteins involved in the regulation of blood clotting. These are: prothrombin (factor II), factors VII, IX, X and proteins C, S and Z. Vitamin K is responsible for the carboxylation of the bone protein, osteocalcin, to its active form. Osteocalcin regulates the function of calcium in bone turnover and mineralisation. Vitamin K is also required for the biosynthesis of some other proteins found in plasma and the kidney.

Dietary sources

See Table 2 for dietary sources of vitamin K.

Metabolism

Absorption

Vitamin K is absorbed into the lymphatic system, predominantly in the upper part of the small intestine (jejunum and ileum), by a process which requires bile salts and pancreatic juice. The absorption of the different forms of vitamin K differs. Vitamin K_1 (phytomenadione) is absorbed by an active energy-dependent process from the proximal portion of the small intestine; menadione is absorbed by a passive non-carrier-mediated process from both the small and large intestines.

There is evidence that bacterially synthesised vitamin K can be a source of vitamin K for humans, although the availability of a sufficient concentration of bile salts for absorption is questionable (plasma levels of menaquinones suggest that some absorption occurs).

Distribution

Vitamin K is transported in the plasma and metabolised in the liver. Vitamin K_1 is concentrated and retained in the liver. Menadione is poorly retained by the liver but widely distributed in all other tissues.

Elimination

Vitamin K is eliminated partly in the bile (30–40%) and partly in the urine (15%).

Table 1 Dietary Reference Values for vitamin K (μg/day)

Age	UK Safe Intake	US AI	Europe PRI
0–6 months	10	2	–
7–12 months	10	12.5	–
1–3 years	–	30	–
4–8 years	–	55	–
9–13 years	–	60	–
14–18 years	–	75	–
Males			
11–14 years	1 μg/kg BW	–	1 μg/kg BW
15–18 years	1 μg/kg BW	–	1 μg/kg BW
19–24 years	1 μg/kg BW	–	1 μg/kg BW
19–70+ years	–	120	–
25+ years	1 μg/kg BW	–	1 μg/kg BW
Females			
11–14 years	1 μg/kg BW	–	1 μg/kg BW
15–18 years	1 μg/kg BW	–	1 μg/kg BW
19–24 years	1 μg/kg BW	–	1 μg/kg BW
19–70+ years	–	90	–
25+ years	1 μg/kg BW	–	1 μg/kg BW
Pregnancy	1 μg/kg BW	90[1]	1 μg/kg BW
Lactation	1 μg/kg BW	90[1]	1 μg/kg BW

[1]age <18 years, 75 μg.
Some of the requirement for vitamin K is met by synthesis in the intestine.
BW = body weight.

Table 2 Dietary sources of vitamin K

Food portion	Vitamin K content (μg)
Broccoli, boiled (100 g)	**175**
Brussels sprouts, boiled (100 g)	**100**
Cabbage, boiled (100 g)	**125**
Cauliflower, boiled (100 g)	**150**
Kale, boiled (100 g)	**700**
Lettuce (30 g)	45
Spinach, boiled (100 g)	**400**
Soya beans, cooked (100 g)	**190**
Meat – average, cooked (100 g)	50
Cheese (100 g)	50
Bread and cereals (100 g)	<10
Fruit (100 g)	<10

Excellent sources (>100 μg/portion) (**bold**).

Bioavailability

The effect of cooking and food processing on vitamin K has not been carefully studied, but vitamin K appears to be relatively stable.

Deficiency

Vitamin K deficiency is rare and usually only occurs in people who have malabsorption problems or liver disease. However, it can occur in newborn babies, and all newborns should be given vitamin K. Deficiency leads to a prolonged prothrombin time which can be corrected by vitamin K supplementation.

Possible uses

Osteoporosis

Vitamin K is not in common use as a dietary

supplement, and few products contain it. However, there is increasing evidence that vitamin K deficiency may contribute to osteoporosis by reducing the carboxylation of osteocalcin in bone. Low serum levels of vitamin K and high levels of under-carboxylated osteocalcin have been reported in both postmenopausal women and individuals who have sustained hip fractures,[1–3] and low intakes of vitamin K may increase the risk of hip fracture.[4] In addition, some studies have shown that patients taking oral anticoagulants (which are vitamin K antagonists) are at increased risk of osteoporosis. Several ongoing studies are investigating the role of vitamin K at higher than usual intakes in the metabolism of bone markers and also for the risk of hip fracture.

Precautions/contraindications

None known (except Interactions – see below).

Pregnancy and breast-feeding

No problems reported.

Adverse effects

Oral ingestion of natural forms of vitamin K is not associated with toxicity. A rare hypersensitivity reaction (occasionally results in death) has been reported after intravenous administration of phytomenadione (especially if rapid).

Interactions

Drugs

Antibiotics: may increase requirement for vitamin K.
Anticoagulants: anticoagulant effect reduced by vitamin K (vitamin K is present in several tube feeds); dosage adjustment of anticoagulant may be necessary, especially when vitamin K has been used to antagonise excessive effects of anticoagulants (see the *British National Formulary*).
Colestyramine or colestipol: may reduce intestinal absorption of vitamin K.
Liquid paraffin: may reduce intestinal absorption of vitamin K (avoid long-term use of liquid paraffin).
Sucralfate: may reduce intestinal absorption of vitamin K.

Nutrients

Vitamin A: under conditions of hypervitaminosis A hypothrombinaemia may occur; it can be corrected by administering vitamin K.
Vitamin E: large doses of vitamin E (1200 mg daily) increase the vitamin K requirement in patients taking anticoagulants, but have no confirmed effect in individuals not taking anticoagulants.

Dose

Vitamin K is not generally available in isolation as a supplement. It is an ingredient in some multivitamin preparations. No dose has been established.

References

1 Binkle NC, Suttie JW. Vitamin K nutrition and osteoporosis. *J Nutr* 1995; 125: 1812–1821.
2 Kanai T, Takagi T, Masuhiro K, *et al.* Serum vitamin K level and bone mineral density in post-menopausal women. *Int J Gynaecol Obstet* 1997; 56: 25–30.
3 Vermeer C, Gijsbers BL, Cracium AM, *et al.* Effects of vitamin K on bone mass and bone metabolism. *J Nutr* 1996; 126 (suppl. 4): 1187S–1191S.
4 Feskanich D, Weber P, Willett WC, *et al.* Vitamin K intake and hip fractures in women: A prospective study. *Am J Clin Nutr* 1999; 69: 74–79.

Zinc

Description

Zinc is an essential trace mineral.

Human requirements

See Table 1 for Dietary Reference Values for zinc.

Intakes

In the UK, the average adult daily diet provides: for men, 11.7 mg; for women, 8.7 mg.

Action

Zinc is an essential component of over 200 enzymes. It plays an important role in the metabolism of proteins, carbohydrates, lipids and nucleic acids, and is involved in gene expression. Zinc is also crucial for maintaining the structure and integrity of cell membranes (loss of zinc results in an increased susceptibility to oxidative damage).

Dietary sources

See Table 2 for dietary sources of zinc.

Metabolism

Absorption

Absorption occurs throughout the length of the small intestine, mostly in the jejunum, both by a carrier-mediated process and by diffusion.

Distribution

Zinc is transported in association with albumin, amino acids and a 2-macroglobulin. About 60% is stored in skeletal muscle and 30% in bone, with 4–6% in the skin. Highest concentrations are found in the iris, retina and choroid of the eye and in the prostate and spermatozoa.

Elimination

Elimination of zinc is mainly in the faeces; smaller amounts are excreted in the urine and via the skin.

Bioavailability

Absorption of zinc is enhanced by certain amino acids such as cysteine and histidine; meat, dairy produce and fish contain zinc which is therefore efficiently absorbed. Zinc from wholegrain cereals, including bran products, and also soy protein, is less available, due, in part, to the presence of phytate. The effect of non-starch polysaccharides (dietary fibre), tannic acid and caffeine is equivocal. High calcium intake may reduce absorption, but this is likely only at higher than recommended intakes of calcium (e.g. >1500 mg daily).

Deficiency

Clinical manifestations of severe zinc deficiency include alopecia, diarrhoea, dermatitis, psychiatric disorder, weight loss, intercurrent infection (due to impaired immune function), hypogonadism in males, and poor ulcer healing. Signs of mild to moderate deficiency include growth retardation, male hypogonadism, poor appetite, rough skin, mental lethargy, delayed wound healing and impaired taste acuity.

Maternal zinc deficiency before and during pregnancy may lead to intrauterine growth retardation and congenital abnormalities in the fetus.

Table 1 Dietary Reference Values for zinc (mg/day)

EU RDA = 15 mg

Age	UK			USA		WHO[1]	Europe PRI
	LNRI	EAR	RNI	RDA	UL		
0–3 months	2.6	3.3	4.0	2.0[2]	4.0	5.0	5.3
4–6 months	2.6	3.3	4.0	2.0[2]	4.0	5.0	3.1
7–12 months	3.0	3.8	5.0	3.0	5.0	5.6	4.0
1–3 years	3.0	3.8	5.0	3.0	7.0	5.5	4.0
4–6 years	4.0	5.0	6.5	–	–	6.5	6.0
4–8 years	–	–	–	5.0	12.0	–	–
7–10 years	4.0	5.4	7.0	–	–	7.5	7.0
9–13 years	–	–	–	8.0	23.0	–	–
Males							
11–14 years	5.3	7.0	9.0	–	–	12.1	9.0
14–18 years	–	–	–	11.0	34.0	–	–
15–18 years	5.5	7.3	9.5	–	–	13.1	9.0
19–50+ years	5.5	7.3	9.5	11.0	40.0	9.4	9.5
Females							
11–14 years	5.3	7.0	9.0	–	–	10.3	9.0
14–18 years	–	–	–	9.0	34.0	–	–
15–18 years	4.0	5.5	7.0	–	–	10.2	7.0
19–50+ years	4.0	5.5	7.0	8.0	40.0	6.5	7.0
Pregnancy	*	*	*	11.0[3]	40.0[4]	7.3–13.3	*
Lactation	–	–	–	12.0[5]	40.0[4]	–	–
0–4 months	–	–	+6.0	–	–	12.7	+5.0
4+ months	–	–	+2.5	–	–	14.0	+5.0

*No increment.
[1]Normative requirement on diet of moderate zinc availability.
[2]Adequate Intakes (AIs).
[3]aged <18 years, 13 mg daily.
[4]aged <18 years, 34 mg daily.
[5]aged <18 years, 14 mg daily.
UL = Tolerable Upper Intake Level.

Possible uses

Anorexia nervosa

It has been suggested that zinc deficiency is involved in the aetiology of anorexia nervosa. Teenage girls who are restricting their food intake during the period of rapid growth may develop a state of zinc deficiency and anorexia nervosa. A daily supplement of 45 mg of zinc, as zinc sulphate, has been reported to result in weight gain in 17 young female patients with long-standing anorexia nervosa.[1] The weight gain continued over a four-year follow-up period. Compared with placebo, a daily dose of 100 mg of zinc gluconate doubled the rate of increase in body mass index in 35 female patients with anorexia.[2]

Wound healing

Zinc deficiency impairs wound repair by reducing the rate of epithelialisation and cellular proliferation. Low zinc levels have been associated with poor wound healing, and supplementation has promoted the healing process.[3,4] In one study, zinc supplementation reduced death rates

Table 2 Dietary sources of zinc

Food portion	Zinc content (mg)	Food portion	Zinc content (mg)
Breakfast cereals		**1 beef steak (155 g)**	**7.0**
1 bowl All-Bran (45 g)	**3.0**	**Minced beef, lean, stewed (100 g)**	**6.0**
1 bowl Bran Flakes (45 g)	*1.5*	*1 chicken leg (190 g)*	*2.0*
1 bowl Corn Flakes (30 g)	0.1	**Liver, lamb's, cooked (90 g)**	**4.0**
1 bowl Muesli (95 g)	*2.0*	**Kidney, lamb's, cooked (75 g)**	**3.0**
2 pieces Shredded Wheat	1.0		
2 Weetabix	1.0	**Fish**	
		Pilchards, canned (105 g)	*1.5*
Cereal products		*Sardines, canned (70 g)*	*2.0*
Bread, brown, 2 slices	0.7	**Crab (100 g)**	**5.5**
white, 2 slices	0.4	**1 dozen oysters**	**78.7**
wholemeal, 2 slices	1.3		
1 chapati	0.7	**Vegetables**	
Pasta, brown, boiled (150 g)	*1.5*	Green vegetables, average,	
white, boiled (150 g)	0.7	boiled (100g)	0.4
Rice, brown, boiled (165 g)	1.0	Potatoes, boiled (150 g)	0.5
white, boiled (165 g)	1.0	1 small can baked beans (200 g)	1.0
		Lentils, kidney beans or other	
Milk and dairy products		pulses (105 g)	1.0
½ pint (280 ml) milk, whole,		*Dahl, chickpeas, lentils (155 g)*	*1.5*
semi-skimmed or skimmed	1.0	Soya beans, cooked (100 g)	1.0
1 pot yoghurt (150 g)	1.0		
Cheese, Brie (50 g)	1.0	**Fruit**	
Camembert (50 g)	1.3	8 dried apricots	0.2
Cheddar (50 g)	1.1	4 figs	0.3
Cheddar, reduced fat (50 g)	1.4	½ an avocado pear	0.3
Cottage cheese (100 g)	0.5	1 banana	0.2
Cream cheese (30 g)	0.2	Blackberries (100 g)	0.2
Edam (50 g)	1.1	Blackcurrants (100 g)	0.3
Feta (50 g)	0.4		
Fromage frais (100 g)	0.3	**Nuts**	
White cheese (50 g)	*1.5*	20 almonds	0.6
1 egg, size 2 (60 g)	0.8	10 Brazil nuts	1.0
		30 hazelnuts	0.7
Meat		1 small bag peanuts (25 g)	1.0
Red meat, roast (85 g)	**4.0**		

Excellent sources (**bold**); good sources (*italics*).

and improved recovery in patients with severe head injury.[5]

Common cold

Several studies have investigated the effect of zinc lozenges on treating the common cold. In a randomised, double-blind, controlled trial carried out in Cleveland, USA,[6] 100 subjects received either a lozenge containing 13.3 mg of zinc every 2 h, or placebo. Duration of cold symptoms in the zinc group was reduced from 7.6 days to 4.4 days. Particular symptoms which improved with zinc included coughing, headache, hoarseness, nasal congestion and sore throat, while resolution of fever, muscle ache, itchy throat and sneezing did not. However, more patients in the zinc group had side-effects, including nausea and bad taste reactions.

Another US study[7] showed that administration of zinc lozenges was associated with reduced duration and severity of cold symptoms, especially cough. In this study, 50 volunteers were recruited within 24 h of developing symptoms of the common cold. Subjects took 12.8 mg zinc acetate every 2–3 h while awake as long as they had cold symptoms. Compared with the placebo group, the zinc group had shorter mean overall durations of cold symptoms (4.5 versus 8.1 days), cough (3.1 versus 6.3 days) and nasal discharge (4.1 versus 5.8 days) and reduced total severity scores for all symptoms.

A study in children and adolescents[8] showed that zinc lozenges (10 mg, five to six times a day depending on age) were not effective in treating cold symptoms. There were no significant differences in the time to resolution of any of the symptoms investigated.

A meta-analysis[9] of six randomised clinical trials of zinc lozenges in the common cold concluded that evidence for effectiveness of zinc in reducing the duration of common colds is lacking. However, two reviews[10,11] concluded that zinc lozenges could reduce the duration and severity of symptoms of the common cold, although side-effects might limit compliance. Formulation appears to be important because the addition of citric acid, tartaric acid, mannitol or sorbitol may reduce efficacy because of binding of zinc.

Miscellaneous

There is limited evidence that zinc may play a role in the treatment of benign prostatic hyperplasia (BPH), male infertility,[12] exercise performance[13] and immune function in the elderly.[14] In AIDS patients receiving zidovudine (azidothymidine (AZT) supplemented with zinc for 30 days, body weight was stabilised and the frequency of opportunistic infections reduced in the following two years.[15] However, further controlled trials are needed. The role of zinc supplements in acne, white spots on the finger nails and treatment of brittle nails is controversial.

> **Conclusion**
> Results from studies investigating the effect of zinc supplements on the common cold are conflicting. There is limited evidence for a benefit of zinc in male infertility and immune function. Further controlled trials are needed.

Adverse effects

Signs of acute toxicity (doses >200 mg daily) include gastrointestinal pain, nausea, vomiting and diarrhoea. Prolonged exposure to doses >50 mg daily may induce copper deficiency (marked by low serum copper and caeruloplasmin levels, microcytic anaemia and neutropenia), and iron deficiency. Doses >150 mg daily may reduce serum high-density lipoprotein levels, depress immune function and cause gastric erosion.

Interactions

Drugs

Ciprofloxacin: zinc reduces absorption of ciprofloxacin.
Oral contraceptives: may reduce plasma zinc levels.
Penicillamine: zinc reduces absorption of penicillamine.
Tetracyclines: reduced absorption of zinc and vice-versa.

Nutrients

Copper: large doses of zinc may reduce absorption of copper.
Folic acid: may reduce zinc absorption (raises concern about pregnant women who are advised to take folic acid to reduce the risk of birth defects).
Iron: reduces absorption of oral iron and vice-versa (raises concern about pregnant women who are often given iron; this may reduce zinc status and increase the risk of intrauterine growth retardation and congenital abnormalities in the fetus).

Dose

Zinc is available in the form of tablets and capsules and as an ingredient in multivitamin preparations.

The dose beyond the RDA is not established.

Dietary supplements contain 5–50 mg (elemental zinc) per daily dose.

The zinc content of some commonly used zinc salts is as follows: zinc amino acid chelate (100 mg/g); zinc gluconate (130 mg/g); zinc orotate (170 mg/g); zinc sulphate (227 mg/g).

References

1 Safai-Kutti S. Oral zinc supplementation in anorexia nervosa. *Acta Psychiatr Scand Suppl* 1990; 361: 14–17.

2 Birmingham CL, Goldner EM, Bakan R. Controlled trial of zinc supplementation in anorexia nervosa. *Int J Eat Disord* 1994; 15: 251–255.

3 Hallbrook T, Lanner E. Serum zinc and healing of various leg ulcers. *Lancet* 1972; 2: 780–782.

4 Thomas AJ, Bunker VW, Hinks LJ. Energy, protein, zinc and copper status of 21 elderly inpatients: Analysed dietary intake and biochemical indices. *Br J Nutr* 1988; 59: 181–191.

5 Young B, Ott L, Kasarkis E, *et al.* Zinc supplementation is associated with improved neurologic recovery rate and visceral protein levels of patients with severe closed head injury. *J Neurotrauma* 1996; 13: 25–34.

6 Mossad SB, Macknin ML, Medendorp SV, *et al.* Zinc gluconate lozenges for treating the common cold: A randomized, double-blind, placebo-controlled study. *Ann Intern Med* 1996; 125: 81–88.

7 Prasad AS, Fitzgerald JT, Bao B, *et al.* Duration of symptoms and plasma cytokine levels in patients with the common cold treated with zinc acetate. *Ann Intern Med* 2000; 133: 245–252.

8 Macknin ML, Piedmonte M, Calendine C, *et al.* Zinc gluconate lozenges for treating the common cold in children: A randomized controlled trial. *JAMA* 1998; 278: 1962–1967.

9 Jackson ML, Peterson C, Lesho E. A meta-analysis of zinc salts lozenges and the common cold. *Arch Intern Med* 1997; 157: 2373–2376.

10 Marshall S. Zinc gluconate and the common cold. Review of randomized controlled trials. *Can Fam Physician* 1998; 44: 1037–1042.

11 Garland ML, Hagmeyer KO. The role of zinc lozenges in the treatment of the common cold. *Ann Pharmacother* 1998; 32: 63–69.

12 Hunt CD, Johnson PE, Herbel J, *et al.* Effects of dietary zinc depletion on seminal volume and zinc loss, serum testosterone concentrations and sperm morphology in young men. *Am J Clin Nutr* 1992; 56: 148–157.

13 Krotiewski M, Gudmundson M, Backstrom P, *et al.* Zinc and muscle strength and endurance. *Acta Physiol Scand* 1982; 116: 309–311.

14 Bodgen JD, Oleske JM, Lavenhar MA, *et al.* Effects of one year supplementation with zinc and other micronutrients on cellular immunity in the elderly. *J Am Coll Nutr* 1990; 9: 214–215.

15 Mocchegiani E. Benefit of oral zinc supplementation as an adjunct to zidovudine (AZT) therapy against opportunistic infections in AIDS. *Int J Immunopharmacol* 1995; 17: 719–727.

Appendix 1

Guidance on daily intakes of vitamins and minerals

Vitamin/mineral	EU RDA	Upper Safe Level	Tolerable Upper Intake Level
Vitamin A (retinol equivalent μg)	800	2300	3000
Vitamin B_1 (thiamine) mg	1.4	100	None
Vitamin B_2 (riboflavin) mg	1.6	200	None
Vitamin B_6 (pyridoxine) mg	2	100	100
Vitamin B_{12} (cobalamin) μg	1	3000	None
Vitamin C (ascorbic acid) mg	60	2000	2000
Vitamin D (cholecalciferol) μg	5	10	50
Vitamin E (tocopherol) mg	10	800	1000
Nicotinic acid mg	18	150	35
Biotin μg	150	2500	None
Folic acid μg	200	400	1000
Pantothenic acid mg	6	1000	None
Calcium mg	800	1500	2500
Iodine μg	150	500	1100
Iron mg	14	15	45
Magnesium mg	300	300	350
Phosphorus mg	800	1500	4000
Zinc mg	15	15	40
Vitamin K	–	–	None
Betacarotene mg	–	20	None
Chromium μg	–	200	None
Copper mg	–	5	10
Manganese mg	–	15	11
Molybdenum μg	–	200	2000
Selenium μg	–	200	400

tba: to be announced.

EU RDA: the Recommended Daily Allowance considered sufficient to prevent deficiency in most individuals in the population.

Upper Safe Levels: defined by the European Federation of Health Product Manufacturers (EHPM) and the UK Council for Responsible Nutrition (CRN) as daily intakes from supplements which could be consumed on a long-term basis. The Upper Safe Levels are made on the assumption that a typical European diet is consumed. These figures are not recommended intakes, but levels of consumption which it would be unwise to exceed.

Tolerable Upper Intake Levels: defined by the Food and Nutrition Board of the US National Academy of Sciences as the highest total level of a nutrient (diet plus supplements) which could be consumed safely on a daily basis, that is unlikely to cause adverse health effects to almost all individuals in the general population. As intakes rise above the UL, the risk of adverse effects increases. The UL describes long-term intakes, so an isolated dose above the UL need not necessarily cause adverse effects. The UL defines safety limits, and is not a recommended intake for most people most of the time.

Appendix 2

Drug and supplement interactions

Drug	Food/nutrient	Effect	Intervention
Drugs acting on the gastrointestinal system			
Antacids	Iron	Aluminium-, magnesium- and calcium-containing antacids and sodium bicarbonate reduce absorption of iron	Separate administration of antacids and iron by at least 2 h
Sulfasalazine	Folic acid	Sulfasalazine can reduce absorption of folic acid	Monitor and give a supplement if necessary
Stimulant laxatives	Potassium	Prolonged use of stimulant laxatives can precipitate hypokalaemia	Avoid prolonged use of laxatives
Liquid paraffin	Fat-soluble vitamins	Liquid paraffin reduces absorption of of vitamins A, D, E and K	Avoid prolonged use of liquid paraffin

Drugs acting in the treatment of diseases of the cardiovascular system			
Thiazide diuretics	Calcium/vitamin D	Excessive serum calcium levels can develop in patients given thiazides with supplements of calcium or vitamin D	Concurrent use of thiazides with calcium and/or vitamin D need not be avoided, but serum calcium levels should be monitored
ACE inhibitors	Potassium	Concurrent use of ACE inhibitors with potassium may induce severe hyperkalaemia	Avoid
Potassium-sparing diuretics	Potassium	Concurrent use of potassium-sparing diuretics and either potassium supplements or potassium-containing salt substitutes may induce severe hyperkalaemia	Avoid concurrent use of potassium-sparing diuretics and potassium supplements unless potassium levels are monitored; warn patients about risks of salt substitutes
Calcium-channel blockers	Calcium	Therapeutic effects of verapamil can be antagonised by calcium	Calcium supplements should be used with caution in patients taking verapamil

Drug	Food/nutrient	Effect	Intervention
Hydralazine	Vitamin B_6	Long-term administration of hydralazine may lead to pyridoxine deficiency	Vitamin B_6 supplement may be needed if symptoms of peripheral neuritis develop
Anticoagulants	Vitamin E	Effects of warfarin may be increased by large doses of vitamin E (>100 units daily)	Avoid high-dose vitamine E supplements
	Vitamin K	Effects of anticoagulants can be reduced or abolished by large intakes of vitamin K	Avoid excessive intake of vitamin K (e.g. check labels of enteral feeds)
	Bromelain Chondroitin	Effects of anticoagulants may be increased by these supplements	Care with these supplements in people taking anticoagulants, aspirin and anti-platelet drugs.
	Fish oils		Avoid if possible. Otherwise monitor
	Garlic		
	Ginkgo biloba		
	Ginseng		
	Grape seed extract		
	Green tea		
	S-Adenosylmethionine		
Colestyramine	Fat-soluble vitamins	Prolonged use of these drugs may result in deficiency of fat-soluble vitamins	Supplements of vitamins A, D, E and K may be needed if these drugs are administered for prolonged periods
Drugs acting on the central nervous system			
Phenothiazines	Evening primrose oil	Evening primrose oil supplements may increase the risk of epileptic side effects	Avoid evening primrose oil supplements
Monoamine oxidase	Brewer's yeast	Brewer's yeast may provoke a hypertensive crisis	Avoid brewer's yeast supplements
Anti-epileptics	Folic acid	Anti-epileptics may casue folate deficiency, but use of folic acid supplements may lead to a fall in serum anticonvulsant levels and reduced seizure control	Folic acid supplements should be given only to those folate-deficient patients on anti-epileptics who can be monitored
	Vitamin B_6	Large doses of vitamin B_6 may reduce serum levels of phenytoin and phenobarbitone	Avoid large doses of vitamin B_6 from supplements (>10 mg daily)

Drug	Food/nutrient	Effect	Intervention
Anti-epileptics (continued)	Vitamin D	Anti-epileptics may disturb metabolism of vitamin D leading to osteomalacia	Susceptible individuals should take 10 μg vitamin D daily
Levodopa	Iron	Iron reduces the absorption rate of levodopa	Separate doses of iron and levodopa by at least 2 h
	Vitamin B_6	Effects of levodopa are reduced or abolished by vitamin B_6 supplements (>5 mg daily), but dietry vitamin B_6 has no effect	Avoid all supplements containing any vitamin B_6. Suggest co-careldopa or co-beneldopa as an alternative to levodopa.
Drugs used in the treatment of infections			
Tetracyclines	Iron	Absorption of tetracyclines is reduced by iron and vice-versa	Separate doses of iron and tetracyclines by at least 2 h
	Calcium/ magnesium/zinc	Absorption of tetracyclines may be reduced by mineral supplements and vice-versa	Separate doses of mineral supplements and tetracyclines by at least 2 h
Trimethoprim	Folic acid	Folate deficiency in susceptible individuals	Folic acid supplement may be needed if drug used for prolonged periods
4-Quinolones	Iron/zinc	Absorption of 4-quinolones may be reduced by mineral supplements and vice-versa	Separate doses of mineral supplements and 4-quinolones by at least 2 h
Cycloserine	Folic acid	Folate deficiency in susceptible individuals	Monitor folate status and give supplement if necessary
Isoniazid	Vitamin B_6	Long-term administration of isoniazid may lead to pyridoxine deficiency	Vitamin B_6 supplement may be needed if symptoms of peripheral neuritis develop
Rifampicin	Vitamin D	Rifampicin may disturb metabolism of vitamin D leading to osteomalacia in susceptible individuals	Monitor serum vitamin D levels
Drugs used in the treatment of disorders of the endocrine system			
Oral hypoglycaemics and insulin	Aloe vera Alpha-lipoic acid Chromium	These supplements could theoretically potentiate the effects of oral hypoglycaemics and insulin	Care in people on medication for diabetes
	Glucosamine	Glucosamine might reduce the effects of oral hypoglycaemics and insulin	Care in people on medication for diabetes
Oestrogens (including HRT and oral contraceptives)	Vitamin C	Concurrent administration of oestrogens and large doses of vitamin C (1 g daily) increases serum levels of oestrogens	Avoid high-dose vitamin C supplements

Drug	Food/nutrient	Effect	Intervention
HRT and oral contraceptives (continued)	DHEA	May potentiate hormonal effects	Care in people using HRT
	Isoflavones	May potentiate hormonal effects	Care in people using HRT
Bisphosphonates	Calcium	May lead to reduced absorption of bisphosphonate	Take 2 h apart
Thyroid medication	Kelp/iodone	May lead to poor control of thyroid condition	Avoid without a doctor's advice
Drugs used in the treatment of musculoskeletal and joint diseases			
Penicillamine	Iron/zinc	Absorption of penicillamine reduced by mineral supplements and vice-versa	Separate doses of mineral supplements and penicillamine by at least 2 h

Appendix 3

Additional resources

Government web sites related to dietary supplements

United Kingdom

UK Food Standards Agency Expert Group on Vitamins and Minerals
A group of independent experts established to consider the safety of vitamins and minerals sold under food law. Provides meeting reports and papers on this group's deliberations on vitamin and mineral toxicity and safe upper dosage levels.
http://www.foodstandards.gov.uk/evm.htm

The Secretariat can be contacted at:

Ministry of Agriculture, Fisheries and Food
Room 306B
Ergon House
C/o Nobel House
17 Smith Square
London SW1P 3JR

Department of Health
Room 652C
Skipton House
80 London Road
Elephant and Castle
London SE1 6LH

Medicines Control Agency (MCA)
The UK body which licenses medicines. Provides information on legislation relating to herbals and supplements.
http://www.opengov.uk/mca/mcahome.htm

Market Towers
1 Nine Elms Lane
London SW8 5NQ
Tel: +44 (0) 20 7273 3000
Fax: +44 (0) 20 7273 0353

USA

US Food and Drug Administration
FDA Center for Food Safety & Applied Nutrition
http://vm.cfsan.fda.gov/list.html

FDA Press Releases & Fact Sheets
http://vm.cfsan.fda.gov/~lrd/press.html

FDA what's new?
http://vm.cfsan.fda.gov/~news/whatsnew.html

Health claims
http://vm.cfsan.fda.gov/~dms/fdhclm.html

Announcements about dietary supplements
Includes details of adverse effects reported to the FDA about individual supplements.
http://vm.cfsan.fda.gov/~dms/supplmnt.html

Overview and history of FDA and the Center for Food Safety and Applied Nutrition
http://vm.cfsan.fda.gov/~lrd/fdahist.html

National Institutes of Health Office of Dietary Supplements
http://www.dietary-supplements.info.nih.gov

National Institutes of Health
Building 31, Room 1B25
31 Cente Drive, MSC 2086
Bethesda, Maryland 20892-2086
Tel: +1 301 435 2920

Associations representing industry

Association of the European Self-Medication Industry
European trade association representing the over-the-counter healthcare products industry.
http://www.aesgp.be

7 Avenue de Tervuren
B-1040 Brussels
Belgium
Tel: +32 2 735 51 30
Fax: +32 2 735 52 22
Email: info@aesgp.be

Council for Responsible Nutrition
Provides member companies with legislative guidance, regulatory interpretation, scientific information on supplement benefits and safety issues and communications expertise.
UK web site: http://www.crn-north.demon.co.uk
US web site: http://www.crnusa.org

St Mary's Centre
Oystershell Lane
Newcastle upon Tyne NE4 5QS
Tel: +44 (0) 191 232 3100
Fax: +44 (0) 191 232 2500
Email: carlrawlings@crn-north.demon.co.uk

European Responsible Nutrition Alliance (ERNA)
http://www.erna.net

Rue de l'Association 50
B-1000 Brussels
Belgium
Tel: +32 2 209 11 50
Fax: +32 2 223 30 64
Email: erna@eas.be

Health Food Manufacturers' Association
A trade association which acts as a voice for the industry; covers food supplements, health foods, herbal remedies, etc.
http://www.hfma.co.uk

Head Office
63 Hampton Court Way
Thames Ditton
Surrey KT7 6CT
Tel: 020 8398 4066
Fax: 020 8398 5402
Email: hfma@hfma.co.uk

International Alliance of Dietary/Food Supplement Associations
Aims to facilitate a sound legislative and political environment to build growth in the international market for dietary supplements based on scientific principles.
http://www.iadsa.org

Proprietary Association of Great Britain (PAGB)
UK Trade association representing the consumer healthcare industry.
http://www.pagb.co.uk

Vernon House
Sicilian Avenue
London WC1A 2QH
Tel: +44 (0) 20 7242 8331
Fax: +44 (0) 20 7405 7719

Journals and newsletters

Alternative Medicine Review: A Journal of Clinical Therapeutics
Published bimonthly.
http://www.thorne.com/altmedrev

Thorne Research Inc.
Tel: +1 208 263 1337

The American Journal of Clinical Nutrition
Official journal of the American Society for Clinical Nutrition. Published monthly.
http://www.ajcn.org

The American Journal of Clinical Nutrition
9650 Rockville Pike
L-2310
Bethesda MD 20814-3998, USA
Tel: +1 301 530 7029
Fax: +1 301 571 5728.
Email: staff@dues.faseb.org

The Dietary Supplement
A quarterly newsletter providing information on the use of dietary supplements (for both professionals and public).
http://www.thedietarysupplement.com

Focus on Alternative and Complementary Therapies (FACT)
Published quarterly. Provides summaries and commentaries on various aspects of complementary medicine, including vitamins, minerals and supplements.
http://www.pharmpress.com

The Pharmaceutical Press
PO Box 151
Wallingford
Oxon OX10 8QU
Tel: +44 (0) 1491 829 272
Fax: +44 (0) 1491 829 292
Email: rpsgb@cabi.org.

Journal of the American Nutraceutical Association
A publication devoted to vitamins, minerals and supplements. Contents pages only available on line.
http://www.nsanet.com/jana/html

Journal of Nutraceuticals, Functional and Medical Foods
A peer-reviewed academic publication, published quarterly, providing the latest information on food ingredients with health-enhancing effects. Covers product development and policy issues relating to nutraceuticals.
http://www.haworthpressinc.com

The Haworth Press Inc
Tel: +1 800 342 9678

Medicinal Foods News
An online magazine devoted to medical and functional foods.
http://www.medicinalfoodnews.com

PRISM
Publication produced by the European Responsible Nutrition Alliance.
http://www.erna.net

Rue de l'Association 50
B-1000 Brussels
Belgium
Tel: +32 2 209 11 50
Fax: +32 2 223 30 64
Email: erna@eas.be

Veris Newsletter
Non-profit organisation, which provides responsible source of information on the role of nutrition in health, with emphasis on antioxidants.
http://www.veris-online.org

Online research information and comment

Arbor Nutrition Guide
Provides regular updates on nutritional issues, including those with relevance to supplements.
http://arborcom.com/

International Bibliographic Information on Dietary Supplements (IBIDS)
The aim of this database is to help health professionals, researchers and the general public in finding scientific literature on dietary supplements.
http://odp.od.nih.gov/ods/databases/ibids.html

Medline
Medline is the US National Library of Medicine's bibliographic database providing extensive coverage of medicine and healthcare from approximately 3900 current biomedical journals, published in about 70 countries.
http://www.ncbi.nlm.nih.gov/pubmed

Nutritiongate
Abstracts and full text articles from a large number of nutrition journals world-wide.
http://www.nutritiongate.com

Nutrition News Focus
Provides a daily online newsletter free of charge, which attempts to bring clarity to confusing nutrition news stories.
http://www.NutritionNewsFocus.com

Tufts Nutrition Commentator
Provides critical commentary on studies published in professional journals, and on forthcoming policy decisions and public health guidelines.
http://www.commentator.tufts.edu/html

Other information

Consumer Lab
Tests content of diet supplements in the USA and provides reports on its work.
http://consumerlab.com/results/same.html

Health Supplement Information Service (HSIS)
Developed by the Proprietary Association of Great Britain (PAGB), HSIS presents the facts about health supplements in a straightforward way. Aims to eliminate confusion and provide reliable data about individual nutrients and supplements.
http://www.hsis.org

Joint Health Claims Initiative (JHCI)
Established as a joint venture by consumer organisations, enforcement authorities and industry trade associations to address concerns relating to health claims and develop a code of practice to regulate the use of health claims on foods and supplements.
http://www.jhci.org.uk

Nutrient information
Information on food sources, diet recommendations, deficiencies, toxicity, clinical uses, recent research and references for further information is provided for the micro- and macronutrients listed.
http://www.nutrition.org./nutinfo/

Quackwatch
A non-profit organisation with the aim of debunking health-related frauds, myths, fads and fallacies. There are sections on dietary supplements.
http://www.quackwatch.com/index.html

Index

Page numbers in *italics* indicate tables.